Adults with Childhood Illnesses

Edited by J. Timothy Bricker, Hatim A. Omar, Joav Merrick

Health, Medicine and Human Development

Edited by
Joav Merrick

Health is a key component of human development, growth and quality of life. The *Health, Medicine and Human Development* book series aim to provide a public forum for book publications from a multidisciplinary group of researchers, practitioners and clinicians for an international professional forum interested in the broad spectrum of health, medicine and human development. We welcome research on a wide variety of substantive areas that will promote and impact healthy human development including prevention, intervention and care also among people in vulnerable conditions.

Adults with Childhood Illnesses

Considerations for Practice

Edited by J. Timothy Bricker, Hatim A. Omar, Joav Merrick

DE GRUYTER

Editors

J. Timothy Bricker, MD
Pediatric Cardiology
University of Texas Medical School
Children's Memorial Hermann Hospital
Houston, Texas
United States
John.T.Bricker@uth.tmc.edu

Hatim A. Omar, MD
Division of Adolescent Medicine
Kentucky Children's Hospital
University of Kentucky, Lexington
United States
haomar2@uky.edu

Joav Merrick, MD, MMedSc, DMSc
National Institute of Child Health and Human Development
Ministry of Social Affairs
Jerusalem
Israel
jmerrick@zahav.net.il

ISBN 978-3-11-025521-8
e-ISBN 978-3-11-025568-3

Library of Congress Cataloging-in-Publication Data

Bricker, J. Timothy.
Adults with childhood illnesses : considerations for practice / by J. Timothy Bricker, Hatim A. Omar, Joav Merrick.
p. ; cm. — (Health, medicine, and human development)
Includes index.
ISBN 978-3-11-025521-8 (alk. paper)
1. Chronic diseases. 2. Adulthood. I. Omar, Hatim A. II. Merrick, Joav, 1950-
III. Title. IV. Series: Health, medicine, and human development.
[DNLM: 1. Chronic Disease—therapy. 2. Adult. 3. Congenital Abnormalities—therapy.
4. Human Development. 5. Patient Care Management. 6. Survivors. WT 500]
RC108.B75 2011
616'.044—dc22 2011002652

Bibliographic information published by the Deutsche Nationalbibliothek
The Deutsche Nationalbibliothek lists this publication in the Deutsche Nationalbibliografie; detailed bibliographic data are available in the Internet at http://dnb.d-nb.de.

Typesetting: RefineCatch Ltd, Bungay, Suffolk
Printing: Hubert & Co. GmbH & Co. KG, Göttingen
Cover image: iStockphoto/Thinkstock

♾ Printed on acid-free paper
Printed in Germany

www.degruyter.com

Contents

Preface

The purpose of this book is to provide a practical resource for clinicians who are encountering new groups of patients with diagnoses that were once exclusive to the care of children. For example, there are now more adults with cystic fibrosis than children due to our successes in pediatric care. This experience is being reproduced with many other diseases.

This book targets the needs of primary care providers for adults who have these conditions as well as trainees who are in pediatric, internal medicine, family practice, and med-peds training programs. Adult subspecialists with low familiarity with the pediatric disorders, and pediatric subspecialists who are involved in transitioning to adult care are groups that will find information contained here of interest.

Coordination of adult and pediatric care has been facilitated at the University of Kentucky and Kentucky Children's Hospital by integration of training programs and a tradition of coordinated care for the "graduates" of our pediatric specialty programs. Most of the authors have board certification in both adult and pediatric care. All have extensive experience with the care of patients with the pediatric diagnoses as well as transition into adult years.

I am sure that confidence, comfort, and information are acquired from this book to improve the care of grown-ups with childhood disease diagnoses and therefore recommend this book for health professionals working in the transition from pediatric to adult care.

Mohammed Morad
May 2011

Abbreviations

ACC	American College of Cardiology
ACE	Angiotensin-converting enzyme
ACTH	Adrenocorticotropic hormone
ADA	American Diabetes Association
ADHD	Attention-deficit/hyperactivity disorder
ADL	Activities of daily living
ADPKD	Autosomal dominant polyscystic kidney disease
AFP	Alpha feto-protein
AHA	American Heart Association
AIDS	Acquired immune deficiency syndrome
AITD	Autoimmune thyroid disease
ALL	Acute lymphoid leukemia
AML	Acute myeloid leukemia
API	Asthma predictive index
aPTT	Activated partial thromboplastin time
ARB	Angiotensin receptor blocker
ARPKD	Autosomal recessive polycystic kidney disease
ASD	Atrial septal defect
BGU	Ben Gurion University of the Negev
BMD	Bone mineral density
BMI	Body mass index
CAH	Congenital adrenal hyperplasia
CBC	Complete blood count
CBT	Cognitive behavioral therapy
CCSS	Childhood Cancer Survivor Study
CF	Cystic fibrosis
CFRDM	Cystic fibrosis-related diabetes mellitus
CGMD	Continuous glucose monitoring devices
CKD	Chronic kidney disease
CPT	Continuous performance tests
CSII	Continuous subcutaneous insulin infusion
CT	Computed tomography
DBA	Diamond–Blackfan anemia
DDAVP	1-deamino-8-D-arginine vasopressin
DHEAS	Dehydroepiandrosterone sulfate
DKA	Diabetic ketoacidosis
D_LCO	Diffusing capacity of the lung for carbon monoxide test

DMR	Division for Mental Retardation
DSCAM	Down syndrome cell adhesion molecule
DXA	Dual-energy absorptiometry
ECG	Electrocardiography
EEG	Electroencephalography
ERT	Enzyme replacement therapy
ESRD	End-stage renal disease
FDA	Food and Drug Administration
FEV_1	Forced expiratory volume in one second
FOHS	Faculty of Health Sciences
FSGS	Focal segmental glomerulosclerosis
FSH	Follicle-stimulating hormone
FVC	Forced vital capacity
GH	Growth hormone
GI	Gastrointestinal
G6PD	Glucose 6 phosphate dehydrogenase deficiency
HCV	Hepatitis C virus
HgbA1c	Glycated hemoglobin
ICE	Intracardiac echocardiography
ICU	Intensive care unit
IDT	Intradermal dilutional testing
IEM	Inborn errors of metabolism
Ig	Immunoglobulin
IGF1	Insulin growth factor-1
IQ	Intelligence quotient
KDOQI	Kidney Disease Outcomes Quality Initiative
LERIC	Late Physical, Psychological and Social Effects of Renal Insufficiency in Children Study
LH	Luteinizing hormone
LNNA	Large neutral amino acid
LVEF	Left ventricular ejection fraction
MCAD	Medium-chain Acyl CoA dehydrogenase disease
MCKD	Multicystic kidney disease
MELAS	Mitochondrial encephalopathy with lactic acid and stroke
MFS	Marfan syndrome
MMA	Methylmalonic aciduria
MOPP	Mechlorethamine, oncovin, procarbazine, and prednisone

MRA	Magnetic resonance angiography
MRI	Magnetic resonance imaging
MRSA	Meticillin-resistant *Staphylococcus aureus*
mtDNA	Mitochondrial DNA
MVP	Mitral valve prolapse
NADPH	Reduced form of nicotinamide adenine dinucleotide phosphate
NAPRTCS	North American Pediatric Renal Trials and Collaborative Study
NBS	Newborn screening
NICHD	National Institute of Child Health and Human Development
NPH	Neutral protamine Hagedorn
NSAID	Non-steroidal anti-inflammatory drug
NYHA	New York Heart Association
OFC	Occipitofrontal head circumference
OMD	Office of the Medical Director
PDA	Patent ductus arteriosus
PFO	Patent foramen ovale
PFT	Pulmonary function test
PKD	Polycystic kidney disease
PKU	Phenylketonuria
PNH	Paroxysmal nocturnal hemoglobinuria
PT	Prothrombin time
PTLD	Post-transplant lymphoproliferative disorder
PUV	Posterior urethral valve
PV	Pyruvate-kinase
PVR	Pulmonary vascular resistance
QoL	Quality of life
RAST	Radioallergosorbent test
RBC	Red blood cell
rhGH	Recombinant human growth hormone
RS	Rett syndrome
RSV	Respiratory syncytial virus
RTx	Renal transplantation
RV	Rhinovirus
SBE	Subacute endocarditis
SCIT	Subcutaneous immunotherapy
SCT	Stem cell transplant
SDA	Shwachman–Diamond anemia
SLIT	Sublingual immunotherapy
SMBG	Self-monitored blood glucose

STI	Sexually transmitted infection
SVC	Superior vena cava
TDI	Total daily insulin
TEE	Transesophageal echocardiography
TGFB-1	Transforming growth factor beta-1
TGFB-2	Transforming growth factor beta-2
TS	Turner syndrome
TTE	Transthoracic echocardiography
T1DM	Type-1 diabetes mellitus
T2DM	Type-2 diabetes mellitus
T3	Triidothyronine
T4	Thyroxine
UTI	Urinary tract infection
VCFC	Velo-cardio facial syndrome
VHL	von Hippel–Lindau disease
VSD	Ventricular septal defect
VUR	Vesicourethral reflux
vWF	von Willebrand factor
V/Q	Ventilation/perfusion
WBS	Williams–Beuren syndrome

Authors index

Jorge R. Alegria, MD
Department of Pediatrics
University of Kentucky
800 Rose Street, Lexington
United States
jorge.alegria@uky.edu
Chapter 5

Craig Alexander, MD
Division of Pediatric Cardiology
University of Kentucky College of Medicine
800 Rose Street, Lexington
United States
chalex0@email.uky.edu
Chapter 7

Michael I. Anstead, MD
Adult Cystic Fibrosis Program and Pediatric Cystic Fibrosis Center
University of Kentucky
740 South Limestone Street, Lexington
United States
mianst0@email.uky.edu
Chapter 3

Shoshana Aspler, RN, BSc
National Institute of Child Health and Human Development
Ministry of Social Affairs
Jerusalem, Israel
shoshiasp@walla.com
Chapter 19

Carolyn Bay, MD
Department of Pediatrics
University of Kentucky
740 South Limestone Street, Lexington
United States
carolyn.bay@uky.edu
Chapter 9

Sherry Bayliff, MD, MPH
University of Kentucky
Kentucky Children's Hospital
740 South Limestone Street, Lexington
United States
sbayl2@uky.edu
Chapter 11

Louis I. Bezold, MD
Division of Pediatric Cardiology
University of Kentucky College of Medicine
800 Rose Street, Lexington
United States
libezo2@email.uky.edu
Chapter 7

J. Timothy Bricker, MD
Pediatric Cardiology
University of Texas Medical School
Children's Memorial Hermann Hospital
Houston, Texas
United States
John.T.Bricker@uth.tmc.edu
Chapter 1, 5, 21, 22

Lee A. Bricker, MD
Adult Endocrine and Diabetes Clinics
Michigan State University College of Human Medicine
1000 Oakland Drive, Kalamazoo
United States
Greydanus@kcms.msu.edu
Chapter 8

Aftab S. Chishti, MD
Division of Nephrology Hypertension and Renal Transplantation
Kentucky Children's Hospital
University of Kentucky
800 Rose Street, Lexington
United States
aftab.chishti@uky.edu
Chapter 10

Zoran Danov, MD
Departments of Pediatrics and Internal Medicine
University of Kentucky Medical Center
800 Rose Street, Lexington
United States
Zoran.danov@uky.edu
Chapter 4

Ashley Daub, RD, LD
University of Kentucky
Department of Pediatrics
740 South Limestone Street, Lexington
United States
ashley.daub@uky.edu
Chapter 9

Brian S. Fuchs, MPH
National Institute of Child Health and Human Development
Ministry of Social Affairs
Jerusalem, Israel
briansethfuchs@gmail.com
Chapter 19

Michelle A. Grenier, MD
University of Kentucky
KY Children's Hospital Department of Pediatrics
800 Rose Street, Lexington
United States
michelle.grenier@uky.edu
Chapter 12

Donald E. Greydanus, MD, DrHC (ATHENS)
Michigan State University College of Human Medicine
1000 Oakland Drive, Kalamazoo
United States
Greydanus@kcms.msu.edu
Chapter 8

Richard C. Haydon, MD
Division of Otolaryngology, Head and Neck Surgery
University of Kentucky College of Medicine
800 Rose Street, Lexington
United States
rhayd1@uky.edu
Chapter 18

Don Hayes, Jr, MD
Departments of Pediatrics and Internal Medicine
University of Kentucky Medical Center
800 Rose Street, Lexington
United States
don.hayes@uky.edu
Chapter 4

Marlene B. Huff, LCSW, PhD
Department of Pediatrics
University of Kentucky
Lexington, United States
marlene.huff@uky.edu
Chapter 16

Manmohan K. Kamboj, MD
Section of Endocrinology, Metabolism and Diabetes
Nationwide Children's Hospital
700 Children's Drive (ED425)
Columbus, Ohio 43205, United States
Manmohan.Kamboj@Nationwidechildrens.org
Chapter 8

Isack Kandel, MA, PhD
National Institute of Child Health and Human Development
Ministry of Social Affairs
Jerusalem, Israel
kandel.isack@gmail.com
Chapter 19

Stefan G. Kiessling, MD
Pediatric Nephrology
Kentucky Children's Hospital
University of Kentucky
800 Rose Street, Lexington
United States
stefan.kiessling@uky.edu
Chapter 10

Meir Lotan, BPT, MScPT, PhD
Department of Physical Therapy
Ariel University Center of Samaria
Ariel, Israel
ml_pt_rs@netvision.net.il
Chapter 19, 20

Joav Merrick, MD, MMedSc, DMSc
National Institute of Child Health and Human Development
Ministry of Social Affairs
Jerusalem, Israel
jmerrick@zahav.net.il
Chapter 1, 19, 20, 21, 24

Mohammed Morad, PhD, MD
Department of Family Medicine
Faculty of Health Sciences
Ben Gurion University of the Negev
Beer-Sheva, Israel
morad62@013.net.il
Foreword, Chapter 19, 20

Jeffrey A. Moscow, MD
Pediatric Hematology and Oncology
Kentucky Children's Hospital
University of Kentucky
740 South Limestone Street, Lexington
United States
jefferey.moscow@uky.edu
Chapter 11, 14, 17

Jacqueline A. Noonan, MD
Kentucky Children's Hospital
University of Kentucky
800 Rose Street, Lexington
United States
jnoonan@uky.edu
Chapter 12, 15

Hatim A. Omar, MD
Division of Adolescent Medicine
Kentucky Children's Hospital
University of Kentucky, Lexington
United States
haomar2@uky.edu
Chapter 1, 21, 23

Dilip R. Patel MD, FAAP, FSAM, FAACPDM, FACSM
Michigan State University College of Human Medicine
1000 Oakland Drive, Kalamazoo
United States
patel@kcms.msu.edu
Chapter 8

Susan M. Peterson, MSN, FNP-C
Pediatric Hematology Oncology
University of Kentucky
740 South Limestone Street, Lexington
United States
susan.peterson@uky.edu
Chapter 17

Vlad C. Radulescu, MD
Pediatric Hematology Oncology
University of Kentucky
740 South Limestone Street, Lexington
United States
vlad.radulescu@uky.edu
Chapter 14, 17

Mordechai Raskas, MD
National Institute of Child Health and Human Development
Ministry of Social Affairs
Jerusalem, Israel
mraskas@gmail.com
Chapter 20

Carol Reid, MPA, MT (ASCP)
Department of Pediatrics
University of Kentucky
740 South Limestone Street, Lexington
United States
mcreid2@uky.edu
Chapter 9

William B. Rogers, MD
Department of Urology
University of Kentucky, Lexington
United States
william.rpgers@uky.edu
Chapter 13

Douglas J. Schneider, MD
Division of Pediatric Cardiology
University of Kentucky College of Medicine
800 Rose Street, Lexington
United States
dsc223@uky.edu
Chapter 6

Stephen E. Strup, MD
Department of Urology
University of Kentucky, Lexington
United States
Stephen.Strup@uky.edu
Chapter 13

Maria C. Veling, MD
Division of Otolaryngology, Head and Neck Surgery
University of Kentucky College of Medicine
800 Rose Street, Lexington
United States
mveli3@email.uky.edu
Chapter 18

Abbas A. Younes, MD
Division of Otolaryngology, Head and Neck Surgery
University of Kentucky College of Medicine
800 Rose Street, Lexington
United States
ayoun5@email.uky.edu
Chapter 18

John A. Yozwiak, PhD
Department of Pediatrics
University of Kentucky College of Medicine
Lexington
United Sates
jayozw00@uky.edu
Chapter 2

Ali M. Ziada, MD
Department of Urology
University of Kentucky, Lexington
United States
ali.ziada@uky.edu
Chapter 13

Introduction

1 Adults with childhood illnesses

J. Timothy Bricker, Hatim A. Omar and Joav Merrick

Just a few decades ago, children born with significant congenital anomalies or genetic and metabolic diseases perished at an early age. Very few survived into their teens and even fewer into adulthood. For example, in Israel in 1979, only 40% of children born with Down syndrome survived after 14 years of age. Congenital heart disease, major errors in metabolism, cancer, cystic fibrosis and many other major diseases were fatal. Hence, many physicians in adult primary care did not have the opportunity to see patients with these problems and thus were unable to learn how to care for them.

With major advancements in medical knowledge, technology, imaging techniques, surgical skills and pharmaceutical products as well as prosthetic devices, many of these patients now live much longer and sometimes even close to the mean life expectancy for the country (at least in the "developed" world). With this increase in life expectancy, a new challenge in medical care was created. Healthcare providers in adult medicine (e.g., family practitioners, internists, cardiologists) have to deal with individuals suffering from unfamiliar diseases. Hence, many pediatric sub-specialists find themselves caring for, for example, 40-year-old subjects with congenital heart disease or cystic fibrosis. It is not usually very pleasant to be admitted to a Pediatric Unit or to be seen in a Pediatric Outpatient Clinic if you are ≥40 years. These patients rarely find a Physician who cares for adults (hereafter termed an "adult physician") who is suitably comfortable to handle their particular problem. Although improvements in postgraduate medical education and the addition of medicine/pediatric residency programs have helped, this is still a major healthcare issue.

In addition to all of the above, there are insufficient resources to help providers care for these patients. We are not aware of a single textbook addressing these illnesses in adults or the problems of transitioning to adult care (including health insurance-related problems). The American Academy of Pediatrics started advocating the medical home concept in the late 1990s. They provided some resources to help physicians with transitioning their chronically ill patients to adult healthcare. However, many adult physicians are not members of the Academy, and may or may not have had exposure to these resources.

In this contribution, we have recruited highly qualified and experienced physicians to compile the first book dealing entirely with children's diseases in adults. Our goal is to provide a resource for all healthcare providers to help in the careof such adult patients. We believe that it will be valuable to all individuals who provide care to adults with children's diseases.

Childhood into Adulthood

2 Attention-Deficit/Hyperactivity Disorder: Epidemiology, assessment, and treatment among children, adolescents, and adults

John A. Yozwiak

2.1 Introduction

Several developmental and behavioral disorders exist among children, adolescents, and adults (▶ Tab. 2.1). Developmental and behavioral disorders are associated with significant impairment in academic, occupational, and interpersonal functioning, and can be challenging to treat and manage. Examples of these disorders include learning disorders, Mental Retardation, pervasive development disorders, and communication disorders. These disorders begin in infancy, childhood, or adolescence, and can persist into adulthood. Other disorders, such as depressive disorders and anxiety disorders may also have an onset in childhood or adolescence, but an early age of onset is not a defining feature (1).

This review focuses on the developmental and behavioral condition Attention-Deficit/Hyperactivity Disorder (ADHD). This disorder is the most frequently encountered neurodevelopmental disorder with a childhood onset in primary care settings (2). Referrals to healthcare providers for assessment and treatment of ADHD occur at a high rate (2, 3), and it is being increasingly recognized in adults. ADHD is a significant public health issue and clinical condition because of its associated morbidity and impairment in multiple domains of functioning (4).

The assessment, diagnosis, and treatment of ADHD among children and adolescents have been widely studied and effective pharmacological and psychosocial treatments have been established. The persistence of ADHD into adulthood has garnered

Tab. 2.1: Disorders usually first diagnosed in infancy, childhood, or adolescence (1).

• Mental Retardation	• Attention-deficit and disruptive behavior disorders (e.g., ADHD, Conduct Disorder)
• Learning disorders	• Feeding and eating disorders of infancy or early childhood
• Motor skills disorders	• Tic disorders
• Communication disorders (e.g., Stuttering)	• Elimination disorders (e.g., Enuresis)
• Pervasive developmental disorders (e.g., Autistic Disorder, Asperger's Disorder)	• Other disorders of infancy, childhood, or adolescence (e.g., Separation Anxiety Disorder)

increased attention. This chapter includes a review of the diagnostic criteria of ADHD and its prevalence, correlates, comorbidities, assessment, and treatment approaches for children and adolescents. The continuity of ADHD and adulthood will be reviewed, including its manifestations, associated features, assessment, and treatment approaches unique to this age group. This review of ADHD across the lifespan highlights issues common to the management of other developmental and behavioral disorders, such as the importance of conducting a thorough and comprehensive assessment that utilizes data from multiple sources and the provision of multimodal treatment.

2.2 Diagnostic criteria, epidemiology, comorbidities, and associated features

ADHD is characterized by inattention, hyperactivity, and impulsivity (1). ▶ Tab. 2.2 lists the diagnostic criteria of ADHD as outlined in the Diagnostic and Statistical Manual of Mental Disorders, Fourth Edition (DSM-IV) (1). The diagnostic criteria are based on empirical research and have high interrater reliability, predict course and response to treatment when used appropriately, and have good face validity (5). Some inattentiveness, impulsivity, and hyperactivity are common among many children and adolescents. Hence, the key to diagnosing ADHD is a demonstration that the symptoms impair functioning (e.g., academic functioning, social functioning), are developmentally inappropriate for the child's age and sex, and are enduring and persistent across different settings (1). ADHD is divided into three types: Predominantly Inattentive Type, Predominantly Hyperactive-Impulsive Type, and Combined Type (1).

Children and adolescents with ADHD can have impairments in many domains of functioning. Academic problems, difficulties making and sustaining peer relationships, behavioral problems at school, and difficulties with parents and siblings are commonly experienced (6). Delays in cognitive, language, motor, and physical development;

Tab. 2.2: DSM-IV diagnostic criteria for Attention-Deficit Hyperactivity Disorder (ADHD) (1).

A. Either (1) or (2):

(1) six (or more) for the following symptoms of **inattention** have persisted for at least 6 months to a degree that is maladaptive and inconsistent with developmental level:

Inattention

(a) often does not give close attention to details or makes careless mistakes in schoolwork, work, or other activities
(b) often has trouble keeping attention on tasks or play activities
(c) often does not seem to listen when spoken to directly
(d) often does not follow instructions and fails to finish schoolwork, chores, or duties in the workplace (not due to oppositional behavior or failure to understand instructions)
(e) often has difficulty organizing tasks and activities
(f) avoids, dislikes, or is reluctant to engage in tasks that require sustained mental effort (such as schoolwork or homework)
(g) often loses things necessary for tasks or activities (e.g., toys, school assignments, pencils, books, or tools)
(h) often easily distracted by extraneous stimuli
(i) often forgetful in daily activities

(2) six (or more) of the following symptoms of **hyperactivity-impulsivity** have persisted for at least 6 months to a degree that is maladaptive and inconsistent with developmental level:

Hyperactivity

(a) often fidgets with hands or feet or squirms in seat
(b) often leaves seat in classroom or in other situation in which remaining seated is expected
(c) often runs about or climbs excessively in situations in which it is inappropriate (in adolescents or adults, may be limited to subjective feelings of restlessness)
(d) often has difficulty playing or engaging in leisure activities quietly
(e) is often "on the go" or often acts as if "driven by a motor"
(f) often talks excessively

Impulsivity

(g) often blurts out answers before questions have been completed
(h) often has difficulty awaiting turn
(i) often interrupts or intrudes on others (e.g., butts into conversations or games)

B. Some hyperactive–impulsive or inattentive symptoms that caused impairment were present before age 7 years.

C. Some impairment from the symptoms is present in two or more settings (e.g., at school [or work] and at home).

D. There must be clear evidence of clinically significant impairment in social, academic, or occupational functioning.

E. The symptoms do not occur exclusively during the course of a pervasive developmental disorder, Schizophrenia, or other psychotic disorder and are not better accounted for by another mental disorder (e.g., mood disorder, anxiety disorder, dissociative disorder, or personality disorder)

Attention-Deficit/Hyperactivity Disorder, Combined Type: if both Criteria A1 and A2 are met for the past 6 months

Attention-Deficit/Hyperactivity Disorder, Predominantly Inattentive Type: if Criterion A1 is met but Criterion A2 is not met for the past 6 months

Attention-Deficit/Hyperactivity Disorder, Predominantly Hyperactive-Impulsive Type if Criterion A2 is met but Criterion A1 is not met for the past 6 months

poor self-regulation of emotion; increased incidents of medical difficulties; and greater proneness to accidents are associated with ADHD (7).

Prevalence estimates for ADHD among children and adolescents vary. Based on a review of studies that examined the prevalence of ADHD, Brown et al. (2) concluded that the prevalence among elementary school children ranges from 4% to 12%, with a higher prevalence in males and in community samples versus school samples. Males have a higher prevalence of ADHD than females in community surveys and even more so in clinic samples (8). This sex difference in clinic samples might be the result of a referral bias in which males are more likely than females to manifest aggressive behavior that warrants a referral (8). However, the higher prevalence for males in community samples suggests that the sex difference may not be accounted for solely by a referral bias (8). Most cases of ADHD are treated by family practitioners (5). In general pediatric settings, at least 10% of behavioral problems may be due to ADHD (9).

ADHD is a heterogeneous disorder with no single etiology. Genetics likely play a role (10), as relatives of children with ADHD are at risk for the disorder, including second-degree relatives (11, 12). Moreover, adopted relatives of children with ADHD are less likely than biological relatives to manifest symptoms of this condition (13). Catecholamine dysfunction has been implicated in the pathophysiology of ADHD, particularly dopaminergic dysfunction, with norepinephrine playing a more indirect role (14). Children with ADHD display deficits in neuropsychological functioning. Impairments in executive functioning and working memory have been identified, which suggest that the frontal cortex, or regions projecting to the frontal cortex, may be dysfunctional in some children with ADHD (15). Barkley (16) proposed that ADHD is a disorder characterized by deficits in behavioral inhibition, motor control, regulation of motivation, and working memory.

Several psychiatric disorders are comorbid with ADHD in youth, and up to 65% of children with ADHD have at least one comorbid condition (17). Comorbid conditions include Conduct Disorder, Oppositional Defiant Disorder, mood disorders, and anxiety disorders. Overlap between ADHD, Conduct Disorder, and Oppositional Defiant Disorder can be as high as 50% (6). Untreated hyperactivity increases the likelihood of later peer problems, antisocial behavior, and social maladjustment (18). Patterns of comorbidity may vary based on the type of ADHD. Individuals with the Combined Type of ADHD are more impaired than individuals with the other types, and have more comorbid psychiatric conditions and substance use disorders. Individuals with the Predominantly Inattentive Type of ADHD have fewer emotional and behavioral problems as compared with individuals with the Predominantly Hyperactive-Impulsive Type or the Combined Type. However, those with the Predominantly Inattentive Type have more academic problems than those with the Combined Type (19). Mood disorders, anxiety disorders, and learning disorders tend to be associated more with the Predominantly Inattentive Type, and externalizing disorders, such as Conduct Disorder and Oppositional Defiant Disorder tend to be associated more with the Predominantly Hyperactive-Impulsive Type (20). The comorbidity of ADHD highlights the importance of comprehensive screening and assessment in primary care settings, which is consistent with the practice guidelines of the American Academy of Pediatrics (21).

2.3 Assessment of ADHD in children and adolescents

The accurate assessment of ADHD hinges on integrating data from various sources. A multidisciplinary approach can enhance the assessment process. One source of data about child and adolescent functioning often comes from behavioral rating scales. Behavioral rating scales are easy to administer, simple to score, cost-effective, and provide a range of information about functioning (2). Parents and teachers are asked to rate the child or adolescent on a variety of symptoms. Rating scales are often designed for multiple informants, which is important given that a diagnostic requirement is that some impairment from the symptoms is present in at least two settings (1). Because the items on behavioral rating scales are transparent, responses may be biased by the prejudices or motivations of the respondent (22).

Behavioral rating scales can be classified into ADHD-specific ratings scales (e.g., Conners' Rating Scale – Revised [23]) or rating scales that assess a variety of difficulties (e.g., Child Behavior Checklist [24]). Brown et al. (2) compared the use of broad-band checklists with rating scales that specifically assess ADHD symptoms. The use of rating scales of specific ADHD symptoms was found to be more useful in the diagnostic process for ADHD than broad-band checklists, but the latter may be effective in the assessment of comorbid conditions (2).

One form of testing that is often used in ADHD evaluations is continuous performance tests (CPTs). A CPT is typically administered via computer. Individuals are instructed to respond only if a certain stimulus appears on the screen. The data gathered include the number of correct responses, omission errors, and commission errors. A CPT appears to assess impulsivity and inattention (25), and is a reliable psychological test that can discriminate children with ADHD from children without ADHD (26). However, if a child performs well on a CPT it does not suggest that the child does not have ADHD (25). Comprehensive neuropsychological assessment batteries which include multiple subtests have also been used in the assessment process, but there appears to be no basis for their routine use (25).

Behavioral rating scales and CPTs can provide useful information in the diagnostic process. It is imperative to integrate the data from these sources with the information obtained from a thorough interview with at least one of the young person's caregivers. Important elements of such an interview include a complete developmental history, a review of academic history, family history, interpersonal functioning, and treatment history. An interview with at least one teacher can also provide clinically relevant information about peer and academic functioning. The assessment process can be further enhanced by meeting with the child or adolescent. The focus of this meeting will vary based on the age of the patient. For older children and adolescents, inquiries can be made into their view of their symptoms, perceptions of the referral, and their functioning in multiple domains of their lives. For younger children, the focus can be on observing their in-session behavior and facilitating their comfort in the treatment setting (22). A thorough medical evaluation to rule out alternative medical and psychological explanations and to assess for comorbid conditions is also necessary.

2.4 Treatment of ADHD in children and adolescents

Pharmacological treatment is the first-line treatment for children and adolescents with ADHD (▶ Tab. 2.3 for a list of common medications used in the treatment of ADHD). Psychostimulants are the most commonly used class of medications (29). Psychostimulants block the reuptake of norepinephrine and dopamine by increasing dopamine in the synapse (27). The short half-life of these medications often necessitates multiple dosing throughout the day, but long-acting formulations have reduced this problem (28). In randomized controlled clinical trials, medication has been shown to reduce hyperactivity, impulsivity, and inattentiveness; improve classroom behavior; reduce oppositional behavior; and improve social functioning (5, 29). Children and adolescents treated with psychostimulants have been found to be less likely to develop depressive disorders, anxiety disorders, and disruptive behavior 10 years later, and less likely to repeat a grade than youth who were not treated (29). Common side effects of

Tab. 2.3: Common medications for ADHD (19, 27, 28, 56).

Medication	Mechanism of action	Possible side effects
CNS stimulants (e.g., methylphenidate, lisdexamfetamine)	Blocks the reuptake of dopamine and norepinephrine	Reduced appetite, weight loss, insomnia, abdominal pain, nausea, headache, jitteriness, dizziness
Atomoxetine	Norepinephrine reuptake inhibitor	Reduced appetite, insomnia, abdominal pain, nausea, vomiting, drowsiness, headache
α2 agonists (clonidine, guanfacine)	Stimulates α2-adrenoceptors; modulates pre-synaptic and post-synaptic norepinephrine	Reduced appetite, dizziness, drowsiness, constipation, dry mouth, headache, insomnia
Bupropion	Blocks the reuptake of dopamine and norepinephrine	Reduced appetite, agitation, weight loss, dizziness, dry mouth, constipation, headache, nausea, insomnia, tremor, excessive sweating, blurred vision
Tricyclic antidepressants (e.g., imipramine, desipramine)	Block the reuptake of norepinephrine	Constipation, dry mouth, weight change, vital sign and electroencephalography changes
Modafinil	Unclear; may affect catecholamine reuptake	Reduced appetite, diarrhea, insomnia, dizziness, dry mouth, headache, loss of muscle strength, nausea, nervousness, prickling or tingling feeling

stimulant medication include a reduced appetite, insomnia, abdominal pain, headache, and jitteriness (5). Psychostimulants have different mechanisms of action, so a patient who does not respond to one stimulant or has an adverse effect can be prescribed another stimulant (19).

Despite the efficacy of stimulant medication, a significant minority may display no effect or have an adverse reaction (5). In addition, concerns have been raised about the misuse of these medications by the child or adolescent, by his or her peers, and the possibility of their illegal distribution (5). Consequently, the use of non-stimulant medications for ADHD has garnered increased attention. An alternative to stimulant medication has been the use of tricyclic antidepressants. These medications were a popular treatment for ADHD in the past, but their use has diminished as more effective agents with fewer side effects have been developed (28). In addition, the use of tricyclic antidepressants was associated with the deaths of six children between the ages of 5 and 14 years (31, 32).

Atomoxetine, bupropion, clonidine, guanfacine, and modafinil are other non-stimulant medications that have shown promise in treating the symptoms of ADHD. Atomoxetine is a selective norepinephrine reuptake inhibitor. Similar to the other non-stimulant agents, this medication has a low potential for abuse. Bupropion is a novel antidepressant that inhibits the reuptake of dopamine, serotonin, and norepinephrine. This medication may be useful in children and adolescents with comorbid ADHD and a depressive disorder. Clonidine and guanfacine are α2 agonists and are generally used to treat the hyperactive and impulsive symptoms of ADHD, as well as aggression and sleep disturbances, especially in young children (19). Clonidine may be a useful adjunct to stimulant treatment if symptoms of impulsivity, hyperactivity, and aggression persist (33). Guanfacine may reduce tics in children with ADHD and tic disorders (34). In addition, modafinil has been used to promote wakefulness. The precise mechanism of action of this drug is unclear, but it is different from psychostimulants and produces fewer side effects. Pharmacological agents can be combined when there is an insufficient response to a single agent, other conditions are comorbid with ADHD, or there is a need to treat adverse side effects (19).

Stimulant medication does not produce lasting changes in functioning after it has been discontinued (5, 29), and significant minorities of youth do not respond to medication (29). Children and adolescents do not learn new skills from taking medication, and the various social, psychological, and educational problems still require clinical attention (29). Furthermore, medication does not alter the parenting styles that may also be contributing to the difficulties of the young patient (6). Therefore, adjunctive psychosocial treatments for ADHD are often necessary.

Behavioral parent training is an empirically supported treatment for ADHD (6). Behavioral parent training involves training parents to implement behavioral techniques such as a point system, time outs for undesirable behavior, and contingent attention (i.e., the provision of attention after the child displays desirable behavior) (6). The evidence supporting behavioral parent training is stronger for younger than for older children (6). In addition, behavioral interventions in classroom settings have empirical support (6). These interventions typically are more intensive than behavioral parent training programs, and often consist of trained professionals working individually with children (35). Studies of classroom interventions have not included adolescents (6). Although these treatments have empirical support they do not produce noticeable improvements in peer relationships and treatment gains are often lost once treatment is withdrawn (6). Cognitive therapy has been used extensively in the treatment of depression and anxiety in youth. When applied to ADHD, this form of treatment is designed partly to reinforce the insufficient internal mediators that characterize the disorder in children and adolescents, but it has not received empirical support (6).

The limitations in pharmacological treatment and psychosocial treatment have resulted in attempts to examine the effectiveness of combined treatment. A large-scale randomized clinical trial compared the effectiveness of pharmacological and psychosocial treatments and their combination for children with ADHD, Combined type (36). More than 500 children were randomized to intensive behavioral treatment that included parent, child, and school components; 14 months of medication management; the two treatments combined; or standard community care including medication administration. Children in the medication management group and the combined treatment group displayed significantly greater improvement for most ADHD symptoms than children who received intensive behavioral treatment and standard community care. Combined treatment produced no benefits beyond what was obtained for medication alone for ADHD symptoms. However, the effects of the combined treatment were obtained with lower medication doses than those used in the medication management condition, which suggests that behavioral treatments can play a role in treating ADHD. In addition, more than 75% of participants who received behavioral treatments were successfully maintained without medication. The combined treatment may also have provided benefits for non-ADHD symptoms, such as aggressive behaviors, internalizing symptoms, reading achievement, peer interactions, and relationship with parents (36).

Strong support has been found for pharmacological treatment of ADHD in children and adolescents, and it is often the first-line treatment. There is evidence that behaviorally focused treatments can also target the symptoms of this condition, but the effects are less robust than for medication. Psychosocial treatments may have some utility in ameliorating some of the associated conditions, comorbid disorders of ADHD, and improving family functioning (36). These treatments tend to be well received by parents (5, 36) and are possibly underused in primary care settings (5).

2.5 ADHD in adulthood: Epidemiology, comorbidities, and associated features

The symptoms of ADHD and the associated functional impairment are not limited to children and adolescents. ADHD is a condition that can impact an adult's academic, occupational, social, and relationship functioning. Controversy has existed regarding the validity of ADHD in adults (37). However, empirical evidence supports the validity of this diagnosis in adults based on similar clinical correlates, psychiatric comorbidity, abnormalities in the structure and function of the brain, response to treatment, and the results of family studies that are shared by adults and children with the disorder (38, 39). In addition, the persistence of the disorder from childhood into adulthood has been supported by long-term follow-up studies (40, 41).

A prevalence of 4.4% was found for ADHD in a nationally representative sample of 18–44-year-old respondents (42). Substantial impairment in role functioning was related to ADHD. Males were more likely to carry the diagnosis than females (42), a pattern mirrored among children (8). Additional correlates of ADHD in this sample included being previously married, unemployed, and non-Hispanic white (42). Adults with ADHD tend to experience a higher prevalence of repeated grades, reading disability, tutoring, and special education placement than adults without ADHD (43). In addition, lower socioeconomic status, more frequent job changes, inefficient work habits, reductions in productivity, difficulties managing the demands of the household and childrearing, poor financial decisions, and a higher prevalence of separation and divorce also characterize adults with ADHD (37, 43).

Adults may be less likely to display hyperactivity and impulsivity than their younger counterparts (37, 44). In a sample of clinically-referred adults with ADHD, over 90% endorsed symptoms of inattention (45). Adult ADHD is comorbid with mood disorders, anxiety disorders, substance use disorders, and Antisocial Personality Disorder (42, 43). Comorbidity with other psychiatric conditions may be more prevalent for adults with hyperactivity and impulsivity than for those with inattention (45). Neuropsychological deficits tend to be nonspecific and manifested across multiple domains. Deficits have been found in behavioral inhibition, attention, and memory, which tend to be exacerbated by comorbid psychopathology (46). Adults and children with ADHD display similarities in neuropsychological functioning, which provides additional support for continuity of the disorder into adulthood (46). To appropriately treat ADHD in adulthood, practitioners must be aware of its manifestations, effective assessment approaches, common comorbidities, and treatment options.

2.6 Assessment of ADHD in adults

The assessment of the symptoms of ADHD in adults can be reliably accomplished by professionals with adequate knowledge of the developmental course of ADHD and its common manifestations in adulthood. The same diagnostic criteria used for diagnosing ADHD in childhood and adolescence are used for diagnosing this condition in adulthood (1) (see Tab. 2.2). However, modifications to the assessment process for adults must be made to arrive at an accurate diagnostic formulation. In the absence of an accurate diagnostic formulation, the choice of treatment may be misguided or inappropriate.

A thorough medical evaluation to rule out various medical conditions that can affect attention, such as diabetes and certain cardiac problems is necessary (47). Stressful life events also need to be ruled out as a cause of inattention or poor self-control (47). Adults may be more likely to suffer from psychiatric conditions than children which may make diagnosis difficult (47). In addition, some of the symptoms of ADHD are also symptoms of other psychiatric conditions (47, 48). For instance, problems with concentration are common for individuals who are suffering from a depressive disorder. Fidgetiness can be related to an anxiety disorder, and hyperactivity and impulsivity can be a manifestation of a manic episode (37). A comprehensive clinical interview would determine if these symptoms have persisted since childhood, and thus might be suggestive of ADHD, or are a recent change in functioning that point to another psychiatric condition. The presence of comorbid psychiatric conditions must be assessed because they can have implications for the choice of treatment.

The diagnostic criteria must not only be met with regard to current functioning, but establishment of the core symptoms of ADHD by at least the middle school years is also necessary (47). The methods by which this information is obtained can affect its accuracy. Information gathered from retrospective reports of childhood functioning may be subject to recall bias (47). Whereas the chronic impairment that is associated with ADHD is likely to be remembered by adults (39), the information obtained by a retrospective report should not constitute the primary basis of diagnosis.

A clinical interview with the parents or siblings of the adult patient can provide information about childhood functioning as well as the patient's current symptoms, educational functioning, occupational functioning, and social functioning (47). In addition, parents can complete behavioral rating scales in which they rate the childhood behavior of the adult patient (49). Historical data, such as school report cards, behavioral rating scales completed by teachers, disciplinary reports, and psychological assessments can also shed light on previous levels of functioning. Parental interviews and historical data circumvent the possibility of recall bias that exists when relying solely on a patient's retrospective report. In the absence of a documented history of chronic inattention and poor self-control, a diagnosis of ADHD is likely to be inappropriate (47, 48).

In addition to documenting the history of symptoms, clinically significant impairment in functioning (e.g., educational, vocational, social, relationship) must also be displayed. Information pertinent to this diagnostic requirement may be obtained from performance reviews from jobs and college transcripts (47). Information gathered from self-report inventories such as the Brown Adult Attention-Deficit Disorder Scales (50) and the Wender Utah Rating Scale (51) can also provide clinically relevant information. The results of psychological testing (e.g., intelligence testing, achievement testing) can be used to support conclusions obtained from the clinical interview and historical information, but should not be the sole diagnostic tool (47).

Assessing ADHD in children, adolescents, and adults requires obtaining information from multiple sources. Documentation of cross-situational persistence of inattention, hyperactivity, impulsivity, and functional impairment are required for the diagnosis to be rendered. Ruling out alternative explanations for the symptoms and assessing for comorbid conditions is necessary. The diagnostic process for adults with ADHD is associated with unique challenges, such as assessing for the presence of the core symptoms of ADHD in childhood. Caution must be exercised to assure that the diagnosis of ADHD is reserved only for those adults whose symptoms are lifelong and impair functioning. This diagnosis is not appropriate for adults whose inattention, hyperactivity, and impulsivity are transient, temporary, or normal variations in these constructs (8, 47).

2.7 Treatment of ADHD in adults

Similar to the treatment of ADHD in children and adolescents, pharmacological agents are frequently used with adults with ADHD. Many of the same medications that are used with young patients are used with adults (see Tab. 2.3). Psychostimulants are the most commonly used class of medications in treating ADHD in adults and are considered the first-line treatment (48, 52). These medications enhance attention and concentration, reduce impulsivity, and improve academic and work functioning in adults (37). The response rate of adults with ADHD to methylphenidate may be as high as 70% (53).

There are unique considerations when using these medications with adults. For instance, the effect on cardiovascular functioning of psychostimulants may be of greater concern than it is for children and adolescents. Adults may also require higher doses of psychostimulants than young patients (48). In addition, the abuse potential of the psychostimulants may preclude their use in adults who have a substance use disorder. If a patient has a comorbid substance use disorder it may be more effective to refer that patient to substance abuse treatment before initiating medication for ADHD. However, concurrent treatment for ADHD and substance abuse can produce improvements in both conditions (47).

Similar to the pharmacological treatment of ADHD in children and adolescents, there is a role for the use of non-stimulant medication in adults with ADHD. Bupropion is an atypical antidepressant with stimulant properties (48). Since this medication is not a controlled substance it may be effective for adults with comorbid ADHD and substance abuse (37). Tricyclic antidepressants (e.g., desipramine, imipramine) have also been used (37), but may not be as effective as other agents (49). The use of antidepressants in conjunction with stimulant medication may improve mood and reduce affective instability for individuals whose ADHD is comorbid with a depressive disorder (48). For patients with comorbid hypertension, the use of an antihypertensive agent such as clonidine or guanfacine may be a better choice (37, 48), although the benefits of clonidine for the treatment of ADHD are less clear in adults than they are in children (48).

As with children and adolescents, not all adults respond favorably to medication (53). Medication may not produce a complete amelioration of symptoms, and it does not provide patients with adaptive coping strategies and skills (54). In addition, some adults may have comorbid psychiatric disorders. Therefore, as with young patients, adjunctive psychosocial treatments are an important component of a comprehensive treatment plan for adults with ADHD. The nature of these treatments for adults can take several forms. Adults with ADHD may benefit from education about their disorder (48) and a review of the role that it has played in their lives (49). Simply having an explanation for the years of difficulty in multiple domains of their functioning, as well as reframing the disorder as neurobiological and not characterological (55), can produce a sense of relief and reduce self-blame. Adults with ADHD may profit from training to improve organizational skills, enhance memory, reduce distractions, and improve task completion (48, 56). They may also benefit from receiving support in adjusting to the effects of medication (57).

Cognitive and cognitive–behavioral approaches have also shown promise for treating the symptoms of ADHD in adults. In a naturalistic study of adults with ADHD that included retrospective chart reviews, cognitive therapy resulted in significant improvements of symptoms of ADHD, anxiety, depression, and overall functioning (58). In addition, a pilot study of group-administered treatment based on the principles of cognitive–behavioral treatment for Borderline Personality Disorder (59) that was tailored to adults with ADHD resulted in a reduction in ADHD symptoms and depressive symptoms, and an increase in general health status (60).

These results from uncontrolled studies have been supported by the findings from a controlled clinical trial (61). Thirty-one adults with residual ADHD symptoms after beginning medication were randomized to a trial of cognitive-behavioral therapy (CBT) or continued medication alone. CBT consisted of psychoeducation about ADHD, instruction in organization and planning, learning strategies to reduce distractibility, cognitive restructuring, and optional training in communication, anger management, and reducing procrastination. Adults who received CBT had lower independently-rated ADHD symptoms, anxiety, depression, and lower self-reported ADHD symptoms and anxiety than adults who did not receive CBT (61). Whereas adults appear to benefit from cognitive-oriented treatments for ADHD, cognitive therapy with children and adolescents for this condition has not received empirical support (6). The benefits of cognitive-oriented treatments for adults may be due to their developed cognitive skills (61). Adults may also be more motivated for this form of treatment than children and young adolescents, who typically are referred by parents or teachers (61). Cognitive–behavioral approaches may be particularly suited for adults with ADHD because the sessions are structured, and the use of an agenda promotes focus and adherence to tasks and goals (54).

There may be a role for additional forms of psychosocial treatment for adults with ADHD. For instance, psychotherapy groups can teach and enhance coping skills, provide a source of support, and address interpersonal functioning (52). Couple and family therapy can also be effective for adults with ADHD (49) in that it can provide partners and family members with information about ADHD, address and attempt to remedy interpersonal deficits that have arisen as a consequence of the core symptoms of ADHD, and harness support from significant others in assisting the adult with ADHD in developing more adaptive coping and compensatory strategies. Support groups for family members can provide education about ADHD and ways to assist the adult with this condition (19).

Pharmacological treatment is effective for the management of the core symptoms of ADHD in adults. In addition, there is a role for adjunctive psychosocial treatment. Candidates for psychosocial intervention include individuals with psychiatric comorbidity (e.g., depressive disorders, anxiety disorders), those who experience psychological distress as a result of a lifetime coping with the sequela of ADHD, such as poor interpersonal functioning and decrements in self-worth (52), and those who continue to manifest functionally impairing residual symptoms after beginning medication.

2.8 Conclusions

ADHD is a neurodevelopmental disorder that has an onset in childhood and can persist into adolescence and adulthood. ADHD is one of several behavioral and developmental disorders that are associated with impairment in functioning across the lifespan. The assessment and treatment of ADHD highlight issues that are pertinent to the management of other developmental and behavioral disorders. Similar to other developmental and behavioral disorders, the assessment of ADHD in childhood, adolescence, and adulthood is based on integrating data from multiple sources utilizing multiple methods. Treatment involves pharmacological and psychosocial intervention. A multidisciplinary approach to assessment and treatment of developmental and behavioral disorders can ensure an accurate diagnostic formulation and the provision of effective treatment.

Acknowledgments

The author is appreciative of the editorial assistance that was provided by Rebecca L. Scotland, PhD.

References

1. American Psychiatric Association. (1994) Diagnostic and statistical manual of mental disorders. 4th ed. Washington DC, USA: American Psychiatric Association.
2. Brown, R. T., Freeman, W. S., Perrin, J. M., Stein, M. T., Amler, R. W., Feldman, H. M., et al. (2001) Prevalence and assessment of attention-deficit/hyperactivity disorder in primary care settings. Pediatrics 107:E43.
3. Offord, D. R., Boyle, M. H., Szatmari, P., Rae-Grant, N. I., Links PS, Cadman DT, et al. (1987) Ontario Child Health Study: II. Six-month prevalence of disorder and rates of service utilization. Arch. Gen. Psychiatry 44:832–836.
4. Biederman, J. (1998) Attention-deficit/hyperactivity disorder: a life-span perspective. J. Clin. Psychiatry 59(Suppl 7):4–16.
5. Goldman, L. S., Genel, M., Bezman, R. J., Slanetz, P. J., Council on Scientific Affairs, American Medical Association. (1998) Diagnosis and treatment of attention-deficit/hyperactivity disorder in children and adolescents. JAMA 279:1100–1107.
6. Pelham, W. E., Jr., Wheeler, T., Chronis, A. (1998) Empirically supported psychosocial treatments for attention deficit hyperactivity disorder. J. Clin. Child Psychol. 27:190–205.

7. Barkley, R. A. (1998) Associated problems. In: Barkley, R. A. Attention-deficit hyperactivity disorder: a handbook for diagnosis and treatment, 2nd ed. New York, USA: Guilford, pp. 97–138.
8. Barkley, R. A. (1998) Primary symptoms, diagnostic criteria, prevalence, and gender differences. In: Barkley, R. A. Attention-deficit hyperactivity disorder: a handbook for diagnosis and treatment, 2nd ed. New York, USA: Guilford, pp. 56–96.
9. Cantwell, D. P. (1996) Attention deficit disorder: a review of the past 10 years. J. Am. Acad. Child. Adolesc. Psychiatry 35:978–987.
10. McGuffin, P., Riley, B., Plomin, R. (2001) Genomics and behavior. Toward behavioral genomics. Science 291:1232–1249.
11. Alberts-Corush, J., Firestone, P., Goodman, J. T. (1986) Attention and impulsivity characteristics of the biological and adoptive parents of hyperactive and normal control children. Am. J. Orthopsychiatry 56:413–423.
12. Faraone, S. V., Biederman, J., Milberger, S. (1994) An exploratory study of ADHD among second-degree relatives of ADHD children. Biol. Psychiatry 35:398–402.
13. Sprich, S., Biederman, J., Crawford, M. H., Mundy, E., Faraone, S. V. (2000) Adoptive and biological families of children and adolescents with ADHD. J. Am. Acad. Child Adolesc. Psychiatry 39:1432–1437.
14. Zametkin, A. J., Liotta W. (1998) The neurobiology of attention-deficit/hyperactivity disorder. J. Clin. Psychiatry 59 (Suppl 7):17–23.
15. Faraone, S. V., Biederman, J. (1998) Neurobiology of attention-deficit hyperactivity disorder. Biol. Psychiatry 44:951–958.
16. Barkley, R. A. (1997) Behavioral inhibition, sustained attention, and executive functions: constructing a unifying theory of ADHD. Psychol. Bull. 121:65–94.
17. Biederman, J., Newcorn, J., Sprich, S. (1991) Comorbidity of attention deficit hyperactivity disorder with conduct, depressive, anxiety, and other disorders. Am. J. Psychiatry 148:564–577.
18. Taylor, E., Chadwick, O., Heptinstall, E., Danckaerts, M. (1996) Hyperactivity and conduct problems as risk factors for adolescent development. J. Am. Acad. Child Adolesc. Psychiatry 35:1213–1226.
19. Wilens, T. E., Biederman, J., Spencer, T. J. (2002) Attention deficit/hyperactivity disorder across the lifespan. Annu. Rev. Med. 53:113–131.
20. Wolraich, M. L., Hannah, J. N., Baumgaertel, A., Feurer, I. D. (1998) Examination of DSM-IV criteria for attention deficit/hyperactivity disorder in a county-wide sample. J. Dev. Behav. Pediatr. 19:162–168.
21. American Academy of Pediatrics. (2000) Clinical practice guideline: diagnosis and evaluation of the child with attention-deficit/hyperactivity disorder. Pediatrics 105:1158–1170.
22. Barkley, R. A., Edwards, G. (1998) Diagnostic interview, behavioral ratings scales, and the medical examination. In: Barkley, R. A. Attention-deficit hyperactivity disorder: a handbook for diagnosis and treatment, 2nd ed. New York, USA: Guilford Press, pp. 263–293.
23. Conners, C. K. (1997) Conners' rating scales – revised: instruments for use with children and adolescents. New York, USA: Multi-Health Systems.
24. Achenbach, T. M. (1991) Manual for the Child Behavior Checklist/4-18 and 1991 profile. Burlington, USA: University Vermont Department Psychiatry.
25. Gordon, M., Barkley, R. A. (1998) Tests and observational measures. In: Barkley, R. A. Attention-deficit hyperactivity disorder: a handbook for diagnosis and treatment, 2nd ed. New York, USA: Guilford, pp. 294–311.
26. Corkum, P. V., Siegel, L. S. (1993) Is the continuous performance task a valuable research tool for use with children with attention-deficit-hyperactivity disorder? J. Child Psychol. Psychiatry 34:1217–1239.
27. Biederman, J., Arnsten, A. F., Faraone, S. V., Doyle, A. E., Spencer, T. J., Wilens, T. E. et al. (2006) New developments in the treatment of ADHD. J. Clin. Psychiatry 67:148–159.

28. Biederman, J., Faraone, S. V. (2005) Attention-deficit hyperactivity disorder. Lancet 366:237–248.
29. DuPaul, G. J., Barkley, R. A., Connor, D. F. Stimulants. (1998) In: Barkley, R. A. Attention-deficit hyperactivity disorder: a handbook for diagnosis and treatment, 2nd ed. New York, USA: Guilford Press, pp. 510–551.
30. Biederman. J., Monuteaux, M. C., Spencer, T., Wilens, T. E., Faraone, S. V. (2009) Do stimulants protect against psychiatric disorders in youth with ADHD? A 10-year follow-up study. Pediatrics 124:71–78.
31. Biederman, J., Thisted, R. A., Greenhill, L. L., Ryan, N. D. (1995) Estimation of the association between desipramine and the risk for sudden death in 5- to 14-year-old children. J. Clin. Psychiatry 56:87–93.
32. Varley, C. K., McClellan, J. (1997) Case study: two additional sudden deaths with tricyclic antidepressants. J. Am. Acad. Child Adolesc. Psychiatry 36:390–394.
33. Wilens, T. E., Spencer, T. J., Swanson, J. M., Connor, D. F., Cantwell, D. (1999) Combining methylphenidate and clonidine: a clinically sound medication option. J. Am. Acad. Child Adolesc. Psychiatry 38:614–619.
34. Scahill, L., Chappell, P. B., Kim, Y. S., Schultz, R. T., Katsovich, L., Shepherd, E. et al. (2001) A placebo-controlled study of guanfacine in the treatment of children with tic disorders and attention deficit hyperactivity disorder. Am. J. Psychiatry 158:1067–1074.
35. DuPaul, G. J., Guevremont, D. C., Barkley, R. A. (1992) Behavioral treatment of attention-deficit hyperactivity disorder in the classroom. The use of the attention training system. Behav. Modif. 16:204–225.
36. The MTA Cooperative Group. (1999) A 14-month randomized clinical trial of treatment strategies for attention-deficit/hyperactivity disorder. The MTA Cooperative Group. Multimodal Treatment Study of Children with ADHD. Arch. Gen. Psychiatry 56:1073–1086.
37. Pary, R., Lewis, S., Matuschka, P. R., Rudzinskiy, P., Safi, M., Lippmann, S. (2002) Attention deficit disorder in adults. Ann. Clin. Psychiatry 14:105–111.
38. Faraone, S. V., Biederman, J., Spencer, T., Wilens, T., Seidman, L. J., Mick, E., et al. (2000) Attention-deficit/hyperactivity disorder in adults: an overview. Biol. Psychiatry 48:9–20.
39. Spencer, T., Biederman, J., Wilens, T. E., Faraone, S. V. (1998) Adults with attention-deficit/hyperactivity disorder: a controversial diagnosis. J. Clin. Psychiatry 59(Suppl. 7):59–68.
40. Mannuzza, S., Klein, R. G., Bonagura, N., Malloy, P., Giampino, T. L., Addalli, K. A. (1991) Hyperactive boys almost grown up. V. Replication of psychiatric status. Arch. Gen. Psychiatry 48:77–83.
41. Mannuzza, S., Klein, R. G., Bessler, A., Malloy, P., LaPadula, M. (1993) Adult outcome of hyperactive boys. Educational achievement, occupational rank, and psychiatric status. Arch. Gen. Psychiatry 50:565–576.
42. Kessler, R. C., Adler, L., Barkley, R., Biederman, J., Conners, C. K., Demler, O., et al. (2006) The prevalence and correlates of adult ADHD in the United States: results from the National Comorbidity Survey Replication. Am. J. Psychiatry 163:716–723.
43. Biederman, J., Faraone, S. V., Spencer, T., Wilens, T., Norman, D., Lapey, K. A., et al. (1993) Patterns of psychiatric comorbidity, cognition, and psychosocial functioning in adults with attention deficit hyperactivity disorder. Am. J. Psychiatry 150:1792–1798.
44. Biederman, J., Mick, E., Faraone, S. V. (2000) Age-dependent decline of symptoms of attention deficit hyperactivity disorder: impact of remission definition and symptom type. Am. J. Psychiatry 157:816–818.
45. Millstein, R. B., Wilens, T. E., Biederman, J., Spencer, T. J. (1997) Presenting ADHD symptoms and subtypes in clinically referred adults with ADHD. J. Atten. Disord. 2:159–166.
46. Hervey, A. S., Epstein, J. N., Curry, J. F. (2004) Neuropsychology of adults with attention-deficit/hyperactivity disorder: a meta-analytic review. Neuropsychology 18:485–503.
47. Murphy, K. R., Gordon, M. (1998) Assessment of adults with ADHD. In: Barkley, R. A. Attention-deficit hyperactivity disorder: a handbook for diagnosis and treatment. New York, USA: Guilford, pp. 345–369.

48. Searight, H. R., Burke, J. M., Rottnek, F. (2000) Adult ADHD: evaluation and treatment in family medicine. Am. Fam. Physician 62:2077–86, 2091–2092.
49. Wender, P. H., Wolf, L. E., Wasserstein, J. (2001) Adults with ADHD. An overview. Ann. NY Acad. Sci. 931:1–16.
50. Brown, T. E. (1996) Brown attention-deficit disorder scales for adolescents and adults. San Antonio, USA: Psychol Corporation.
51. Ward, M. F., Wender, P. H., Reimherr, F. W. (1993) The Wender Utah Rating Scale: an aid in the retrospective diagnosis of childhood attention deficit hyperactivity disorder. Am. J. Psychiatry 150:885–890.
52. Wilens, T. E., Spencer, T. J., Biederman, J. (1998) Pharmacotherapy of adult ADHD. In: Barkley, R. A. Attention-deficit hyperactivity disorder: a handbook for diagnosis and treatment. New York, USA: Guilford, pp. 592–606.
53. Spencer, T., Wilens, T., Biederman, J., Faraone, S. V., Ablon, J. S., Lapey, K. (1995) A double-blind, crossover comparison of methylphenidate and placebo in adults with childhood-onset attention-deficit hyperactivity disorder. Arch. Gen. Psychiatry 52:434–443.
54. Safren, S. A. (2006) Cognitive-behavioral approaches to ADHD treatment in adulthood. J. Clin. Psychiatry 67(Suppl. 8):46–50.
55. Murphy, K. R. (1998) Psychological counseling of adults with ADHD. In: Barkley, R. A. Attention-deficit hyperactivity disorder: a handbook for diagnosis and treatment. New York, USA: Guilford, pp. 582–591.
56. Wilens, T. E., Faraone, S. V., Biederman, J. (2004) Attention-deficit/hyperactivity disorder in adults. JAMA 292:619–623.
57. Bemporad, J. R. (2001) Aspects of psychotherapy with adults with attention deficit disorder. Ann. NY Acad. Sci. 931:302–309.
58. Wilens, T. E., McDermott, S. P., Biederman, J., Abrantes, A., Hahesy, A., Spencer, T. (1999) Cognitive therapy in the treatment of adults with ADHD: a systematic chart review of 26 cases. J. Cogn. Psychother. 13:215–226.
59. Linehan, M. M. (1993) Cognitive-behavioral treatment of borderline personality disorder. New York, USA: Guilford.
60. Hesslinger, B., Tebartz van Elst, L., Nyberg, E., Dykierek, P., Richter, H., Berner, M. et al. (2002) Psychotherapy of attention deficit hyperactivity disorder in adults: a pilot study using a structured skills training program. Eur. Arch. Psychiatry Clin. Neurosci. 252:177–184.
61. Safren, S. A., Otto, M. W., Sprich, S., Winett, C. L., Wilens, T. E., Biederman, J. (2005) Cognitive-behavioral therapy for ADHD in medication-treated adults with continued symptoms. Behav. Res. Ther. 43:831–842.

3 Adults with cystic fibrosis

Michael I. Anstead

Adults with cystic fibrosis (CF) will soon outnumber children with CF. Hence, adult and pediatric physicians must understand CF. Adults with CF face a very difficult challenge: to have a career and/or a family while still finding the time to keep up the often demanding treatment regimen required to maintain their health in the face of a complicated multisystem disease. It is our duty as physicians to help them meet this challenge by providing effective and compassionate care. Increasingly effective treatments for CF are gradually becoming available that may markedly enhance the quality-of-life (QoL) and improve survival for patients with CF. Intelligently integrating these new therapies with existing therapies to minimize treatment burden while maximizing the benefit of these therapies to maintain lung function and prolong life is perhaps the greatest challenge we face as caregivers to patients with CF.

3.1 Introduction

"Children are not merely little adults" is a mantra professed by many pediatricians. Conversely, physicians caring for adults with CF realize that adults are not just big children, but face a different set of challenges in their care. Improvements in care have significantly increased life expectancy for CF patients. The mean lifespan for patients with CF improves every year. The median predicted survival age for CF was 37.4 years based on the recent CF Foundation registry (▶ Fig. 3.1). Improvements in survival for adults with CF have lead to changes in the CF population. Almost half of patients with CF are adults now, and within the next few years adults will outnumber children with CF.

CF is an autosomal recessive genetic disease that results from a mutation in the gene that codes for the cystic fibrosis transmembrane conductance regulator (CFTR), which is a membrane-associated chloride channel. The most common mutation in the worldwide is ΔF508, a deletion of a three base pair that results in deletion of a phenylalanine at amino acid position 508. Worldwide, ~90% of patients with CF have at least one copy of the ΔF508 mutation, and 45% are homozygous for this mutation (1). The frequency of this mutation is even higher in Northern Europe and in the USA. However, > 1.600 different mutations have been discovered so far. These many different mutations have different degrees of effect on CFTR function, which accounts for some of the variations in illness severity inCF patients. In addition, other genes separate from the CF locus may act as modifier genes, and have significant effects on the severity of illness.

Although the discovery and cloning of the CF gene in 1989 was a landmark achievement, it has not led to the dramatic new therapies that many then thought were just around the corner. The realization that cures for all chronic diseases are elusive has led the Cystic Fibrosis Foundation and CF Care Centers to move away from the "cure" paradigm to a more pragmatic paradigm to improve care and treatments for CF

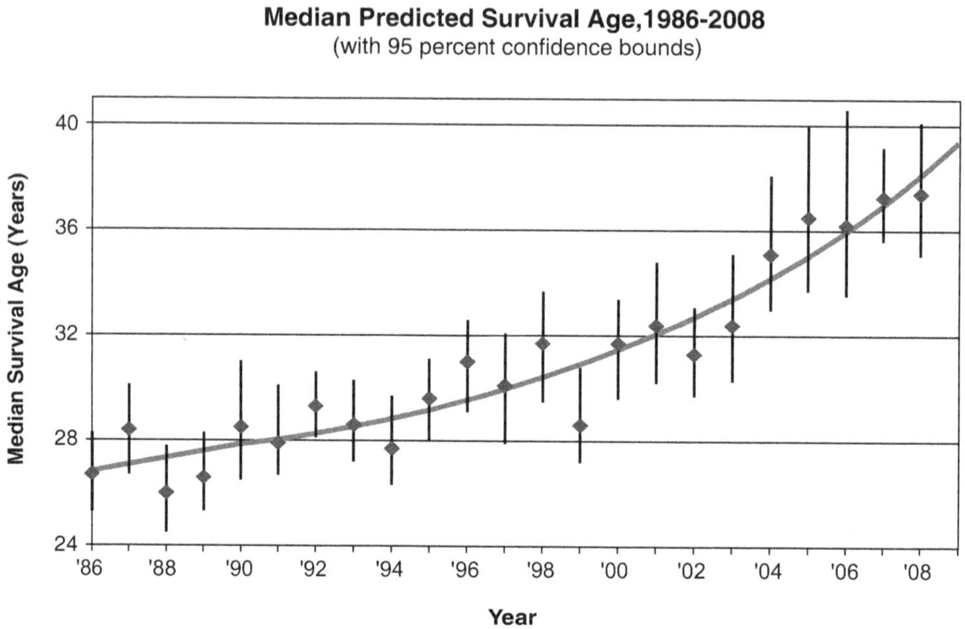

Fig. 3.1: Median predicted survival age 1986–2008 (with 95% confidence intervals). The median predicted survival age by life table analysis was 37.4 years for 2008. This represents the age by which half of the current CF Registry population would be expected to die given the ages of CF patients in the Registry and the mortality distribution of deaths in 2008. The whiskers represent the 95% confidence intervals for the survival estimates, indicating that the 2008 median predicted survival is between 35.0 years and 40.1 years.

across the entire spectrum of the disease. In addition, expansion of newborn screening for CF to all states in the USA has provided new opportunities to improve care. By utilizing newborn screening, nearly all patients with CF will be diagnosed before the age of 1 month and before they have significant nutritional or pulmonary sequelae. It is well established that infants with CF diagnosed by newborn screening have better nutritional outcomes (2). Although improvement in pulmonary outcomes is less well established, newborn screening provides may potentially prevent (or eradicate) initial infection with pathogens such as *Pseudomonas aeruginosa* or methicillin-resistant *Staphylococcus aureus* (MRSA) that may be associated with more rapid decline of lung function and a worse prognosis in CF. In the long-run, this improved nutrition and prevention (or eradication) of infection with more virulent pulmonary pathogens may result in improvements in lung function and the prognosis for patients with CF.

3.2 CF care paradigm

There are several potential therapies that are under development that have the potential to directly or indirectly improve the expression or function of the CFTR (the basic defect in CF). Until these therapies become reality, a paradigm for CF care has evolved based on the availability of newborn screening and better utilization of proven therapies.

1. Utilize newborn screening to diagnose most patients before they have malnutrition or chronic lung disease:
   - Optimize nutrition from initial diagnosis by providing adequate caloric intake, treatment of malabsorption with pancreatic enzymes, and supplementation with fat-soluble vitamins.
   - Initiate airway clearance therapies from initial diagnosis.
   - Monitor airway cultures from birth and utilize therapies to prevent (or eradicate) initial respiratory-tract infection with pathogens associated with a more rapid decline in lung function such as *Pseudomonas aeruginosa* or MRSA.
2. Early initiation and further development of therapies that incrementally improve the airway environment or function of airway cells at the cellular level preserve airway function. Examples of these therapies include hypertonic saline that is currently available or denufosol (which is currently in Phase III trials and hopefully will be available soon). Both of these therapies improve hydration of the airway surface layer, hypertonic saline by osmotic movement of water from the airway cells to the surface fluid layer and denufosol through increased secretion of chloride and water form the cells through activation of non-CFTR alternative chloride channels. This increase in airway surface fluid improves ciliary function and mucociliary clearance. Another example is dornase alpha (a nebulized therapy that cleaves DNA macromolecules in sputum from DNA extruded from the nuclei of disintegrating cells), which reduces sputum viscosity (3).
3. Continued aggressive treatment with nebulized, oral, and intravenous antibiotics to help control the burden of infection in CF patients chronically infected with airway pathogens (especially *Pseudomonas aeruginosa*) utilizing accepted treatment guidelines (3, 4).
4. Continual quality improvement efforts to establish best practices and to more uniformly apply them across CF Care Centers across the USA and the world.
5. Efforts to simultaneously enhance adherence in all patients with CF to recommended therapies while simultaneously being cognizant of the impact of treatment burden from all the therapies utilized on the QoL for patients with CF.
6. Continued research into therapies to correct the underlying defect. This can involve inserting a normal gene for CFTR into the cell. It could also involve pharmacologic therapies to improve the function of mutant CFTR by, for example, increasing its transport to the membrane, or increasing chloride ion flow once it reaches the membrane.

   The quality improvement efforts of the Cystic Fibrosis Foundation and CF Care Centers (as well as the development of this paradigm to optimize CF care)may lead to healthier young adults with much better lung function transitioning to adult CF programs and a further increase in survival.

3.3 Transition from pediatric to adult care

To ensure the best care for all CF patients, the Cystic Fibrosis Foundation mandated that all accredited CF Care Centers must have an adult program to provide age-appropriate care for adults with CF. Transition of CF teens and young adults to adult care is about the smooth transfer of patients to the adult care team. However, it should involve a planned, purposeful preparation of patients to move to care from the adult CF team. There is no universal formula for successful transition of CF adolescents and young adults into adult care. Although true outcome-based literature on effective transition strategies is generally not available, several elements of the transition strategy seem to be associated with a more successful transition (5).

Most importantly, the idea of transition should be introduced early to patients and their families. This reinforces the idea to patients and their families that someday they will grow up and have adult responsibilities. Patients and their families should know when transition will occur. This could be a defined age (e.g., 18 years) or a milestone. We transition our patients when they graduate from high school or by the age of 19 years if they are no longer in school.

It is a good practice for the adult team (or at least some members of the adult team) to see the patient at the Pediatric Clinic prior to transfer. This will make the initial visit at the Adult Clinic less stressful. Another potentially useful strategy would be to have CF patients and their families visit the adult inpatient facility prior to transfer. This allows patients to work out some of the anxieties of transition at a time they are feeling well. It also reduces the stress of the first admission to this new facility if they are also facing the stress of an acute on chronic illness.

Communication between the Adult and Pediatric Care Teams is essential to ensure a successful transition. Ideally, the Adult and Pediatric CF Care Teams should meet regularly to discuss patients to be transitioned and discuss recently transitioned patients. These meetings ensure that there is appropriate sharing of necessary clinical information about patients and also encourages a more common approach to CF care between the Adult and Pediatric CF Care Teams.

3.4 Challenges of treatment burden and adherence to maintain lung function

Adults with CF face many challenges in maintaining lung function and health. One of the greatest challenges involves trying to keep up with the tremendous burden of medications (as well as nebulizer and airway clearance therapies) they must undertake everyday to maintain their health. The emergence of many new therapies in CF has given patients more treatment options and has resulted in better overall health for CF patients. Availability of these therapies to preserve lung function in CF (and more appropriate utilization of these therapies) has played a major part in the significant improvements in overall QoL and median lifespan that has been achieved for patients with CF over the previous 15–20 years.

Unfortunately, most of these treatments involve nebulized medications and can be very time-consuming, taking increasing amounts of time out of the patient's lives and impacting significantly on QoL. A recent study of adults with CF showed that the median number of nebulizer and airway clearance therapies per day was 7 and the mean time spent per day was 108 min (6). It is not surprising that the prevalence of treatment adherence for many CF patients is not as high as we would hope, and the overall prevalence of adherence was < 50% among CF patients (7). Poor adherence such treatment in other chronic diseases has resulted in a reduced QoL for patients, increased prevalence of drug resistance and drug reactions, and an increase in morbidity and mortality. It has also been estimated to have a huge impact on healthcare costs; a study published in 2004 estimated that > US $300 billion were wasted annually due to poor adherence (8). Although not well quantified, it is certain that poor adherence in our CF patients results in these same negative impacts on QoL, cost of care, and morbidity and mortality.

Improving treatment adherence is one of the greatest challenges we face as CF caregivers. Improving treatment adherence involves two major efforts. Firstly, we must enhance patients' efforts to carry out all recommendations from the CF Team to maintain and optimize their health. This involves providing them with adequate education, clear treatment plans, and working with them to overcome barriers to adherence. Secondly, through research, we can provide more effective therapies while simultaneously attempting to reduce the treatment burden imposed by these therapies.

Providing more effective therapies while decreasing treatment burden as CF caregivers is a very complex issue. We want to provide the best possible therapies to enhance our patient's lives. We know many medications are helpful, but we are often unsure how these treatments interact and whether these treatments are additive or synergistic (or even potentially antagonistic with each other). A good example is dornase alpha and hypertonic saline. Both of these nebulized medications improve mucociliary clearance in CF via different mechanisms. Dornase alpha cleaves DNA macromolecules in sputum from DNA extruded from the nuclei of disintegrating cells, thereby reducing sputum viscosity. Hypertonic saline is deposited on the airway surface layer of fluid and pulls water from the cells lining the airway by osmosis, helping to augment the diminished airway surface fluid that is characteristic of CF. Dornase is generally a once-daily medication requiring 15–20 minutes to nebulize. Hypertonic saline is recommended twice daily and each nebulizer treatment takes 15–20 minutes. Some patients with CF have bronchospasm as a result of hypertonic saline, so it is recommended that patients administer a bronchodilator inhaler or nebulizer treatment before the hypertonic saline, thereby further increasing therapy time. There have been no randomized controlled studies to determine the effectiveness of these therapies in combinationas opposed to individually. We have no data to help us evaluate if these therapies are synergistic, additive, or antagonist. Some patients combine these therapies, others alternate these therapies, whereas others do hypertonic saline nebulizers once daily instead of twice daily and do dornase once daily instead of the second hypertonic saline nebulizer. It is extremely important that we carry out research to look at some of these therapy combinations to determine the best way to utilize these medications. These sorts of studies will become increasingly important as more therapies emerge for the treatment of CF. Additionally, developing new devices to deliver drug to the airways more efficiently and quickly is also important to optimize adherence for our patients. Hopefully, some new delivery devices such as dry powder-inhaled tobramycin will be available soon, providing patients with options to enhance adherence.

Regardless of our efforts to establish optimal treatment regimens and decrease treatment burdens on adults with CF, adherence ultimately lies with the patient or the patient and his family. Some patients will adhere with very complex time-consuming treatment regimens, whereas others will not adhere with very simple treatment regimens that can be completed in a few minutes. There are many variables that effect adherence in CF patients: their maturity level, their perception of illness, time constraints due to work or other activities, family support, psychological stresses (e.g., depression)as well as the patient–Physician relationship (9). Enhancing a patient's ability to adhere with therapy can be complex and must be individualized. Working with each patient and family to help identify barriers to adherence can be important for individual patients, and should be an important component of the clinic visit for adults with CF.

Although many of the interventions to improve treatment adherence for adults with CF are individualized for each patient, there are some general considerations to improve adherence in all patients with CF. First, measuring adherence and addressing adherence at each clinic visit is important. How to best measure and assess adherence remains controversial, and may change as electronic monitors to assess adherence to therapy become more available. We utilize a combination of adherence self-reporting from an assessment of therapies carried out by the pharmacist or nurse before the patient sees the Physician, along with review of pharmacy refill records in circumstances if we feel self-reporting seems incongruous with our impression of adherence. However you measure adherence, the effort to routinely assess and measure adherence at each clinic visit sends a message to patients how important adherence is and has some beneficial effects. Another important aspect of adherence is adequate education for the patient and family. We must provide patients with appropriate education if we initiate a new therapy. This education must involve not only how to carry out the therapy and how to clean and maintain the device, but also the *rationale* for the therapy and the expected benefits. Understanding the many medications, nebulizer treatments, inhalers, and airway-clearance techniques should be assessed regularly at clinic visits. Lastly, patients should all be given a written comprehensive treatment plan. We must be clear on exactly what we are asking patients to do and that they are clear on exactly what is expected of them. A comprehensive treatment plan defines the expectations for therapy and the ideal goal for adherence. It may be seen as a "contract" between the CF team and the patient.

Improving adherence in patients is an important opportunity for CF caregivers to further improve outcomes in CF. Finding better ways to assess adherence in our patients, reduce the burden of treatment, and facilitate adherence to the recommended therapies must be one of the main priorities for CF care for the foreseeable future.

3.5 Diseases of aging in CF: diabetes, osteoporosis and malignancy

CF is not just a disease of the lungs and exocrine pancreas, but a multisystem disease that affects the lungs, exocrine and endocrine pancreas, intestine, liver, and reproductive tract. As we become better able to control lung disease and improve lifespan in CF, certain complications of CF will become more prevalent as a result of longer-term organ dysfunction in other organs and the consequences of chronic disease. There are three principal disease states/complications that we must address as adult CF physicians to promote and maintain the gains in QoL and quantity-of-life from improved treatment of pulmonary disease: cystic fibrosis-related diabetes mellitus (CFRDM), osteoporosis, and malignancies (▶ Fig. 3.2).

CFTR dysfunction in the pancreas results in impaired secretion of salt and water into the pancreatic ducts. This leads to progressive scarring and eventual destruction of the pancreas. This results in exocrine pancreatic insufficiency very early in life for most CF patients. Despite the extensive scarring and destruction of the pancreas, the β-islet cells are initially relatively preserved. However, as patients get older, fibrosis of the islets occurs, resulting in a reduction in the number of insulin-producing cells (10). This loss of insulin-producing cells and relative insulin deficiency is the primary cause

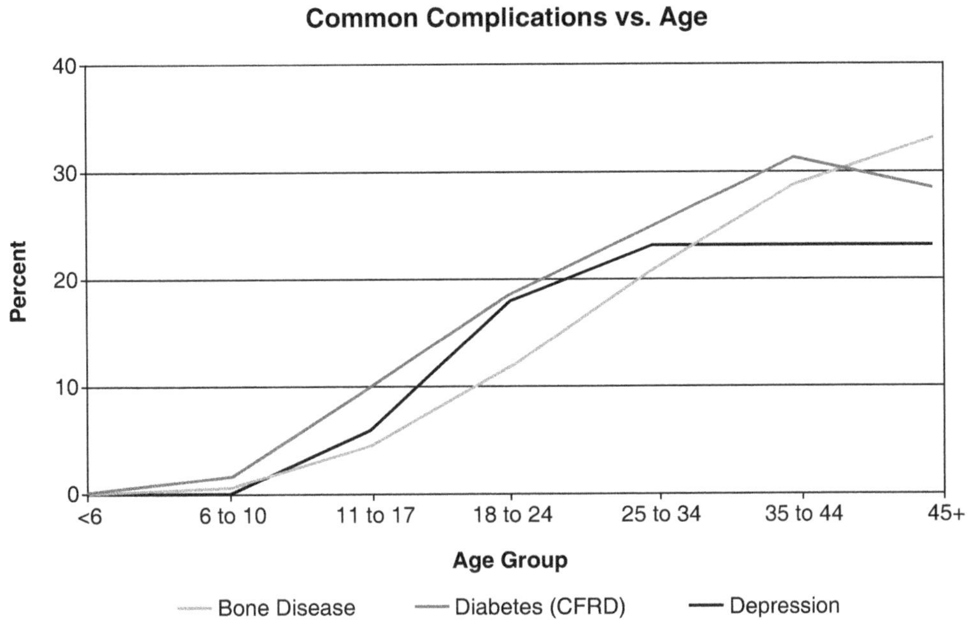

Fig. 3.2: Common complications versus age.

of CFRDM. In general, patients with CF secrete less insulin in response to an oral or intravenous glucose load (11). This insulin secretion is more impaired in CF subjects with CFRDM. In addition, insulin sensitivity seems to be decreased in patients with CF, thereby increasing the risk for CFRDM (12). The cause of insulin resistance in CF is incompletely understood, but probably related to the cytokine environment induced by chronic infection.

The prevalence of CFRDM increases with age in CF. In patients with CF aged≤10 years, the prevalence of CFRDM is ~5%. Based on registry data, by the time patients reach 40 years of age, ≥30% will have CFRDM (13). Until therapies are available for CF that affect CFTR function throughout the body, the prevalence of CFRDM in adults will continue to increase as we have more effective treatments for CF lung disease.

Aggressive detection and treatment of CFRDM is a very important part of maintaining lung function and improving overall health and survival in adults with CF. Adults with CF should be screened at least yearly for CFRDM. Oral glucose tolerance testing is the preferred method for yearly screening. Adults should have a fasting blood sugar drawn, and then drink a glucose solution containing 1.5 g/kg of glucose (maximum, 75 g). Blood sugar should be repeated 2 hours after finishing the glucose solution. Those with normal glucose tolerance will have a fasting glucose < 126 mg/dL and a 2-hour glucose of < 140 mg/dL. Impaired glucose tolerance is classified as a normal fasting glucose (< 126 mg/L), but a 2-hour post-glucose load blood sugar of 140–199 mg/dL. Patients are classified as having CFRDM if their 2-hour post-glucose load blood sugar is 200 mg/dL. CFRDM can also be diagnosed if patients have two documented fasting blood sugars of 126 mg/dL, one fasting blood sugar of 126 mg/dL, a random blood sugar of 200mg/dL, or two random blood sugars of 200 mg/dL (14).

In general, hemoglobin A1c (HgbA1c) is not useful for screening[10]. HgbA1c levels may not be elevated early in CFRDM due to the predominantly post-prandial nature of the disease. The duration of abnormal glucose may be sufficiently transient not to significantly impact HgbA1c. In addition, RBC survival may be shortened in CF, limiting the time for the glycosylation of Hgb, and decreasing the level of HgbA1c related to a given level of hyperglycemia. Nonetheless, once diagnosed, HgbA1c is used as an overall measure of glucose control along with pre- and post-prandial fingerstick blood sugar monitoring.

Management of overt CFRDM predominantly involves insulin therapy (mainly with meals). In general, patients are dosed with a form of short-acting insulin at 1unit of insulin for every 5–20 g of carbohydrate ingested along with a sliding-scale adjustment for initial blood sugar before the meal. Use of some form oflong-acting insulin (usually Lantus) to maintain basal insulin activity may also be necessary (especially if patients have fasting hyperglycemia). For patients with impaired glucose tolerance, dietary measures such as avoiding concentrated sweets and exercise may be enough to control blood sugars. These measures are also useful adjuncts for blood-sugar control for patients with CFRDM. Oral hypoglycemics have not been demonstrated to be useful for treatment of CFRDM (10). However, further studies are warranted, especially as new and novel oral hypoglycemics are developed for use in type-2 diabetes.

Treatment of CFRDM with insulin is associated with improvement in lung function and the body mass index (BMI). Each CF Adult Center must have adult endocrinologists with interest and expertise in CFRDM to help with optimal management of patients with CFRDM. Adult endocrinologists and their staff must understand that CFRDM is distinct with respect to management from type-1 and type-2 diabetes. Managing their diabetes is one of the greatest challenges faced by adults with CF. Having a supportive and knowledgeable adult endocrinologist and staff is crucial for these patients to help them manage their blood sugars through appropriate insulin and diet to optimize their nutrition and lung function. As the lifespan and mean age for CF patients continues to increase, further integrating diabetes care into adult CF care through optimizing cooperation between the Adult CF Team, the Adult Endocrinology Team, and the adult CF patient will be vital to the continued success of the Adult CF Center and the continued improvement in QoL and quantity-of-life for adults with CF.

Promoting/maintaining good bone health in patients with CF is another key challenge Adult CF Teams face as the CF population continues to age. Bone disease can be extremely debilitating to patients with CF, with fractures related to reduced bone mineral density (BMD) causing pain, limiting mobility, and reducing effectiveness of cough and airway-clearance techniques. Although adults with CF suffer most of the complications related to increased bone fragility, CFRBD starts in childhood, so any strategy to prevent it must start then.

BMD appears to be comparable in healthy, well-nourished patients with CF to the general population in early childhood (15). However, during adolescence, the prevalence of decreased BMD begins to rise. This is primarily because of decreased bone formation due to decreased calcium deposition in bones during adolescence (16). In addition, adolescents and young adults with CF may suffer from increased bone loss (especially in CF patients with frequent pulmonary exacerbations). This increased bone loss appears to result from the increased activity and number of osteoclasts induced by inflammatory cytokines released during the exacerbation.

Adult CF Teams must identify patients with CFRBD early to allow nutritional and pharmacologic interventions to prevent further bone loss. According to the Bone Health Consensus Committee Guidelines published by the Cystic Fibrosis Foundation in 2005, baseline BMD should be measured in all adults with CF at age 18 years (17). If children > 8 years of age are at high risk for CFRBD, BMD should be measured earlier. Risk factors include poor nutrition (ideal body weight < 90%), severe lung disease (forced expiratory volume in 1 second (FEV_1) < 50%), frequent treatment with oral corticosteroids, delayed puberty, and history of previous fractures. Dual-energy X-ray absorptiometry (DXA) is the primary method of screening. For patients with normal DXA scans (T or Z-score > –1.0), DXA scanning need not be repeated for 5 years. If bone density is mildly decreased from normal (T or Z score > –1.0 < –2.0), DXA should be followed every 2–4 years. For patients with a significant reduction in BMD (T or Z score < –2.0), annual DXA is recommended for monitoring (17).

Strategies to prevent CFRBD include good nutrition and a good BMI, maintaining lung function through aggressive therapy, regular weight-bearing exercise, early detection and treatment of CFRDM, minimizing exposure to oral and inhaled corticosteroids, and supplementation with calcium and vitamin D. Vitamin K is also an important co-factor for bone formation and should be supplemented. Hypogonadism or delayed puberty should be treated appropriately. Utilizing these preventive strategies and finding further strategies to prevent CFRBD is the key to establishing better overall bone health in adults with CF. Although further deterioration in BMD may be attenuated by bisphosphonates and other medications, none of the currently available medications can truly correct the altered bone formation that occurs in childhood in patients with significant CFRBD. Bisphosphonates should be utilized for treatment of patients with severely reduced BMD (T or Z score < –2.0), in patients with a more mildly reduced BMD (T or Z score < –1.0 > –2.0), if fragility fractures have occurred, or if the patient has rapidly reduced BMD or is awaiting a lung transplant. Oral agents are preferred to IV bisphosphonates, since they are equally efficacious, but have a lower risk of significant side effects, primarily post-infusion bone pain for IV bisphosphonates (10). Administered subcutaneously, the synthetic human parathyroid hormone Teriparatide can be utilized to increase BMD in patients with osteoporosis, and may be useful for some CF patients with severe osteoporosis (18).

Another potentially significant problem for the aging CF population is an increased risk of gastrointestinal (GI) malignancies. Although the overall risk of malignancy does not appear to be increased in CF, there does appear to be a higher than expected prevalence of GI malignancies. Malignancies have been diagnosed at multiple sites throughout the GI tract, including the esophagus, stomach, small intestine, large intestine, and biliary tract. However, the greatest increased risk appears to be for cancers of the small intestine, colon, and biliary tract (19). Lung transplantation appears to confer additional risk, probably as a result of immunosuppressive therapy. As the CF population survives to older ages, this prevalence of malignancy is likely to increase. Determining appropriate screening strategies to detect GI malignancies early in CF is a very important consideration as CF patients survive longer. This is particularly important in light of the many chronic GI symptoms related to CF, which may mask early symptoms of GI malignancy. The Cystic FibrosisFoundation must work with experts in GI malignancy to develop screening guidelines for adults with CF. This is especially true for malignancies such as colon cancer, where effective screening strategies for the general and high-risk populations have developed and have had a significant impact in preventing cancer. We had one colon cancer at age 40 years and one patient with multiple colonic polyps at age 50 years in our population in the last year. Based on this experience and the current evidence of increased colon cancer risk in CF, we are working with our adult gastroenterology specialists to develop colon screening guidelines for CF patients with initial screening colonoscopy at 35 years of age.

3.6 Depression and its impact on CF

Chronic illness is a significant risk factor for depression in adults. A community-based study showed that individuals with chronic medical conditions had a 41% increase in the risk for psychiatric illness (20). The demands of the treatment regimen requiring several hours each day to take medications and do treatments, and the multiple symptoms associated with the disease take an emotional toll and significantly affect QoL. Single-center studies have consistently shown evidence of elevated rates of depression in children, adolescents, and adults with CF (21). The most recent CF registry data show a prevalence of depression of 20.9% in CF patients aged >18 years (13). However, no prospective large-scale systematic studies have been done to determine the true prevalence of depression in the CF population.

Effectively diagnosing and treating adults with CFwho may be depressed is very important to help improve outcomes and QoL. Although studies have not definitely defined a negative impact of depression on lung function in adults with CF, it is likely that depression worsens disease severity by impacting on disease management by decreasing adherence and efforts at disease management. This worsening health may lead to worsening depression. Health-related QoL appears to be significantly affected by depression in CF. Patients with CF who were depressed score lower on questionnaires for emotional functioning, eating disturbances, and body image (22).

The best way to diagnose depression in CF is to be aware of it and screen for it. All Adult CF Centers must develop screening protocols to identify adults with CF with depression. Several screening questionnaires are available, and can be utilized on a yearly basis as part of the patient's yearly comprehensive visit. If elevated symptoms are endorsed, further evaluation by a counselor or psychiatrist may be indicated. CF adults with significant depressive symptoms may benefit from pharmacologic therapy and/or cognitive behavioral therapy. Identifying adults with CF with depression and providing effective treatment would be expected to improve QoL and potentially have an impact on outcome by improving adherence and attention to their medical regimen. Further studies are needed on the impact of depression in adults with CF on QoL and health outcomes.

3.7 Achieving a "normal" life

Although improving lifespan in CF is obviously of great importance, it is just as important to continually work to enhance the QoL for adults with CF. It is important for adults with CF to be able to pursue the normal activities of adult life and aspire to go to school, have a good job, fall in love, and have children and a family. Fortunately, simple goals of life that many of us take for granted can be attained by most adults with CF. The most recent

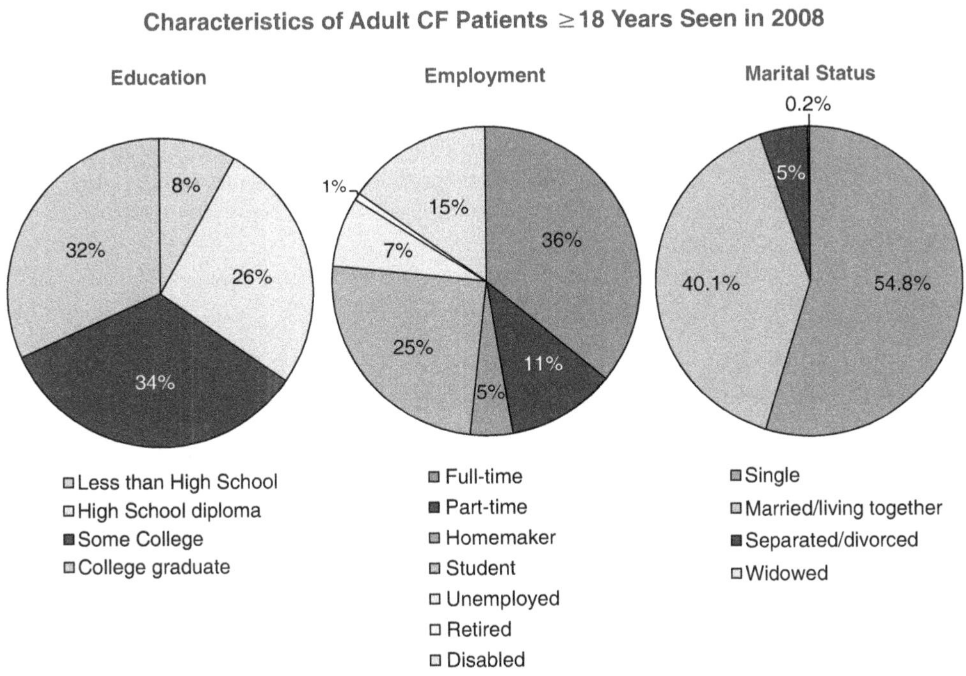

Fig. 3.3: Characteristics of adult CF patients aged ≤18 years seen in 2008.

registry data demonstrate that most adults with CF are able to work or go to school (▶ Fig. 3.3), with ~75% employed or in school.

It is important for the CF Team to work with children and adults with CF throughout their life to help them to find a job when they attain adulthood. Career planning counseling from the CF Team social worker is extremely important in CF adolescents as they prepare to go to college and/or pursue a career. Additional assistance is also available through the Division of Vocational Rehabilitation, which has offices in every state. It is important for patients to find a job that will allow them to care for themselves and not aggravate their respiratory symptoms by exposing them to infection or inhaled irritants or toxins. Work with significant exposure to dust or solvents is potentially hazardous and should be avoided. Another potentially hazardous field is healthcare. CF patients employed in healthcare may be exposed to CF pathogens such as MRSA, which may increase their frequency or exacerbations and antibiotic use and confer a worse prognosis. Conversely, adults with CF who are employed in healthcare could harbor pathogens in the respiratory tract such as MRSA or *Burkholderia cepacia*, which could be transmitted to patients for whom they are caring. This could be particularly problematic if they have to care for other patients with CF. Nonetheless, each CF adult has to make his/her own choices. All we can do is offer advice and try to do our best to help them find a job that maximizes their talents, but avoids hazards to their health and allows them enough time to care for themselves.

It is especially important for adults with CF to consider healthcare insurance when considering a job. It is vital for all CF patients to have healthcare insurance to maintain their health. An older study at one CF Center of 189 CF adults demonstrated a median survival of only 6.1 years for adults with CF without healthcare insurance compared with 20.5 years for those with Medicaid or private insurance (23). The CF Team should work with all CF patients to anticipate insurance needs (especially as CF patients transition to adulthood). Those in school can often be maintained on their parent's policy, at least until age 26 years. All CF adults should be counseled to consider healthcare benefits when considering a job. Those unable to work should be assisted in applying for disability or exploring other potential state programs that may be available to meet their healthcare needs. Hopefully the new healthcare initiative in the US Congress will eventually make it easier for patients with CF and other lifetime chronic illnesses to maintain insurance coverage throughout their lives.

Adults with CF are interested in relationships with others just like everyone else. CF patients usually start dating as adolescents. Counseling may be necessary to help them to overcome insecurities and low self-esteem when trying to establish relationships. According to the CF registry, ~39% of CF adults are married or living together (13), compared with~64% of all adults in the population. This percentage has slowly risen as adults with CF achieve better health and longer lives.

Adults with CF frequently have children. In adult CF men, this is complicated by a high prevalence of azoospermia related to CF. However, assisted reproductive techniques (including testicular sperm extraction and intra-cytoplasmic sperm injection) provide the opportunity for some men with CF to father children. Women with CF have a fertility rate approaching that of the general population. There are many challenges associated with pregnancy for women with CF to maintain their health during pregnancy (especially with regards to unmasking or worsening CFRDM and achieving adequate weight gain). Nonetheless, CF women are not, in general, negatively impacted by pregnancy. Remarkably, CF women who become pregnant and carry a child to term appear to have better survival compared with age-matched CF controls, even when corrected for lung function, frequency of exacerbation, and nutritional status (24). If CF patients are interested in having children, it is important for the Adult CF Team to optimize planning and provide appropriate counseling. Only ~1 person in 25 in the general population is a CF carrier, so most CF adults are not at risk to have offspring with CF, although all their offspring will be carriers of the gene. Nonetheless, partners of CF patients should undergo carrier screening to accurately assess the risk of CF in a potential child. Once women with CF become pregnant, it is important that they are monitored by obstetricians with experience with pregnancy in CF. Aggressive supportive obstetric care is vital to promote optimal outcome for mother and baby (25). It is also important for members of the Adult CF Team to discuss with CF adults the challenges they will face to find time to care for themselves once the baby is born.

With the improved health and increasing lifespan of CF patients and the availability of assisted reproductive techniques for males with CF, increasing numbers of adults with CF will have the opportunity to have children. Although there is an increased risk of premature birth for women with CF who have children, the potential for CF patients to have healthy children is excellent. With appropriate medical care and counseling, CF adults can enjoy a "normal" family life and have healthy children while maintaining their own health.

3.8 Conclusions

Adults with CF will soon outnumber children with CF. Hence, adult and pediatric physicians must understand CF. Adults with CF face a very difficult challenge: to have a career and/or a family while finding time to keep up the often demanding treatment regimen required to maintain their health in the face of a complicated multisystem disease. It is our duty as physicians to help them meet this challenge by providing effective and compassionate care.

Increasingly effective treatments for CF are gradually becoming available that will markedly enhance the QoL and improve survival for patients with CF. Intelligently integrating these new therapies with existing therapies to minimize treatment burden while maximizing the benefit of these therapies to maintain lung function and prolong life is the greatest challenge we face as CF caregivers.

References

1. Cystic Fibrosis Genetic Analysis Consortium. (1994) Population variation of common cystic fibrosis mutations. Hum. Mutat. 4:167–177.
2. Farrell, P. M., et al. (2001) Early diagnosis of cystic fibrosis through neonatal screening prevents severe malnutrition and improves long-term growth. Wisconsin Cystic Fibrosis Neonatal Screening Study Group. Pediatrics 107:1–13.
3. Flume, P. A., et al. (2007) Cystic fibrosis pulmonary guidelines: chronic medications for maintenance of lung health. Am. J. Respir. Crit. Care Med. 176:957–969.
4. Flume, P. A., et al. (2009) Cystic fibrosis pulmonary guidelines: treatment of pulmonary exacerbations. Am. J. Respir. Crit. Care Med. 180:802–808.
5. Flume, P. A. (2009) Smoothing the transition from pediatric to adult care: lessons learned. Flume PA. Curr. Opin. Pulm. Med. 2009 Aug. 19.
6. Sawicki, G. S., Sellers, D. E., Robinson, W. M. (2009) High treatment burden in adults with cystic fibrosis: challenges to disease self-management. J. Cyst. Fibros. 8:91–96.
7. Modi, A. C., et al. (2006) A multi-method assessment of treatment adherence for children with cystic fibrosis. J. Cyst. Fibros. 5:177–185.
8. Bender, B. G., Rand, C. (2004) Medication non-adherence and asthma treatment cost. Curr. Opin. Allergy Clin. Immunol. 4:191–195.
9. Modi, A. C., Quittner, A. L. (2006) Barriers to treatment adherence for children with cystic fibrosis and asthma: what gets in the way? J. Pediatr. Psychol. 31:846–858.
10. Curran, D. R., McArdle, J. R., Talwalkar, J. S. (2009) Diabetes mellitus and bone disease in cystic fibrosis. Semin. Respir. Crit. Care Med. 30:514–530.
11. Lanng, S., et al. (1994) Insulin sensitivity and insulin clearance in cystic fibrosis patients with normal and diabetic glucose tolerance. Clin. Endocrinol. (Oxf.) 41:217–223.
12. Hardin, D. S., et al. (1997) Insulin resistance is associated with decreased clinical status in cystic fibrosis. J. Pediatr. 130:948–956.
13. Patient Registry Annual Data Report for the Center Directors 2008. Bethesda, MD: Cystic Fibrosis Foundation, 2009.
14. Moran, A. et al. (1999) Diagnosis, screening and management of cystic fibrosis related diabetes mellitus: a consensus conference report. Diabetes Res. Clin. Pract. 45:61–73.
15. Buntain, H. M. et al. (2004) Bone mineral density in Australian children, adolescents and adults with cystic fibrosis: a controlled cross sectional study. Thorax 59:149–155.
16. Elborn, J. S. (2007) How can we prevent multisystem complications of cystic fibrosis? Semin. Respir. Crit. Care Med. 28:303–311.

17. Aris, R. M. et al. (2005) Guide to bone health and disease in cystic fibrosis. J. Clin. Endocrinol. Metab. 90:1888–1896.
18. Saag, K. G., et al. (2007) Teriparatide or alendronate in glucocorticoid-induced osteoporosis. N. Engl. J. Med. 357:2028–2039.
19. Maisonneuve, P. et al. (2003) Cancer risk in nontransplanted and transplanted cystic fibrosis patients: a 10-year study. J. Natl. Cancer Inst. 95:381–387.
20. Wells, K. B., Golding, J. M., Burnam, M. A. (1989) Chronic medical conditions in a sample of the general population with anxiety, affective, and substance use disorders. Am. J. Psychiatry 146:1440–1446.
21. Cruz, I, et al. (2009) Anxiety and depression in cystic fibrosis. Semin. Respir. Crit. Care Med. 30:569–578.
22. Havermans, T, Colpaert, K., Dupont, L. J. (2008) Quality of life in patients with cystic fibrosis: association with anxiety and depression. J. Cyst. Fibros. 7:581–584.
23. Curtis, J. R. et al. (1997) Absence of health insurance is associated with decreased life expectancy in patients with cystic fibrosis. Am. J. Respir. Crit. Care Med. 155:1921–1924.
24. Goss, C. H. et al. (2003) The effect of pregnancy on survival in women with cystic fibrosis. Chest 124:1460–1468.
25. Tonelli, M. R., Aitken, M. L. (2007) Pregnancy in cystic fibrosis. Curr. Opin. Pulm. Med. 13:537–540.

4 Childhood asthma into adult years

Don Hayes, Jr. and Zoran Danov

The incidence and prevalence of asthma have increased in recent decades, and the underlying reason is not known. Most cases of persistent wheezing and asthma begin in early childhood, which primarily defines the subjects' respiratory health throughout their lifetime. Nearly half of wheezing preschoolers "outgrow" their symptoms and commonly demonstrate reduced pulmonary function early in life. Their pulmonary function typically improves by age 6 years but not to the levels of normal function as seen in those children that never wheezed. Inhaled corticosteroids are the primary first-line therapy for asthma with improvement in symptoms, but there is failure to prevent the development of airway dysfunction later in life. Clearly, the pathogenic mechanisms have not been identified in this process, so research needs to target this important area by going beyond inflammation. Asthma research needs to address whether corticosteroid insensitivity has a role or whether other physiological mechanisms are involved.

4.1 Introduction

Multiple studies have indicated that the incidence and prevalence of asthma have increased in the recent decades, the underlying reason remains unclear. Most cases of persistent wheezing and asthma begin in early childhood, which primarily defines the individuals' respiratory health throughout their lifetime (1–3). Wheezing is a relatively common occurrence in preschoolers, but predicting if the wheezing child will go on to develop asthma is often very difficult and complex. Nearly half of wheezing preschoolers outgrow their symptoms and commonly demonstrate reduced pulmonary function early in life. Their pulmonary function typically improves by age 6 years but not to the levels of normal function as seen in those children that never wheezed (1). Children with asthma as defined with persistent wheezing have ongoing chronic inflammatory processes, resulting in lower airway alterations and loss of pulmonary function early in childhood (4). This period during infancy or early childhood seems to be very important in asthma development because aeroallergen sensitization in the first 3 years of life affects later outcomes (5). Adults with significant airway obstruction by age 30–40 years previously demonstrated reduced pulmonary function by 10 years of age (1). This review discusses the natural history of asthma and the disease course as seen in children and adults.

4.2 Pathogenesis and pathophysiology of asthma

Airway inflammation is the central pathophysiologic process in asthma. It involves many inflammatory cells and inflammatory mediators. These include chemokines, cytokines, cysteinylleukotrienes and immunoglobulin E (IgE). The inflammatory cells that are involved are lymphocytes, eosinophils, neutrophils, mast cells and local-airway dendritic cells. There is a shift in the lymphocyte population from a normal predominantly Th1 response to a predominantly Th2 response that includes a production of pro-inflammatory cytokines (6–7). Airway inflammation is variable and leads to bronchial hyperresponsiveness and airway obstruction, resulting in various asthma phenotypes (8, 9). Airway inflammation, if long-standing, may lead to irreversible remodeling of the airways (8, 10).

The pathogenesis of asthma is complex and incompletely understood. The most widely accepted hypothesis is that asthma originates in early life as a result of intricate interactions between genetic and environmental factors (11). Simply said, in genetically predisposed children, exposure to environmental factors during the "developmentally vulnerable period" in early childhood steer the maturation of the immune and respiratory system away from normal development towards the asthma phenotype (including airway hypersensitivity and reduced pulmonary function) (▶ Fig. 4.1).

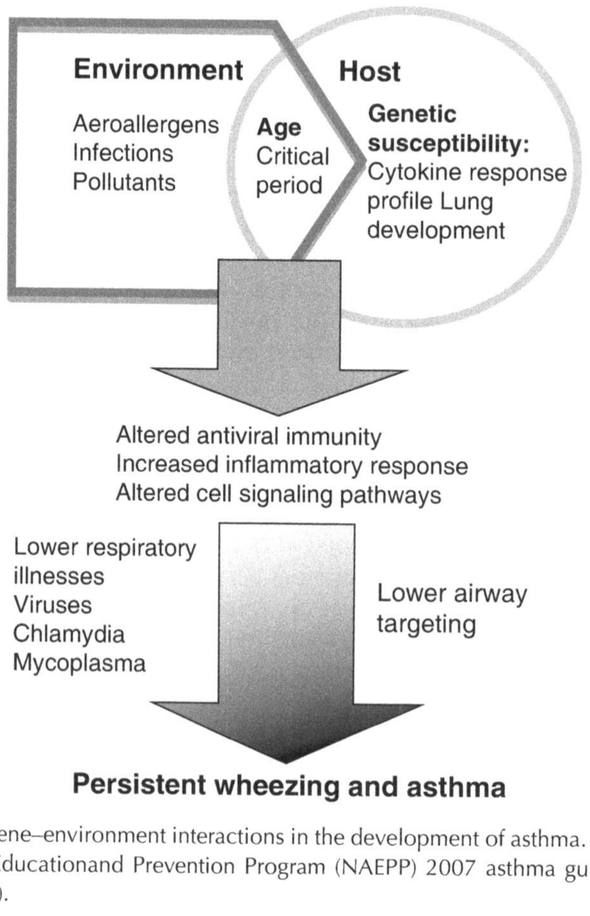

Fig. 4.1: Possible gene–environment interactions in the development of asthma. Modified from the National Asthma Educationand Prevention Program (NAEPP) 2007 asthma guidelines. Modified from reference (11).

4.2.1 Environmental factors

Viruses and allergens are the most commonly implicated environmental factors in asthma. Respiratory infections with the respiratory syncytial virus (RSV) and rhinovirus (RV) in early childhood, and sensitization to aeroallergens (particularly perennial allergens such as dust mites, cat dander and Alternaria) have been associated with the development of asthma later in life (12, 13). Individuals who had severe RSV infection in early life requiring hospitalization were significantly more likely to have asthma in later childhood than children with mild or no RSV infection/bronchiolitis (14). Children at risk of atopy or asthma who had RV-induced wheezing in the first 3 years were more likely to be diagnosed with asthma at 6 years of age compared with children without RV infection in early life (15). Respiratory infections and aeroallergens function interactively in the eventual development of asthma, but the exact mechanism of how this occurs (or its influence upon an individual's immune system) remains unknown.

In contrast, some environmental factors may be protective against the development of asthma. Certain respiratory infections and exposure to non-pathogenic microorganisms early in life are associated with protection against asthma (16). This led to the development of the "hygiene hypothesis". This postulates that commensal microbes are normal stimulants for the maturation towards a balanced immune response, a predominately Th1 response (17, 18). The lack of exposure to bacterial endotoxins and lipopolysacharides in early life allows exposure to certain viruses and allergens to steer the infant's immune system to Th2-driven pro-inflammatory responses (17, 18). The hygiene hypothesis explains the significantly lower prevalence of asthma in infants from large families living on farms. The theory is that immunological maturation occurs through the exposure of more infectious agents from more siblings or through exposure of infectious agents from contact with large animals while residing on the farm. There are other environmental factors such as the "Mediterranean diet" that possibly offer some protection against asthma development. In epidemiological studies, a lack of foods that contain antioxidants and omega-3 fatty acids has been associated with asthma development.

Smoking and secondhand exposure to tobacco have been shown to cause infant wheezing (19) and to lead to more severe asthma with more acute exacerbations in children (20). However, a direct causative effect on asthma development has not been documented. Air pollutants are known to cause asthma exacerbation (especially during heavy exercise) (21), but no direct causative association has been described with asthma pathogenesis.

4.2.2 Host factors (genes and sex)

Asthma clearly is an oligo- or multi-genetic disorder. Genes that may play a part in asthma pathogenesis include those that regulate the development and maturation of innate and adaptive immunity, including IgE production, airway hyperresponsiveness, and regulation of inflammatory mediators. Genes and gene modifiers may be involved not only in the development of asthma but also in determining its severity and an individual's response to treatment, such as the genes for beta adrenergic and corticosteroid receptors. After the Human Genome Project was completed, the study of asthma genetics intensified. Several genes have been identified as having a possible role in asthma development, but most of the genes involved in the development of asthma are unknown.

The prevalence of asthma is higher in boys prior to puberty. However, at puberty, the sex ratio shifts, and in adulthood asthma appears predominantly in women (22). The mechanisms by which sex and possibly sex hormones are linked to asthma are not known.

4.3 Natural history of asthma

The course of asthma over time is commonly referred to as the "natural history of the disease". This may pertain to asthma symptoms, lung function or bronchial hyperresponsiveness. ▶ Tab. 4.1 outlines the definition, pathophysiology, pathogenesis and natural history of asthma. The natural course of asthma varies between individuals and varies in different stages, ranging from childhood to adulthood. Alterations in asthma symptoms over time are not necessarily reflected in changes in pulmonary function or bronchial hyperresponsiveness. The persistence or increase in the severity of asthma symptoms is not always accompanied by a progressive decline in pulmonary function over time.

4.3.1 Natural history of asthma symptoms

In early childhood, there are three phenotypes of children with recurrent wheeze (▶ Fig. 4.2). These are "transient wheezers" who wheeze during viral illnesses during the first 3 years of life; "non-atopic wheezers" who wheeze throughout the first 6 years of life; and "persistent atopic wheezers" who wheeze throughout the first 6 years of life and have personal and family histories of asthma/atopy (1). More than 60%

Tab. 4.1: Pathophysiology, pathogenesis and natural history of asthma: key points.

- Asthma is a chronic inflammatory disorder of the lower airways
- Airway inflammation contributes to airway hyperresponsiveness, airway obstruction, respiratory symptoms and disease chronicity
- Airway inflammation is variable, indicates phenotypic differences, and may influence response to treatment
- Airway remodeling occurs in some patients
- The onset of asthma for most patients begins early in life
- Gene–environmental interactions are important in the development and expression of asthma
- Atopy is the strongest predisposing factor for asthma development
- Viral respiratory infections are frequent causes of asthma exacerbation, and may contribute to the development of asthma
- Current asthma treatment with anti-inflammatory therapy does not prevent progression of the underlying disease severity

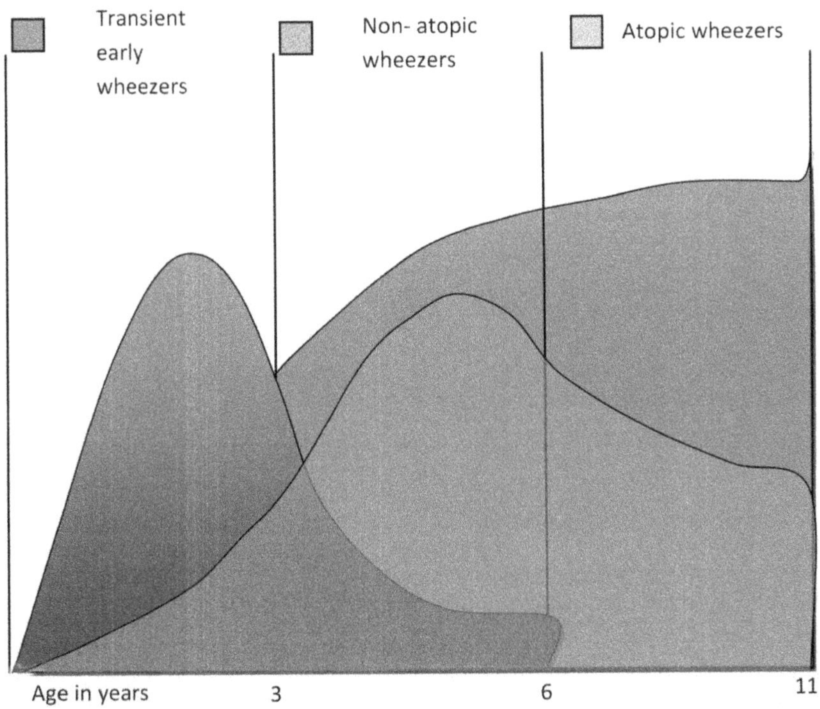

Fig. 4.2: Wheezing phenotypes in childhood and their relative yearly peak prevalence. Prevalence for each age interval is the sum of the areas under each curve. The phenotypes are not exclusive. Modified from Ref. (23).

of children who wheeze only during their first 3 years of life do not wheeze later in life, and do not develop asthma. Approximately 50% of non-atopic persistent wheezers continue to have recurrent wheezing and asthma in adolescence/adulthood. Most atopic wheezers have persistent symptoms and develop atopic asthma, and have asthma throughout childhood and into adulthood (23). The asthma predictive index (API) was developed to help identify those preschool children with recurrent wheezing who may progress to develop asthma later in life. The API (▶ Tab. 4.2) includes risk factors such as personal and parental allergies, and has a positive predictive value of 77% (24).

In school-age children, the course of asthma into adulthood depends mostly on asthma severity. Followed for 5 years, 80% of children with mild asthma demonstrated an improvement, with 23% having remission; for children with severe asthma, 60% had improvement in their symptoms and only 14% had remission (25). In a long-term longitudinal study, 86% of children who had mild infrequent asthma at age 7 years had mild or no asthma at age 42 years, whereas 71% of children with severe and frequent asthma continued to have frequent asthma symptoms (26). In our anecdotal experience, compared with children, adults with asthma typically have less remission over time.

Tab. 4.2: Asthma predictive index.

The Asthma Predictive Index (API) for children younger than 3 years of age with ≥3 episodes of recurrent wheezing. The API is positive if the child has at least one major or two minor criteria.	
Major criteria	Minor criteria
• Parental asthma • Atopic eczema	• Wheezing outside of viral illnesses • Allergic rhinitis • Peripheral eosinophils≥4%

Modified from reference (24)

4.3.2 Natural history of lung function and bronchial hyperreactivity

Transient wheezers, who are more likely to have mothers who smoked during pregnancy, have decreased lung function at birth and decreased lung function at 6 years of age (1). Persistent atopic wheezers have normal lung function at birth but have abnormal lung function by 6 years of life (1). Studies have shown that children who developed asthma-like symptoms before age 3 years had reduced lung function by 6 years of age and continued to have deficits in pulmonary function at 11–16 years of age compared with children who experienced no symptoms in the first 6 years of life, but there was no further loss in the FEV_1 from 6 years of age to 11–16 years of age (24, 27).

A longitudinal study of children with asthma at 8–10 years of age revealed a decline in pulmonary function associated with the degree of bronchial hyperresponsiveness but not with active asthma symptoms (28). Having airway hyperresponsiveness and recent wheeze were associated with lower growth in the FEV_1 but not with subsequent growth in forced vital capacity (FVC) (28). A longitudinal, population-based, cohort study in children from 9 years to 26 years of age found that children with asthma had persistently lower FEV1/FVC ratio levels (29). Regardless of the severity of their symptoms, no further loss of lung function was observed after 9 years of age (29).

Most of the deficits in lung function in children occur in children if symptoms begin during the first 3 years of life (24). The onset of symptoms after 6 years of age is usually not associated with significant deficit in lung function (24). It is, however, clinically important to distinguish this group of early wheezers from the majority of children who wheeze before 3 years of age and who do not experience any more symptoms after 6 years of age (24).

In adults, it is not clear if accelerated loss of lung function occurs. Adult patients with asthma who were followed up over 15–18 years of age had significantly greater average declines in the FEV_1 (30) and a greater slope of decline of the FEV_1 (31). However, other studies have not found a decline in the $FEV_1$to be any different from normal subjects. James et al. (32) found significantly lower lung function with the differences being due to a deficit of lung function present at the beginning of their study when subjects were 19 years of age. In elderly patients aged > 65 years with asthma who were followed up for 7 years, the rate of decline in the FEV_1 was not statistically different between patients with and without asthma (33).

4.4 Prognostic factors of childhood asthma

The outcomes of childhood asthma can be defined in terms of asthma symptoms but also in terms of bronchial hyperresponsiveness and pulmonary function. The prognosis of childhood asthma may therefore vary from complete remission in adulthood (i.e., no symptoms or need for asthma treatment, normal lung function and absence of bronchial hyperresponsiveness) to the development of irreversible airway obstruction and accelerated decline in pulmonary function resulting from airway remodeling. Although there is a fair chance of "remission" or reduction in asthma symptoms between the ages of 10 years and 20 years, the relapse rate after a symptom-free interval is relatively high, and almost 80% of adult asthma may originate in childhood. The length of the symptom-free period may vary from a few years to several years. Even in the absence of asthma symptoms, patients may have obstructed airflow limitation and increased bronchial hyperresponsiveness (34–36).

4.4.1 Childhood predictors of asthma

Age: In general, children who develop asthma by 6 years of age tend to outgrow their asthma more often when compared with children that developed asthma after 6 years of age. The favorable prognosis for children with wheezing in early life may be because this group includes children with wheezing illnesses other than asthma. However, a subset of these children, in which early onset may be an indicator of asthma severity, may have unfavorable outcome.

Sex: Asthma prevalence before puberty is higher in boys, whereas the prevalence is higher in adult females. Despite the sex difference in asthma prevalence, the effect of sex on asthma prognosis is not clear. A commonly held view is that the prognosis is worse in girls, especially in adult females (37). Studies in children have found no difference in the prognosis of asthma between girls and boys from age 10 years to 20 years (38), or have found male sex as a risk factor for disease progression (39–40).

Severity of the disease and lung function abnormality: More severe and more frequent asthmatic symptoms as well as childhood degree of bronchial responsiveness have been consistently shown to be associated with persistence of symptoms into adulthood and lower pulmonary function (41). Severe childhood asthma is a well-known risk factor for the persistence of asthma in adulthood (42). As wheezing frequency increases, airway obstruction becomes more common, and patients with frequent and persistent asthma in childhood continue to have abnormal lung function in mid-adulthood (43).

Atopic manifestations: Asthma in children is associated with allergy to inhaled allergens and a family history of asthma in ≥75% of children. Atopy was found to be a major risk factor for asthma persisting into adulthood. Furthermore, patients with more severe atopy (numbers of positive skin tests or diameter of the reactions) have a greater risk for relapse after a period of symptom-free remission (44). Significant association with persistent symptoms and sensitivity to house dust mite, molds, pollen and milk protein assessed by radioallergosorbent test (RAST) have been demonstrated (45). However, atopy was not associated with the development of irreversible airway obstruction, with low FEV_1 or accelerated decline in the FEV_1 in asthmatic patients, or with the presence of bronchial hyperresponsiveness in patients with remission of asthma (39, 44, 46). Clinical studies of the effect of atopic eczema and/or allergic rhinitis on the progression of childhood asthma have been inconclusive. Gerritsen et al. (46) demonstrated that skin test-reactivity allergens and the number of subjects with positive skin tests to more than one allergen increased from childhood to adulthood. However, the authors demonstrated that the outcome of childhood asthma as defined by current symptoms was not predicted by skin reactivity to allergens, eosinophilia, atopic dermatitis or allergic rhinitis in childhood (46). Childhood atopy is associated with symptoms in adulthood but not with the level of airway obstruction or bronchial hyperactivity.

Lung function: Lower lung function in childhood (measured before or after treatment with bronchodilators to compensate for the reversible part of the disturbance in lung function) is associated with more severe asthma and an unfavorable prognosis. Lower pulmonary function in childhood has been associated with the persistence or relapse of symptoms, development of irreversible airflow limitation, and a low FEV_1/FVC ratio in adulthood (39, 40, 47). There is a strong correlation between the level of pulmonary function in childhood and adulthood. Adults who had severe symptoms had the most serious disturbance in pulmonary function in childhood, and the steepest decline in lung function towards adulthood (48).

Bronchial hyperresponsiveness: Although bronchial hyperresponsiveness is often used as an indicator of asthma severity, its prognostic significance is not clear. Childhood bronchial hyperresponsiveness was one of the few significant variables that predicted persistent symptoms in adulthood (49). Strong association can be found between the presence and degree of bronchial hyperresponsiveness and the need for medication in adulthood. The degree of bronchial hyperresponsiveness during childhood in combination with a low FEV_1 was associated with asthma outcomes in adulthood (41). With longstanding disease, bronchial hyperresponsiveness may become less severe due to airway remodeling and thus may signify a worse prognosis.

Effect of inhaled corticosteroids: The use of anti-inflammatory therapy with inhaled corticosteroids is widespread and is the first-line therapy for treating asthma. Long term (> 10 years) effects of inhaled corticosteroids are not known. However, given for 2–6 years, they improve symptoms and lung function in children with asthma, early at 2–3 years of age and later after 5 years of age. After 12 months of use, use of inhaled corticosteroids decreased the thickness of the subepithelial reticular basement membrane (a marker of airway remodeling) (49). However, there are variable individual responses after discontinuing treatment of inhaled corticosteroids, so these medications do not seem to prevent the natural course of asthma and the associated decline in progressive pulmonary function (50–51).

Genetic factors: Although asthma has a strong genetic component, the role of heredity on asthma progression is unclear. Studies have found no effect of family history of asthma on outcomes in childhood. Genetic markers have been scarcely investigated in relation to disease progression. The ADAM33 gene is not only important in the development of asthma but also in disease progression, and is possibly related to enhanced airway remodeling (52).

4.5 Clinical differences of asthma in childhood versus adulthood

Childhood asthma differs from adult asthma in numerous ways (even including childhood-onset adult asthma) (53). ▶ Tab. 4.3 outlines some of these differences in

Tab. 4.3: Characteristic differences of asthma in children versus adults.

	Children	Adults
Female sex	↓	↑
Male sex	↑	↓
African–American race	↑	↓
Duration of oral glucocorticoid use (years)	↓	↑
Lung function	↑	↓
Symptoms	Episodic	Persistent
IgE levels	↑	↓
Hyperinflation (total lung capacity and residual volume)	↑ Tendency	↓ Tendency
Airway resistance to airflow	↓	↑

children and adults with asthma. Jenkins and colleagues (53) published an important retrospective analysis of 275 patients (125 children and 250 adults) with severe asthma who were admitted to a tertiary Asthma Care Referral Center. Asthma was more prevalent in female adult patients compared with a higher prevalence in males in the pediatric age range, and a greater percentage of children were African–American as compared with adults (53). Asthma is typically more episodic in children and persistent in adults. In fact, the younger the child the more episodic the symptoms are (53). In comparison with adults, children are more hyperinflated with increases in total lung capacity and residual volume with less airway resistance to airflow (54). Children with asthma at all levels of severity can have unimpaired pulmonary function based on FEV_1 measurements when they are clinically stable (50, 53, 55–57).

Hogg and colleagues (58) described peripheral airway resistance in the absence of or before involvement of the large airways, which can explain the normal FEV_1 that occurs in children with asthma. There is a suggestion of a shift in the degree of involvement of the small airways rather than the large airways in asthma between early childhood compared with later childhood, adolescence, and adulthood (5). In children with severe asthma, profound structural changes of the airway with significant thickening of the basement membrane were found in the absence of airway inflammation (59). These same authors demonstrated normal to nearly normal lung function despite the presence of significant remodeling (59). In contrast to asthma severity leading to thickening of the basement membrane, this may not result in irreversible airway obstruction in children.

4.6 Predicting adult asthma

Despite extensive research, correctly predicting if asthma will persist into adulthood during childhood remains unfeasible. Although recent studies have added to our knowledge of the outcomes of childhood asthma in adulthood, we cannot predict if an asthmatic child will outgrow his or her disease. A complicating factor in the investigation of this important question is the different definitions of asthma for children and adults used in research. With the use of standard definitions for asthma, impairment of lung function is associated with asthma duration in asthmatic children and adults with childhood-onset asthma, but there is no relationship between disease severity and asthma duration in adult-onset asthma (53). The Tucson Birth Cohort characterized different wheezing phenotypes, with some of these phenotypes not going on to develop classic asthma or persistent wheezing (27). Even if childhood asthma remits with complete resolution of symptoms, it often does so before or during adolescence; however, many of these patients can experience relapses during young adulthood (60).

Limited studies exist that assess the impact of childhood asthma upon pulmonary function in the adult years. With a longitudinal study assessing lung function in 286 subjects from a 28-year follow-up of childhood asthma, Oswald and colleagues (42) demonstrated that airway obstruction in mid-adult life was present mainly in those with moderately severe asthma. Subjects without wheezing for ≥ 3 years (including those patients with persistent asthma in childhood) had normal lung function and no increased bronchial reactivity (42). There were 2 subjects with persistent asthma during childhood who failed to show an improvement in the FEV_1 of > 10% after inhalation of a beta-adrenergic agonist (42).

4.7 Asthma symptoms in childhood and adulthood

Regarding the persistence of asthma symptoms, a group of 323 subjects with childhood wheezing and 48 control subjects of the same age were studied prospectively from 7 years to 28 years of age (47). Using a classification system centered on wheezing frequency that correlated well with clinical and spirometric findings of airway obstruction, the investigators determined that the amount of wheezing in early adolescence seemed to be a guide for severity in adulthood, with 73% of those with few symptoms at 14 years of age continuing to have little or no asthma at 28 years of age (47). This same study found 68% of those with frequent wheezing at 14 years of age continued to have recurrent asthma at 28 years of age (47). Between 21 and 28 years of age, there was no substantial difference in asthma, so participants with frequent wheezing at 21 years of age continued to have comparable asthma at 28 years of age (47). Approximately one-third of patients who had persistent asthma at 21 years of age improved whereas 44% had worsened symptoms at 28 years (47). Looking at sex differences in this cohort between 21 years and 28 years of age, women fared better, with 19% having worse symptoms compared with 28% of men (47).

4.8 Impact of environmental factors

The role of allergen exposure and allergic sensitization early in life on the course of asthma was studied in the very important German Multicenter Allergy Study Group (61). The large group followed 1,314 children from birth to 13 years of age who had early wheezing as reported by any parent in the first 3 years of life (61). Allergen exposure for the cohort was assessed at 6 months and 18 months and at 3, 4, and 5 years of age with lung function assessed at 7, 10, and 13 years of age (61). The authors demonstrated that 90% of children with wheeze by 3 years of age without atopy lost their symptoms by school age with normal lung function at puberty (61). However, sensitization and exposure to allergens such as dust mites, cat hair or dog hair in the first 3 years of life was associated with a loss of lung function at school age and concomitant exposure to high levels of allergens early in life aggravated this process (61). More importantly, sensitization and exposure to allergens later in life had weaker effects (61). Children with non-atopic wheezing in the first 3 years of life had complete resolution of symptoms by school age and had normal lung function at puberty (61).

4.9 Asthma and development of chronic obstructive pulmonary disease (COPD)

Asthma has been considered to be a distinctly different disease entity than COPD. Asthma is most frequently diagnosed during childhood whereas COPD is typically diagnosed in mid-to-late adulthood. The inflammatory process in COPD is very different from that in asthma. The airway inflammation in asthma is characterized by eosinophilic inflammation affecting all the airways but not lung parenchyma, leading to reversible airway hyperresponsiveness (62). In contrast, COPD has predominantly neutrophilic inflammation in the airways and parenchymal destruction is an important irreversible feature, which leads to airflow obstruction (62). Despite these distinctive physiologic features, there is growing evidence that these two disease entities are related to to each other (31, 63–67). Compared with non-asthmatics, asthma patients with active symptoms had a tenfold higher risk for acquiring symptoms of chronic bronchitis, 17 times-higher risk of receiving a diagnosis of emphysema, and 12.5 times-higher risk of fulfilling COPD criteria, after adjusting for smoking history and other confounders (68). An interesting concept is the loss of reversibility of airway obstruction in asthma over time in some patients with moderate or severe asthma to the point of irreversible or only partially reversible airway obstruction (64–67). Due to overlap of many signs and symptoms of asthma and COPD, attempting to make a distinction between the two diseases is difficulty, especially in the elderly (69).

4.10 Impact of therapy upon the natural course of asthma

Inhaled corticosteroids are the proposed first-line therapy for asthma (including for children aged < 4 years of age). Four independent studies in children have demonstrated that inhaled corticosteroids do not alter the progressive loss of lung function despite controlling: symptoms, need for urgent medical care, and the need for rescue therapy (50, 51, 70, 71). In their longitudinal study, Oswald et al. (41) monitored childhood asthmatics into their adult years. There was no significant difference in the FEV_1 between control subjects and participants with mild wheezy bronchitis, wheezy bronchitis, asthma and severe asthma (42). The FEV_1 was significantly reduced in subjects with wheezy bronchitis, asthma and severe asthma who received inhaled corticosteroids as compared with controls (42). The authors evaluated FEV_1 measurements at 21, 28, and 35 years of age according to original groups and whether inhaled corticosteroids were used at those ages (42). The results demonstrated similar findings with a reduction in

Tab. 4.4: Factors to consider in suboptimal control of asthma.

Poor adherence to drug therapy
Incorrect diagnosis of asthma
Insufficient treatment regimen (including incorrect maintenance therapy)
Insufficient drug dosage
Inadequate technique for aerosol treatment
Inadequate delivery of drug to the lower airways
Poor understanding by the patient of the treatment regimen
Insensitivity of target cell or pathway to corticosteroids

the FEV_1 only in the asthma group receiving inhaled corticosteroids and in the severe asthma group who were or were not receiving inhaled corticosteroids (42).

The role of inhaled corticosteroids during the early period of sensitization in childhood asthma remains unclear. The lack of impact on pulmonary function by inhaled corticosteroids may be due to delayed onset of treatment, insufficient dosing or failure to deliver the aerosol correctly to the distal airways (5). Another potential explanation includes the inability of corticosteroids to suppress the allergic immune response and allergen sensitization (5). Based on our current understanding, inhaled corticosteroids are very effective in reducing asthma symptoms that result from airway inflammation but do not impact the development of airway dysfunction. Compliance and inadequate delivery of aerosol are problems often seen in the treatment of asthma, and may contribute to the development of airway dysfunction. However, other factors may also play a part in poor control of asthma. ▶ Tab. 4.4 lists some potential factors to consider in suboptimal control of asthma. Regarding the effectiveness of corticosteroids, there is a definite difference in how children and adults are treated and their response to corticosteroids. Jenkins and colleagues (53) described that children were as likely to require high-dose inhaled corticosteroids and long-term therapy with oral corticosteroids as adults. Children were more likely to have had prior intubation despite significantly less airway obstruction, less resistance to airflow and larger lung volumes compared with adults (53). Children displayed greater responsiveness to corticosteroids therapy *in vitro* (53).

4.11 Conclusions

Asthma remains a very heterogeneous disorder. The heterogeneity can exist in the same patient from the transition of childhood into adulthood. There have been pleas to abandon asthma as a disease concept due this complexity and heterogeneity (72). The phenotype of asthma during childhood is very different from that in adulthood. Inhaled corticosteroids are the primary first-line therapy for asthma, helping physicians gain control of clinical symptoms. However, research is demonstrating that these therapies do not prevent the development of airway dysfunction later in life. In fact, asthma is now described as a risk factor for COPD. Clearly, the pathogenic mechanisms have not been identified in this process, so research needs to target this very important issue and look beyond inflammation. To make a significant impact upon asthma prevalence as well as morbidity and mortality, research needs to address whether corticosteroid insensitivity plays a part or whether other physiological mechanisms are involved.

References

1. Martinez, F.D., Wright, A.L., Taussig, L.M., Holberg, C.J., Halonen, M., Morgan, W.J., The Group Health Medical Associates. (1995) Asthma and wheezing in the first six years of life. N. Engl. J. Med. 332:133–138.
2. Dezateux, C., Stocks, J. (1997) Lung development and early origins of childhood respiratory illness. Br. Med. Bull. 53:40–57.
3. Stick, S. (2000) Pediatric origins of adult lung disease. 1. The contribution of airway development to paediatric and adult lung disease. Thorax 55:587–594.
4. Gelfand, E. W. (2009) Pediatric asthma: a different disease. Proc. Am. Thorac. Soc. 6:278–282.
5. Gelfand, E. W. (2008) Is asthma in childhood different from asthma in adults? Why do we need special approaches to asthma in children? Allergy Asthma Proc. 29:99–102.
6. Barnes, P. J. (2002) Cytokine modulators as novel therapies for asthma. Annu. Rev. Pharmacol. Toxicol. 42:81–98.
7. Zimmermann, N., Hershey, G. K., Foster, P. S., Rothenberg, M. E. (2003) Chemokines in asthma: cooperative interaction between chemokines and IL-13. J. Allergy Clin. Immunol. 111: 227–243.
8. Busse, W. W., Lemanske, R. F., Jr. (2001) Asthma. N. Engl. J. Med. 344:350–362.
9. Cohn, L., Elias, J. A., Chupp, G. L. (2004)Asthma: mechanisms of disease persistence and progression. Annu. Rev. Immunol. 22:789–815.
10. Holgate, S. T., Polosa, R. (2006) The mechanisms, diagnosis, and management of severe asthma in adults. Lancet 368:780–793.
11. Expert Panel Report 3 (EPR-3): Guidelines for the diagnosis and management of asthma – summary report 2007. J. Allergy Clin. Immunol. 120(Suppl. 5):S94–S138.
12. Huss, K., Adkinson, N. F., Jr., Eggleston, P. A., Dawson, C., Van Natta M. L., Hamilton, R. G. (2001) House dust mite and cockroach exposure are strong risk factors for positive allergy skin test responses in the Childhood Asthma Management Program. J. Allergy Clin. Immunol. 107:48–54.
13. Wahn, U., Lau, S., Bergmann, R., Kulig, M., Forster, J., Bergmann, K., et al. (1997) Indoor allergen exposure is a risk factor for sensitization during the first three years of life. J. Allergy Clin. Immunol. 99(6 Pt 1):763–769.
14. Sigurs, N., Bjarnason, R., Sigurbergsson, F., Kjellman, B. (200) Respiratory syncytial virus bronchiolitis in infancy is an important risk factor for asthma and allergy at age 7. Am. J. Respir. Crit. Care Med. 161:1501–1507.
15. Jackson, D. J., Gangnon, R. E., Evans, M. D., Roberg, K. A., Anderson, E. L., Pappas, T. E., et al. (2008) Wheezing rhinovirus illnesses in early life predict asthma development in high-risk children. Am. J. Respir. Crit. Care Med. 178:667–672.
16. Illi, S., von Mutius, E., Lau, S., Bergmann, R., Niggemann, B., Sommerfeld, C., et al. (2001) Early childhood infectious diseases and the development of asthma up to school age: a birth cohort study. BMJ 322:390–395.
17. Strachan, D. P. (1989) Hay fever, hygiene, and household size. BMJ 299:1259–1260.
18. Strachan, D. P. (2000) Family size, infection and atopy: the first decade of the "hygiene hypothesis". Thorax 55(Suppl. 1):S2–S10.

19. Dezateux, C., Stocks, J., Dundas, I., Fletcher, M. E. (1999) Impaired airway function and wheezing in infancy: the influence of maternal smoking and a genetic predisposition to asthma. Am. J. Respir. Crit. Care Med. 159:403–410.
20. Chilmonczyk, B. A., Salmun, L. M., Megathlin, K. N., Neveux, L. M., Palomaki, G. E., Knight, G. J., et al. (1993) Association between exposure to environmental tobacco smoke and exacerbations of asthma in children. N. Engl. J. Med. 328:1665–1669.
21. McConnell, R., Berhane, K., Gilliland, F., London, S. J., Islam, T., Gauderman, W. J., et al. (2002) Asthma in exercising children exposed to ozone: a cohort study. Lancet 359:386–391.
22. Horwood, L. J., Fergusson, D. M., Shannon, F. T. (1985) Social and familial factors in the development of early childhood asthma. Pediatrics 75:859–868.
23. Wilson N.M. (1994) The significance of early wheezing. Clin Exp Allergy 24:522–529.
24. Castro-Rodriguez, J. A., Holberg, C. J., Wright, A. L., Martinez, F. D. (2000) A clinical index to define risk of asthma in young children with recurrent wheezing. Am. J. Respir. Crit. Care Med. 162(4 Pt 1):1403–1406.
25. Ernst, P., Cai, B., Blais, L., Suissa, S. (2002) The early course of newly diagnosed asthma. Am J Med 112:44–48.
26. Horak, E., Lanigan, A., Roberts, M., Welsh, L., Wilson, J., Carlin, J. B., et al. (2003) Longitudinal study of childhood wheezy bronchitis and asthma: outcome at age 42. BMJ 326:422–423.
27. Morgan, W. J., Stern, D. A., Sherrill, D. L., Guerra, S., Holberg, C. J., Guilbert, T. W., et al. (2005) Outcome of asthma and wheezing in the first 6 years of life: follow-up through adolescence. Am. J. Respir. Crit. Care Med. 172:1253–1258.
28. Xuan, W., Peat, J. K., Toelle, B. G., Marks, G. B., Berry, G., Woolcock, A. J. (2000) Lung function growth and its relation to airway hyperresponsiveness and recent wheeze. Results from a longitudinal population study. Am. J. Respir. Crit. Care Med. 161:1820–1824.
29. Sears, M. R., Greene, J. M., Willan, A. R., Wiecek, E. M., Taylor, D. R., Flannery, E. M., et al. (2003) A longitudinal, population-based, cohort study of childhood asthma followed to adulthood. N. Engl. J. Med. 349:1414–1422.
30. Peat, J. K., Woolcock, A. J., Cullen, K. (1987) Rate of decline of lung function in subjects with asthma. Eur. J. Respir. Dis. 70:171–179.
31. Sherrill, D., Guerra, S., Bobadilla, A., Barbee, R. (2003) The role of concomitant respiratory diseases on the rate of decline in FEV1 among adult asthmatics. Eur. Respir. J. 21:95–100.
32. James, A. L., Palmer, L. J., Kicic, E., Maxwell, P. S., Lagan, S. E., Ryan, G. F., et al. (2005) Decline in lung function in the Busselton Health Study: the effects of asthma and cigarette smoking. Am. J. Respir. Crit. Care Med. 171:109–114.
33. Griffith, K. A., Sherrill, D. L., Siegel, E. M., Manolio, T. A., Bonekat, H. W., Enright, P. L. (2001) Predictors of loss of lung function in the elderly: the Cardiovascular Health Study. Am. J. Respir. Crit. Care Med. 163:61–68.
34. van den Toorn, L. M., Overbeek, S. E., de Jongste J. C., Leman, K., Hoogsteden, H. C., Prins, J. B. (2001) Airway inflammation is present during clinical remission of atopic asthma. Am. J. Respir. Crit. Care Med. 164:2107–2113.
35. Ferguson, A. C. (1998) Persisting airway obstruction in asymptomatic children with asthma with normal peak expiratory flow rates. J. Allergy Clin. Immunol. 82:19–22.
36. Jenkins, M. A., Hopper, J. L., Bowes, G., Carlin, J. B., Flander, L. B., Giles, G. G. (1994) Factors in childhood as predictors of asthma in adult life. BMJ 309:90–93.
37. Nicolai, T., Pereszlenyiova-Bliznakova, L., Illi, S., Reinhardt, D., von Mutius, E. (2003) Longitudinal follow-up of the changing gender ratio in asthma from childhood to adulthood: role of delayed manifestation in girls. Pediatr. Allergy Immunol. 14:280–283.
38. Covar, R. A., Spahn, J. D., Murphy, J. R., Szefler, S. J. (2004) Progression of asthma measured by lung function in the childhood asthma management program. Am. J. Respir. Crit. Care Med. 170:234–241.
39. Rasmussen, F., Taylor, D. R., Flannery, E. M., Cowan, J. O., Greene, J. M., Herbison, G. P., et al. (2002) Risk factors for airway remodeling in asthma manifested by a low postbronchodilator

FEV1/vital capacity ratio: a longitudinal population study from childhood to adulthood. Am. J. Respir. Crit. Care Med. 165:1480–1488.

40. Ulrik, C. S. (1999) Outcome of asthma: longitudinal changes in lung function. Eur. Respir. J. 13:904–918.
41. Roorda, R. J., Gerritsen, J., Van Aalderen, W. M., Schouten, J. P., Veltman, J. C., Weiss S. T., et al. (1993) Risk factors for the persistence of respiratory symptoms in childhood asthma. Am. Rev. Respir. Dis. 148(6 Pt. 1):1490–1495.
42. Oswald, H., Phelan, P. D., Lanigan, A., Hibbert, M., Carlin, J. B., Bowes, G., et al. (1997) Childhood asthma and lung function in mid-adult life. Pediatr. Pulmonol. 23:14–20.
43. Tuchinda, M. (1990) Childhood asthma in Thailand. Acta Paediatr. Jpn. 32:169–172.
44. Roorda, R. J., Gerritsen, J., van Aalderen, W. M., Knol, K. (1993) Skin reactivity and eosinophil count in relation to the outcome of childhood asthma. Eur. Respir. J. 6:509–516.
45. Mazon, A., Nieto, A., Nieto, F. J., Menendez, R., Boquete, M., Brines, J. (1994) Prognostic factors in childhood asthma: a logistic regression analysis. Ann. Allergy 72:455–461.
46. Gerritsen, J., Koeter, G. H., de Monchy, J. G., Knol, K. (1990) Allergy in subjects with asthma from childhood to adulthood. J. Allergy Clin. Immunol. 85(1 Pt. 1):116–125.
47. Kelly, W. J., Hudson, I., Raven, J., Phelan, P. D., Pain, M. C., Olinsky, A. (1998) Childhood asthma and adult lung function. Am. Rev. Respir. Dis. 138:26–30.
48. Godden, D. J., Ross, S., Abdalla, M., McMurray, D., Douglas, A., Oldman, D., et al. (1994) Outcome of wheeze in childhood. Symptoms and pulmonary function 25 years later. Am. J. Respir. Crit. Care Med. 149:106–112.
49. Sont, J. K., Willems, L. N., Bel, E. H., van Krieken, J. H., Vandenbroucke, J. P., Sterk, P. J., AMPUL Study Group. (1999) Clinical control and histopathologic outcome of asthma when using airway hyperresponsiveness as an additional guide to long-term treatment. Am. J. Respir. Crit. Care Med. 159(4 Pt. 1):1043–1051.
50. Childhood Asthma Management Program Research Group. Long-term effects of budesonide or nedocromil in children with asthma. (2000) N. Engl. J. Med. 343:1054–1063.
51. Guilbert, T. W., Morgan, W. J., Zeiger, R. S., Mauger, D. T., Boehmer, S. J., Szefler, S. J., et al. (2006) Long-term inhaled corticosteroids in preschool children at high risk for asthma. N. Engl. J. Med. 354:1985–1997.
52. Jongepier, H., Boezen, H. M., Dijkstra, A., Howard, T. D., Vonk, J. M., Koppelman, G. H., et al. (2004) Polymorphisms of the ADAM33 gene are associated with accelerated lung function decline in asthma. Clin. Exp. Allergy 34:757–760.
53. Jenkins, H. A., Cherniack, R., Szefler, S. J., Covar, R., Gelfand, E. W., Spahn, J. D. (2003) A comparison of the clinical characteristics of children and adults with severe asthma. Chest 124:1318–1324.
54. Spahn, J. D., Covar, R. A., Jain, N., Gleason, M., Shimamoto, R., Szefler, S. J., et al. (2006) Effect of montelukast on peripheral airflow obstruction in children with asthma. Ann. Allergy Asthma Immunol. 96:541–549.
55. Fuhlbrigge, A. L., Kitch, B. T., Paltiel, A. D., Kuntz, K. M., Neumann, P. J., Dockery, D. W., et al. (2001) FEV(1) is associated with risk of asthma attacks in a pediatric population. J. Allergy Clin. Immunol. 107:61–67.
56. Spahn, J. D., Cherniack, R., Paull, K., Gelfand, E. W. (2004)Is forced expiratory volume in one second the best measure of severity in childhood asthma? Am. J. Respir. Crit. Care Med. 169:784–786.
57. Bacharier, L. B., Strunk, R. C., Mauger, D., White, D., Lemanske, R. F., Jr., Sorkness, C. A. (2004) Classifying asthma severity in children: mismatch between symptoms, medication use, and lung function. Am. J. Respir. Crit. Care Med. 170:426–432.
58. Hogg, J. C., Macklem, P. T., Thurlbeck, W. M. (1968) Site and nature of airway obstruction in chronic obstructive lung disease. N. Engl. J. Med. 278:1355–1360.
59. Jenkins, H. A., Cool, C., Szefler, S. J., Covar, R., Brugman, S., Gelfand, E. W., et al. (2006) Histopathology of severe childhood asthma: a case series. Chest 124:32–41.

60. Vonk, J. M., Boezen, H. M. (2006) Predicting adult asthma in childhood. Curr. Opin. Pulm. Med. 12(1):42–47.
61. Illi, S., von Mutius, E., Lau, S., Niggemann, B., Gruber, C., Wahn, U. (2006) Perennial allergen sensitisation early in life and chronic asthma in children: a birth cohort study. Lancet 368:763–770.
62. Barnes, P. J. (2000) Mechanisms in COPD: differences from asthma. Chest 117(Suppl. 2):10S–14S.
63. Lange, P., Parner, J., Vestbo, J., Schnohr, P., Jensen, G. (1998) A 15-year follow-up study of ventilatory function in adults with asthma. N. Engl. J. Med. 339:1194–1200.
64. Hudon, C., Turcotte, H., Laviolette, M., Carrier, G., Boulet, L. P. (1997) Characteristics of bronchial asthma with incomplete reversibility of airflow obstruction. Ann. Allergy Asthma Immunol. 78:195–202.
65. Reed, C. E. (1999) The natural history of asthma in adults: the problem of irreversibility. J. Allergy Clin. Immunol. 103:539–547.
66. Ulrik, C. S., Backer, V. (1999) Nonreversible airflow obstruction in life-long nonsmokers with moderate to severe asthma. Eur. Respir. J. 14:892–896.
67. Vonk, J. M., Jongepier. H., Panhuysen, C. I., Schouten, J. P., Bleecker, E. R., Postma, D. S. (2003) Risk factors associated with the presence of irreversible airflow limitation and reduced transfer coefficient in patients with asthma after 26 years of follow up. Thorax 58:322–327.
68. Silva, G. E., Sherrill, D. L., Guerra, S., Barbee, R. A. (2004) Asthma as a risk factor for COPD in a longitudinal study. Chest 126:59–65.
69. Fanta, C. H. (1989) Asthma in the elderly. J Asthma 26:87–97.
70. Murray, C. S., Woodcock, A., Langley, S. J., Morris, J., Custovic, A. (2006) Secondary prevention of asthma by the use of Inhaled Fluticasone propionate in Wheezy INfants (IFWIN): double-blind, randomised, controlled study. Lancet 368:754–762.
71. Bisgaard, H., Hermansen, M. N., Loland, L., Halkjaer, L. B., Buchvald, F. (2006) Intermittent inhaled corticosteroids in infants with episodic wheezing. N. Engl. J. Med. 354:1998–2005.
72. *The Lancet* (2006) A plea to abandon asthma as a disease concept. Lancet 368(9537):705.

5 Cyanotic congenital heart defects in adulthood

J. Timothy Bricker and Jorge R. Alegria

Cyanotic heart defects are fatal in infancy and childhood without surgical treatment. However, there are rare circumstances in which a cyanotic individual may survive into adult years with fairly good health. Prolonged survival in non-surgically treated cyanotic heart defect cases is dependent upon a well-balanced circulation with pulmonary blood flow that is near normal but not excessive. Physicians may encounter cases in which the diagnosis was missed in childhood or patients who had a diagnosis of a cardiac malformation but are recent immigrants from a part of the world in which surgical treatment was not possible. These unusual survivors have a different spectrum of anatomic malformations than the cyanotic defects found in newborn babies. Even with a well-balanced circulation, chronic ventricular volume overload is likely to lead to myocardial dysfunction over time. The evaluation by a Cardiac Team with expertise in the treatment of congenital cardiac defects in adult patients is important to the long-term health and survival of the patients.

5.1 Introduction

Most cyanotic heart defects are fatal in infancy and childhood without surgical treatment. However, there are rare circumstances in which a cyanotic individual may survive into adult years with fairly good health. When in Montreal, William Osler demonstrated a heart specimen of a non-transposed form of a single ventricle to medical students from McGill University. The case was a farmer who died in a pitchfork accident. Dr. Osler's successor in Pathology at McGill University, Dr. Maude Abbott, began her illustrious career cataloging congenital cardiac defects with an interest in the very same specimen.

5.2 Presentation in adult years

Prolonged survival in non-surgically treated cyanotic heart defect cases is dependent upon a well-balanced circulation with pulmonary blood flow that is near normal but not excessive. Physicians may encounter cases in which the diagnosis was missed in childhood or patients who had a diagnosis of a cardiac malformation but are recent immigrants from a part of the world in which surgical treatment was not possible. These unusual survivors have a different spectrum of anatomic malformations than the cyanotic defects found in newborn babies. Even with a well-balanced circulation, chronic ventricular volume overload is likely to lead to myocardial dysfunction over time. The evaluation by a Cardiac Team with expertise in the treatment of congenital cardiac defects in adult patients is important for the long-term health and survival of the patients. The presenting features of non-surgically treated cyanotic heart disease in older individuals is often from a cardiac murmur. The murmur of tricuspid regurgitation in a patient with Ebstein's anomaly or the posterior thoracic murmur of collaterals supplying pulmonary blood flow in an adult with untreated pulmonary atresia may be how these patients attract attention. Seemingly healthy college students, middle-aged individuals, and even elderly adults have presented with a cyanotic heart defect that was evaluated only because of the murmur. Individuals with obvious cyanosis and clubbing of the nailbeds are much less likely to be unrecognized into adult years.

Definitive and complete anatomic diagnosis can generally be provided by transthoracic echocardiography at a Congenital Heart Center. Selected questions may require transesophagal cardiac ultrasound imaging or cardiac magnetic resonance imaging (MRI). Cardiac catheterization is used to answer specific questions prior to surgery or, in selected cases, for interventional procedures to improve hemodynamics. This is a group of patients with increased risk of cardiac catheterization compared with other adult patients. Cardiac catheterization is not routinely needed and often contributes little other than risk when pursued by those with limited experience of treating cyanotic congenital heart disorders. Polycythemia is characteristic of prolonged hypoxemia. As with infants, 5 g of desaturated hemoglobin is required for an adult patient to appear cyanotic. Therefore, a hypoxemic individual who is anemic may not appear particularly blue on examination. The wide availability of pulse oximetry has led to occasional recognition of cyanotic congenital heart patients with subtle physical findings.

The most commonly seen cyanotic heart defects compatible with prolonged survival without surgery are unique cases of tetralogy of Fallot or pulmonary atresia that have adequate pulmonary blood flow. A persisting patent ductus arteriosus (PDA), aorticopulmonary collaterals, or reversed flow in an anomalous coronary artery originating from the pulmonary trunk are among the ways that this can happen. Pulmonary valve stenosis with an atrial septal defect (ASD) was recognized by Fallot as another rare type of cyanosis in adult patients who develop cyanosis late when progressive right ventricular dysfunction results in right-to-left shunting at the atrial level. Ebstein's anomaly of the tricuspid valve or congenital tricuspid valve stenosis may also cause cyanosis in adult years from an atrial right-to-left shunt. Non-surgically treated patients with congenital heart defects that formerly had increased pulmonary blood flow may develop cyanosis as adults if pulmonary vascular changes from chronic increased flow ("Eisenmenger" physiology) progress over time. Patients in this category can include those with a large ventricular septal defect (VSD) or PDA or ASD, transposition with VSD, tricuspid atresia, or even the truncus arteriosus.

Another category of adult patients with non-surgically treated cyanotic heart defects are individuals with an accurate anatomic diagnosis and a previous decision that surgical intervention is not possible or carries an excessive risk. Medical follow-up of patients in this group should include periodic reconsideration about this assumption in light of advances in care and current congenital surgical results.

5.3 Complications of right-to-left shunts

Cyanotic patients are at risk of paradoxical embolization. The small clot or air bubble that would cause an insignificant and unrecognized pulmonary embolism in an adult with a structurally normal heart is a major risk for a stroke in the cyanotic patient. We minimize intravenous infusions, eliminate "keep-open" intravenous infusions, use air filters on intravenous infusions, a meticulously monitor intravenous drips. Paradoxical embolization is also a risk with venous thromboembolic disease. We caution patients about prolonged sitting (e.g., on long automobile trips or on aeroplanes) without walking and remain attuned to other risks for thromboembolic disease. Most of our adult cyanotic patients are on a low dose of salicylate if there is not a contraindication. There is a low threshold for anti-coagulation of cyanotic congenital heart patients with risks for thromboembolic disease. The risks of paradoxical embolization must be considered and communicated if sending the patient to an Emergency Room or to an anesthesiologist.

Significant desaturation is likely to be associated with polycythemia. Increased iron turnover places the cyanotic adult at risk for the sequelae of iron deficiency even if they are not found to be anemic. Erythrocyte production in the setting of iron deficiency results in stiff red cells that are microcytic and which then exacerbate microcirculatory difficulties. GI and neurologic complications of iron deficiency can also be a factor in these cyanotic patients with iron deficiency without anemia. Moderate polycythemia is a physiologic advantage because of increased oxygen-carrying capacity in people with hyposmia. However, at the extremes of polycythemia, hyperviscosity of the blood results in diminished perfusion in tissue. The threshold for this is generally a hematocrit in the 65–70% range. Symptoms include lethargy, fatigue, and neurologic symptoms. Cautious isovolumic partial exchange transfusion has been used in selected circumstances to decrease viscosity and improve flow. Hemodynamic changes with volume depletion of phlebotomy (such as with donating 1 unit of blood in a Blood Bank) can be hazardous. Care is required to present paradoxical embolization with isovolumic partial exchange procedures.

Cyanotic adult patients are at increased risk for brain abscesses. These may be present without fever. Headache, especially with symptoms or findings of intracranial hypertension, should raise this possibility in a cyanotic adult. Polycythemic patients are at risk for hyperuricemia because of the high turnover of cells. Gout with joint symptoms and with renal manifestations may develop if this is not recognized and treated early. Most do well with allopurinol.

Vasodilation will usually make a cyanotic patient more intensely desaturated. This may occur with fever, with a generalized rash, with a sedative that is a vasodilator, or with a vasodilator used for the intention of afterload reduction or anti-hypertensive therapy. The reason for the further decrease in oxygen saturation is due to the pulmonary blood flow dropping because of lower systemic arteriolar resistance. Drugs which increase systemic vascular resistance may increase arterial saturation if pulmonary blood flow is improved (although possibly at the expense of deterioration of ventricular function). Oxygen administration is unlikely to be effective in improving desaturation due to diminished pulmonary blood flow.

Adult patients who have had palliative surgery for congenital heart disease may be cyanotic. A patient with an aortapulmonary shunt for tetralogy of Fallot, for pulmonary atresia, or for tricuspid atresia would fall into this category. The shunt may have been undertaken as a definitive palliation because of factors (such as pulmonary arteries which are too small) which precluded separation of the pulmonary and systemic circulation. Some cases of d-transposition of the great arteries with a large VSD and pulmonary vascular obstructive disease are improved by an atrial-switch procedure without VSD closure (palliative Mustard procedure). Pulmonary artery banding may result in diminished pulmonary flow over time if the band becomes too tight or migrates distally on the pulmonary arteries. Risks and complications for patients with cyanotic heart disease physiology after surgery are similar to the unoperated group. Surgical procedures that divide the systemic and pulmonary circulations in cyanotic patients are traditionally called "corrections" or "repairs." Families and sometimes practitioners have the mistaken impression that the heart is normal after procedures named in this way. Significant residual problems and late complications may occur. A "corrected" cyanotic heart defect should not mean that the abnormalities of cardiac function can be considered very unlikely by the practitioner treating such a patient.

5.4 Patients who have had surgery for a right-to-left shunt

The most common repaired congenital heart defect is tetralogy of Fallot. Repair is usually done in early childhood. Most are healthy in adult years with mild or no symptoms. A soft systolic murmur at the left upper sternal border is common. A low-frequency diastolic decrescendo murmur in the same area is also common from pulmonary insufficiency in patients who required pulmonary valvotomy and a transanuler patch. Although chronic pulmonary regurgitation is tolerated better than residual obstruction on a long-term basis, some patients may develop progressive right ventricular dilation and right ventricular dysfunction over time. Repair or replacement of the pulmonary valve may be needed for some of these patients in adult years. Most patients will have a prolonged QRS with a right bundle branch block pattern on electrocardiography (ECG) after repair of tetralogy of Fallot. Ventricular arrhythmias are a concern in patients with repair of tetralogy of Fallot and, particularly in the presence of significant residual hemodynamic abnormalities, represent a risk of sudden cardiac death.

Most adults with transposition of the great arteries underwent surgical repair in the era when atrial-switch procedures (Mustard or Senning procedures) were standard. This approach re-routed the atrial blood from the systemic venous return to the subpulmonary left ventricle and the pulmonary venous blood return to the subaortic left ventricle. Obstruction of the systemic venous pathway or the pulmonary venous pathway was an occasional complication of these procedures, and may be found in adult survivors. A major long-term problem has been atrial arrhythmia (particularly atrial flutter) which is associated with a risk of late sudden death. Sinus node dysfunction with bradycardia also occurs. The right ventricle is the systemic ventricle pumping to the aorta in these patients. Dilation of the right ventricle with right ventricular failure may develop in adult years. While some adult patients have been treated with the "double-switch" procedure that includes take-down of the atrial pathways and arterial switch, surgical procedures to induce the development of left ventricular hypertrophy are required before the double-switch. This approach is hazardous and quite controversial. Cardiac transplantation is preferred at most centers for advanced right ventricular failure after atrial-switch procedures. The aorta in transposition repair with an atrial-switch procedure remains very anterior, which results in a loud single second heart sound (A2). This finding in association with the expected right ventricular lift on palpation and expected right ventricular hypertrophy on ECG lead the uninitiated to the mistaken diagnosis of pulmonary hypertension in the atrial-switch patient who has a good result. Transposition patients who underwent the arterial switch procedure are increasingly entering the adult population. Possible late issues for these adults include supravalvar aortic obstruction, supravalvar pulmonic obstruction. As a group, the arterial switch patients are doing much better long-term than the Mustard or Senning atrial-switch groups. Truncus arteriosus adult patients carry the risk of developing progressive truncal valve regurgitation over time and may develop conduit obstruction or regurgitation of their conduit valve. Congenital coronary abnormalities in the truncus arteriosus may rarely be a source of late concern. The major cardiac complications for adult patients who had surgical correction of total anomalous pulmonary venous return in infancy or childhood is late pulmonary venous obstruction. This is another group of repaired cyanotic defects at risk for atrial arrhythmias.

The Fontan approach for patients with single-ventricle physiology utilizes the single ventricle to pump systemic flow and relies on passive flow through the pulmonary circulation with venous connections directly to the pulmonary arteries. The original Fontan approach was for tricuspid atresia, but it is now used for many types of single ventricle. Although the presumption was that a single left ventricle would do better in the long run than an anatomic right ventricle, many postoperative Fontan patients with a single right ventricle are doing very well. Atrial flutter, sinus node dysfunction, and other atrial arrhythmias are of concern for these patients. Chronic elevation of systemic venous pressure results in a risk of cirrhosis, renal abnormalities, and intenstinal lymphangiectasia. Obstruction of the systemic venous pathways may develop over time. Most Fontan patients are on salicylate or anti-coagulation to decrease the risk of thrombosis if flow is sluggish. On average, Fontan patients are more limited than the other adult patients who have had surgery to correct the cyanosis. A residual fenestration is frequently left intentionally at surgery for a right-to-left "pop-off" if needed. The fenestration may close spontaneously, might be closed in the Catheterization Laboratory, or could be left open indefinitely depending upon patient status. Ventricular dysfunction of the single ventricle is a long-term concern. Most patients will be on afterload reduction with the intent to minimize myocardial work and to preserve ventricular function as much as possible.

5.5 Other cardiac complications in adults survivors of cyanotic heart defects in childhood

Pulmonary vascular obstructive changes with elevated pulmonary vascular resistance (PVR) can contribute greatly to morbidity and mortality in adults with cyanotic heart defects. This occurs to a great degree in the left-to-right lesions that develop Eisenmenger physiology with late cyanosis. However, elevated pulmonary resistance in transposition patients who have had surgical repairs, tetralogy patients who once had a large shunt, and single-ventricle patients who now have a Fontan can be a major problem. Some adult cardiac patients will benefit from pulmonary vasodilators (e.g., sidenifil) on a chronic basis. Sleep apnea and nocturnal hypoventilation increase pulmonary resistance. Sleep disorders have been under-recognized as contributors to morbidity in adult patients with congenital cardiac malformations.

Experimental studies have suggested that hypoxemia in early development might increase the risk of late atherosclerosis. While convincing epidemiologic evidence of this in adult patients with cyanotic heart defects would not be available for some time, an emphasis on prevention of coronary artery disease is very important for adults with cyanotic heart defects whether they underwent surgery for repair or not. Prevention or cessation of smoking, blood-pressure control, obesity prevention, treatment of elevated lipids, and moderate but regular physical activity are recommended for these patients.

5.6 Conclusion

Guidelines for the evaluation and management of adult patients with childhood heart disease at Cardiac Centers are becoming more available. Familiarity with the primary-care aspect of these disorders may improve the future health of these individuals.

References

1. McNamara, D. G., Bricker, J. T. (1989) Congenital heart disease in the adult. In: Adams, F. H., Emmanouilides, G. C., Reimenschneider, T. A., eds. The adult with Postoperative Congenital Heart Disease, 4th ed. Baltimore, USA: Williams Wilkins, pp. 670–684.
2. Warnes, C. A., Williams, R. G., Bashore, T. M., Child, J. S., Connolly, H. M., Dearani, J. A., et al. (2008) ACC/AHA 2008 guidelines for the management of adults with congenital heart disease: A report of the American College of Cardiology/American Heart Association Task Force on Practice Guidelines (Writing Committee to Develop Guidelines on the Management of Adults With Congenital Heart Disease). Developed in Collaboration With the American Society of Echocardiography, Heart Rhythm Society, International Society for Adult Congenital Heart Disease, Society for Cardiovascular Angiography and Interventions, and Society of Thoracic Surgeons. J. Am. Coll. Cardiol. 52:e1–e121.
3. Silversides, C. K., Marelli, A., Beauchesne, L., Dore, A., Kiess, M., Salehian, O., et al. (2010) Canadian Cardiovascular Society 2009 Consensus Conference on the management of adults with congenital heart disease: executive summary. Can. J. Cardiol. 26:143–150.

6 Obstructive and regurgitant cardiac lesions in adults who had childhood heart disease

Douglas J. Schneider

Adults with congenital heart disease can have some degree of cardiac obstruction or valve regurgitation even after repair or intervention. Because many such patients will benefit from medical therapy, catheter intervention, or surgery as adults, long-term follow-up with coordination of care between primary-care providers and adult congenital heart disease specialists is important. In this review, left ventricular outflow tract obstruction, aortic valve regurgitation, coarctation of the aorta, mitral valve stenosis, mitral valve regurgitation, tricuspid stenosis, tricuspid valve regurgitation, pulmonary stenosis and pulmonary regurgitation will be discussed from the perspective of childhood or adolescent cardiac lesions entering adulthood as well as the interventions and management.

6.1 Introduction

Many adults with congenital heart disease have some degree of cardiac obstruction or valve regurgitation even after repair or intervention. Because many such patients will benefit from medical therapy, catheter intervention, or surgery as adults, long-term follow-up with coordination of care between primarycare providers and Adult Congenital Heart Disease Specialists is important. In this review, the approach to care of adults with significant obstructive or regurgitant lesions will be discussed.

6.2 Left ventricular outflow tract obstruction

Congenital left heart obstructions may occur in several locations from the left atrium to the descending aorta in isolation or in combination, and may be associated with other congenital heart defects, including complex lesions such as hypoplastic left heart syndrome. In this review, the various left heart obstructions are primarily discussed in the context of primary lesions with otherwise relatively normal cardiac anatomy. Aortic stenosis may occur at the level of the aortic valve (valvular), in the aortic root above the valve leaflets (supravalvar), and/or in the left ventricular outflow tract below the valve (subvalvar). Because even with current excellent interventional and surgical techniques most patients with aortic stenosis are not rendered completely normal, residual valve dysfunction is frequently present throughout adult life.

6.2.1 Aortic valve stenosis and the bicuspid aortic valve

The normal aortic valve has three cusps that hinge along three commissures (▶ Fig. 6.1), with thin pliable leaflets that open fully during systole. The most common congenital

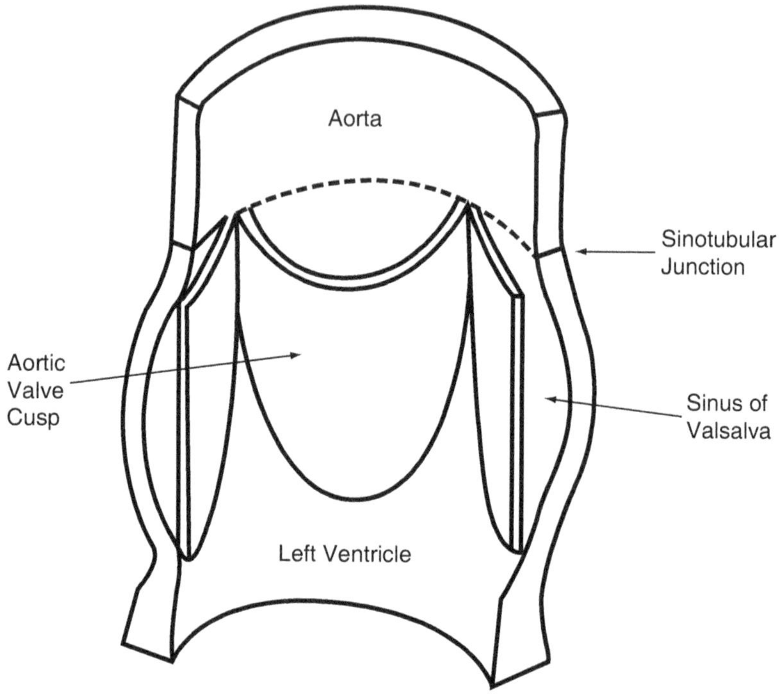

Fig. 6.1: Anatomy of the aortic valve.

abnormality is a bicuspid aortic valve (▶ Fig. 6.2). This accounts for 95% of congenital aortic valve abnormalities (1–3), and results from the fusion of two of the valve cusps during development (4). The remainder are unicuspid valves (with no commissure or a single commisure) and tricuspid (or, rarely, quadracuspid) valves with thickened and dysplastic leaflets. Although there is strong evidence that genetic factors are involved, the etiology of congenital aortic valve abnormalities is probably multifactorial. The male-to-female ratio is ~4:1 (5). In addition to aortic valve pathology, many patients have a dilated aortic root due to an inherent abnormality of the aortic wall (6) and abnormal aortic wall stress from high-velocity and turbulent flow distal to the stenotic valve.

Aortic valve anomalies are the most common congenital cardiac malformation (although many of these lesions are undetected in childhood). Approximately 1.3% of newborns have a bicuspid aortic valve (2, 4), but only ~2% of patients with a congenital aortic valve abnormality will have significant aortic valve stenosis or regurgitation by adolescence. Accordingly, most adults with congenital aortic valve disease have native lesions that have not required intervention or surgery during childhood. The natural history is one of gradual progression of valve dysfunction, and a high percentage of patients with a congenital aortic valve abnormality will require intervention and/or surgery during their lifetime (5, 7, 8). In general, the prognosis is related to the age of onset of valve dysfunction and the pressure gradient (degree of stenosis) at the time of diagnosis.

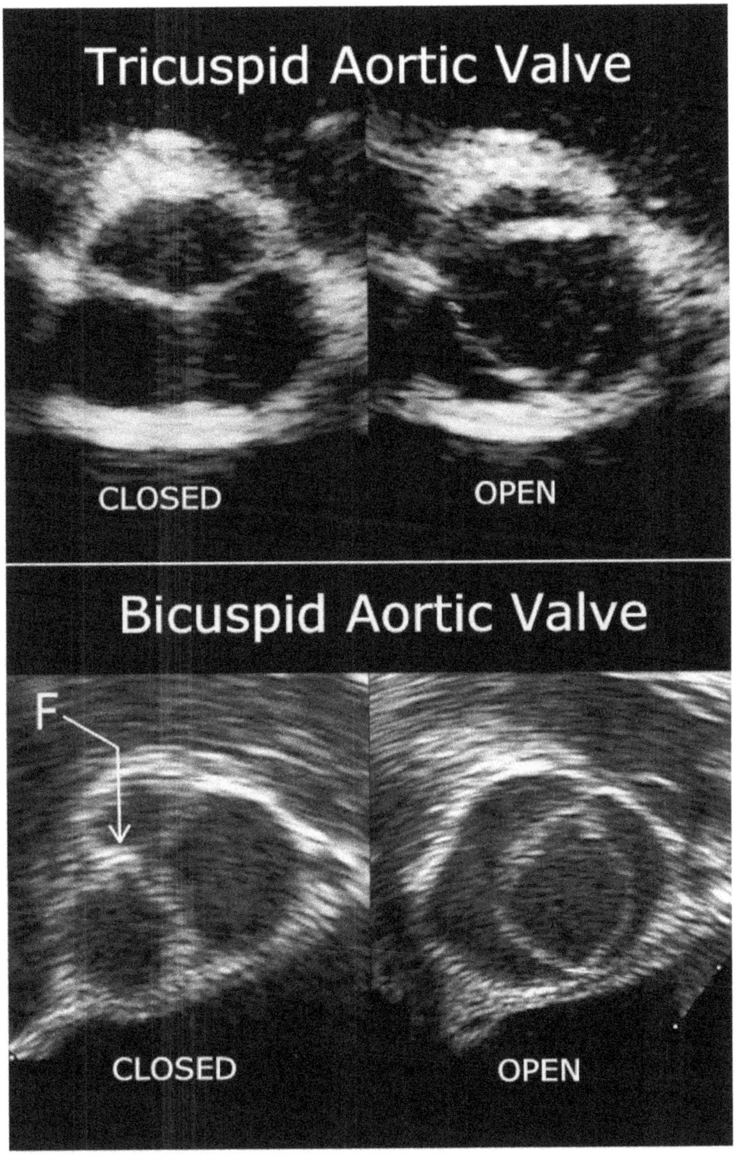

Fig. 6.2: Short-axis echocardiographic views of a normal tricuspid aortic valve and bicuspid aortic valve. Fusion of two cusps (F) results in abnormal opening of the valve along two commissures instead of the normal three.

Most patients are asymptomatic until the stenosis is severe, and the diagnosis is usually made on the basis of detection of a heart murmur on examination of an asymptomatic patient. Patients may present with symptoms, including anginal chest pain (especially if there is concomitant coronary artery disease), syncope, dyspnea with exertion, atrial fibrillation, and rarely (in end-stage disease) pulmonary hypertension and right heart failure. Occasionally, patients present with aortic valve endocarditis without prior knowledge of a bicuspid or otherwise abnormal aortic valve. Physical examination reveals an early systolic ejection click followed by an ejection murmur loudest at the upper right sternal border, with radiation into the neck. A thrill in the suprasternal notch is frequently present. If significant aortic regurgitation is also present, a decrescendo diastolic murmur will be heard along the left sternal border and at the apex. The cardiac impulse may be prominent and/or displaced laterally.

ECG may be normal if the stenosis is mild, but will frequently demonstrate left ventricular hyperterophy. In more severe cases, there may be ST segment and T-wave changes that are sometimes referred to as a "strain" pattern. Except in advanced cases in symptomatic patients, chest radiography usually demonstrates normal heart size and a prominent aortic root.

Echocardiography usually establishes the diagnosis (▶ Fig. 6.3) and defines the anatomy of the aortic valve. The presence or absence of left ventricular hypertrophy is also determined, and left ventricular systolic function is also appraised. In addition, echocardiography is used to evaluate for other potential associated anomalies such as coarctation of the aorta, VSD, and mitral valve anomalies. Doppler is used to quantify the degree of stenosis. Peak instantaneous and mean pressure gradients are calculated, and the aortic valve area can also be calculated. Care needs to be taken to measure the Doppler signal in multiple views to avoid underestimating the gradient due to a suboptimal angle of interrogation. In the absence of left ventricular dysfunction, the Doppler-derived pressure gradient is used to determine the degree of stenosis. Doppler is also used to detect and quantify the degree of aortic valve regurgitation.

Cardiac MRI or computed tomography (CT) angiography may also be used to non-invasively image the aortic valve, quantify hypertrophy and function of the left ventricle, estimate pressure gradients, evaluate aortic regurgitation, and provide excellent imaging of the aortic root and ascending aorta for quantification of dilation of the aortic root.

Cardiac catheterization may be undertaken to help quantify the degree of stenosis and guide management decisions, and also to carry out balloon valvuloplasty if deemed necessary. The left ventricular end-diastolic pressure can be measured as an indicator of diastolic ventricular function which may be impaired from hypertrophy and potentially from subendocardial ischemia/fibrosis. The valve area can also be calculated as an indication of stenosis severity but, in general, if ventricular systolic function is normal, the pressure gradient is used to define the severity of the stenosis. Angiography with injection into the ascending aorta can also be done to help quantify the degree of aortic valve regurgitation (if present).

Management of aortic stenosis in adults is dependentupon age, severity, and symptoms (9, 10). In older adults, replacement of the aortic valve is indicated in those with symptoms. After symptoms develop, mean survival is 2–3 years (11) and the risk of sudden death is high. Provocation of symptoms or hypotension by exercise testing is also considered an indication for aortic valve replacement. In older patients, most experts do not recommend aortic valve replacement unless symptoms develop because the probability of hospital mortality or important late complication from aortic valve replacement is significantly higher than the risk of sudden death in asymptomatic patients. In patients with symptomatic severe aortic stenosis who are deemed to be high-risk surgical candidates, balloon angioplasty may be considered. However, the results are generally suboptimal due largely to the severe degree of valve calcification in this age group. A more promising treatment, currently under investigation in clinical trials, is transcatheter aortic valve replacement.

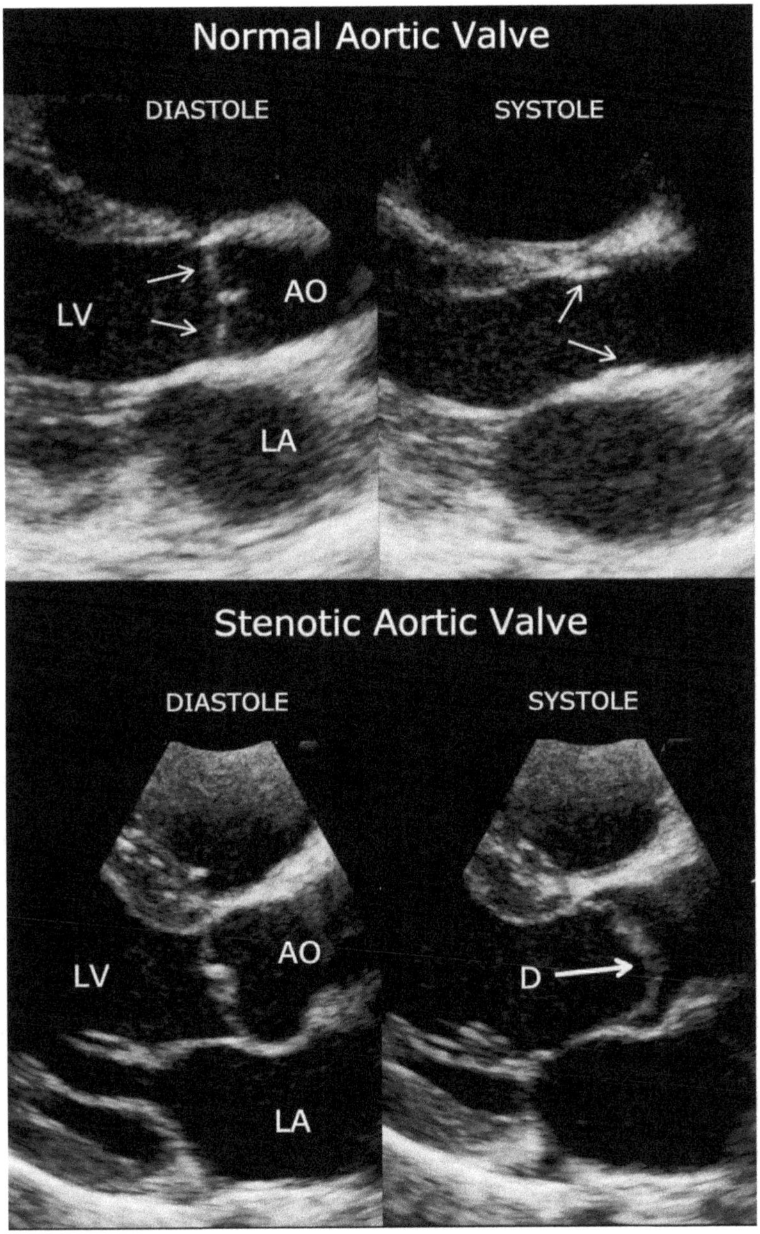

Fig. 6.3: Long-axis echocardiographic views of normal (top) and stenotic (bottom) aortic valves. The cusps of the normal valve open completely such that they are oriented parallel to the aortic wall, whereas the stenotic valve cusps "dome" (D) during systole. LV, left ventricle; AO, aorta; LA, left atrium.

In younger adults and adolescents, the indications for surgery or balloon valvuloplasty are more liberal. Irreversible myocardial dysfunction and fibrosis may develop if intervention is delayed until symptoms develop (12–14), and long-term preservation of myocardial function needs to be the primary goal of therapy. In general, adolescents and young adults with mild or moderate stenosis can be observed and followed up, and those with severe stenosis are candidates for intervention. Exercise stress testing may be used to help determine the timing of intervention in cases with otherwise borderline findings. Anginal chest pain, ischemic ECG changes, or exercise-induced hypertension are considered indications for intervention. Compared with older adults with highly calcified valves that do not respond well to balloon valvuloplasty, younger aortic valves are more pliable and amenable to balloon valvuloplasty. Unless there is significant valve regurgitation, balloon valvuloplasty is usually attempted to delay the need for surgery. If balloon valvuloplasty fails or is precluded by significant regurgitation, surgical aortic valve replacement is undertaken.

Surgical therapy consists of repair or replacement of the aortic valve. Valve repair is possible in many situations: if there is only mild regurgitation, surgical valvotomy may provide relief of obstruction and significantly delay the need for valve replacement. More extensive leaflet repair is necessary if there is significant regurgitation and, although such repairs may be excellent, frequently the repair is not durable for the long-term. Options for aortic valve replacement include the Ross procedure (translocation of the pulmonary valve to the aortic position and pulmonary valve replacement with a xenograft or homograft valve), replacement of the aortic valve with a tissue valve (xenograft or homograft), and aortic valve replacement with a prosthetic valve. Xenograft valves are constructed using tissue from other species, whereas homograft valves are harvested from human cadavers.

The major advantage of the Ross procedure is that anti-coagulation is not required, desirous for those who want to participate in sports or contemplating pregnancy, and also eliminating the risks associated with long-term anti-coagulation. The Ross procedure is often preferred in infants and children because the autograft (native pulmonary valve now in the aortic position) will grow as the patient grows, unlike prosthetic valves and aortic homograft valves which do not grow. The major disadvantage is that the durability of pulmonary valve replacement (homograft or xenograft) is limited, resulting in potential right heart dysfunction and necessitating further surgeries to replace the pulmonary valve.

Prosthetic valves in the aortic position are durable for many years (even decades) but require chronic anti-coagulation. Tissue valves are not as durable as prosthetic valves, and usually require replacement within a decade, but do not require anti-coagulation and are a good choice in some situations. Newer designs of prosthetic valves that would not require anti-coagulation are currently under investigation, and this might become a very attractive option for adolescents and young adults in the future. The role of transcatheter aortic valve replacement in adolescents and young adults has not been explored. However, as technology improves, it is very possible that replacement of the aortic valve via catheterization may become a preferred treatment in the future.

Although many patients with congenital aortic stenosis do not require treatment until adolescence or adulthood, a significant number of adults with aortic stenosis will have had balloon angioplasty or surgery during childhood. These patients require long-term follow-up. Those who have had balloon valvuloplasty, surgical valvuloplasty, or surgical repair have a very high incidence of progressive recurrent stenosis or progressive regurgitation. Similarly, those with the Ross procedure or aortic valve replacement with a tissue valve will very probably require further surgery because tissue valves tend to develop progressive dysfunction over time (usually the neo-pulmonary valve in the case of the Ross procedure, but autograft failure also occurs). Patients with prosthetic valves need close follow-up of their anti-coagulation status, and smaller prosthetic valves placed during childhood may require replacement when the patient is fully grown. Prophylaxis against subacute bacterial endocarditis is recommended for patients with prosthetic valves.

In addition to attention to valve function, follow-up of patients with native or postoperative aortic valve disease requires attention to the status of the aortic root, which may become aneurysmally dilated even in the absence of significant valve dysfunction. Such patients are at risk of aortic dissection, and the size of the aortic root should be monitored. Beta blockers or angiotensin receptor blockers may be helpful in slowing the progression of enlargement of the aortic root. Surgical replacement of the aortic root is indicated in patients with large aneurysms or rapid change in their clinical situation. The possibility of aortic root dissection should be considered in any patient with congenital aortic valve disease that presents with acute chest pain or other symptoms of aortic dissection.

Activity restrictions are recommended in patients with more-than-mild aortic stenosis. Detailed recommendations are outlined in the Bethesda Conference Guidelines (15). Intense exercise, particularly isometric activities such as weightlifting, is associated with increased risk of sudden death from subendocardial ischemia due to increased ventricular pressure, hypertrophy, and increased oxygen demand. Chronic intermittent subendocardial ischemia may lead to fibrosis and further increased risk of arrhythmia. Patients with prosthetic valves on anti-coagulation therapy should not participate in activities that are associated with significant risk of impact (e.g., football) even if their aortic prosthesis is functioning very well due to the risk of bleeding.

Pregnancy is not advisable in patients with moderate or severe aortic stenosis, and may be associated with clinical deterioration. The demand for increased cardiac output with fixed outflow obstruction results in higher pressure gradients, which increase myocardial oxygen demand. Simultaneous vasodilation may impair myocardial perfusion. Angina, heart failure, and/or arrhythmia may develop. Accordingly, patients with significant aortic stenosis should defer pregnancy until the stenosis is alleviated.

6.2.2 Subvalvular aortic stenosis

Subvalvular aortic stenosis may occur in isolation but frequently occurs in combination with other cardiovascular malformations such as VSD, coarctation of the aorta, valvular aortic stenosis, or atrioventricular septal defect. It may occur as a discrete subaortic membrane, fibromuscular ridge, or as a diffuse tunnel-like left ventricular outflow tract. Physical findings are similar to valvular aortic stenosis except with absence of an ejection click and that the murmur at the mid-left sternal borderis louder. The diagnosis is confirmed by echocardiography, with quantitative assessment of the pressure gradient by Doppler evaluation.

Subaortic stenosis is rarely evident during infancy but progresses over time. However, the rate of progression is highly variable. Frequently, subaortic stenosis is accompanied by aortic valve regurgitation, and this may be a consequence of turbulent high-velocity flow directed at the aortic valve leaflets. For this reason, and because progression of subaortic stenosis may be rapid (16), many advocate surgery at the time of the diagnosis or when aortic regurgitation first appears (17). However, many patients have stable mild obstruction and mild regurgitation for many years, and in adolescents and adults with only mild obstruction, observation with periodic follow-up is a prudent strategy in most patients (18).

Treatment involves resection of obstructive tissue, as well as repair or replacement of the aortic valve if it is significantly regurgitant. Aortic regurgitation is likely to progress even after resection of the stenosis, and recurrence of stenosis may occur in ≤15% of cases. Therefore, long-term follow-up is important even after surgery.

6.2.3 Supravalvular aortic stenosis

Supravalvular aortic stenosis is the least common type of aortic stenosis. It is seen primarily as a result of elastin gene mutation on chromosome 7 in association with Williams syndrome or non-syndromic familial supravalvular aortic stenosis. Genetic transmission is autosomal dominant. The physiology of supravalvular aortic stenosis is similar to other forms of left ventricular outflow tract obstruction with the important additional factor of impaired diastolic coronary artery flow because the stenosis is between the ascending aorta and the origins of the coronary artery (▶ Fig. 6.4). Ostial coronary artery lesions have also been described. Aortic valve abnormalities may also be present, and the aorta itself may be slightly diffuse with decreased elasticity.

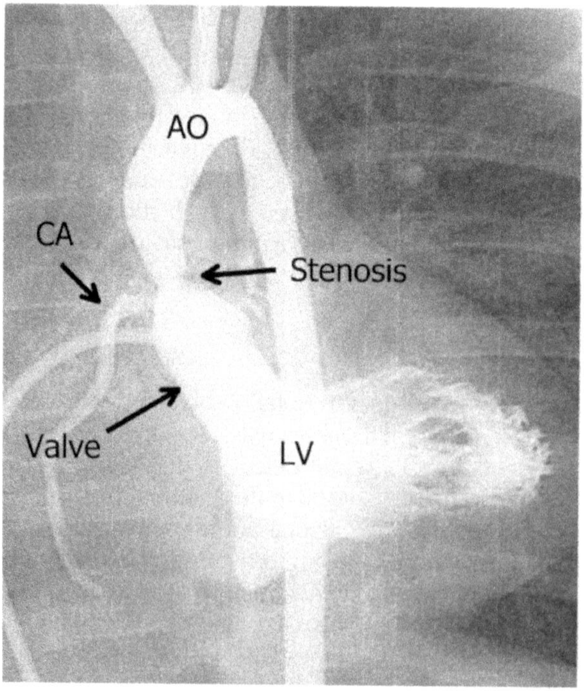

Fig. 6.4: Angiogram of supravalvular aortic stenosis. The stenosis is above the origin of the coronary artery, potentially limiting diastolic flow from the aorta to the coronary circulation. LV, left ventricle; CA, coronary artery; AO, aorta.

The symptoms and signs of supravalvular aortic stenosis are as with valvular aortic stenosis. Because coronary blood flow may be impaired by the stenosis and/or ostial lesions, angina, syncope, and cardiac arrest occur with relatively high frequency.

Echocardiography confirms the diagnosis, and Doppler evaluation is useful to quantify the degree of stenosis. Cardiac MRI or CT angiography has become routine to evaluate the anatomy of the entire thoracic aorta and coronary artery origins. Cardiac catheterization with angiography may also be done. Because coronary blood flow may be impaired, and the myocardial oxygen demand is increased due to the obstruction and hypertrophy, sedation and anesthesia should be administered cautiously such that excessive vasodilation is avoided; systemic hypotension may quickly lead to ischemia and cardiac arrest.

Treatment involves enlargement of the surgical patch of the stenotic area. Long-term follow-up is advisable due to the incidence of aortic valve dysfunction and the possibility of recurrence of aortic obstruction.

6.3 Aortic valve regurgitation

Aortic valve regurgitation may occur as the primary manifestation of a congenitally abnormal aortic valve (frequently in combination with aortic stenosis), after balloon valvuloplasty for aortic stenosis, or after surgical repair or replacement of the aortic valve. Aortic valve regurgitation may also occur with dilation of the aortic root without intrinsic valve leaflet abnormality, such as in Marfan syndrome (MFS). Other causes include subarterial VSD with distortion of a valve cusp by the VSD flow, subaortic stenosis, postoperative arterial switch and tetralogy of Fallot (usually with aortic root dilation), truncus arteriosus, and infective endocarditis.

Isolated chronic aortic valve regurgitation is generally well tolerated, but it is progressive and leads to left ventricular enlargement and eventually left ventricular dysfunction. Symptoms develop late, frequently after left ventricular dysfunction develops, and include dyspnea with exertion, orthopnea, and fatigue. Angina may also occur. Physical findings are the presence of a wide pulse pressure with "bounding" pulses, lateral displacement of the cardiac impulse, and a diastolic decrescendo murmur. The wide pulse pressure is the result of increased systolic stroke volume (increased systolic pressure) and diastolic runoff into the left ventricle (decreased diastolic pressure). Physical signs associated with the resultant bounding pulses include Quincke's sign (nailbed pulses that are visible), Corrigan's "water hammer" pulse, and Duroziez' sign (to-and-fro murmur generated by compression of the femoral artery). A systolic ejection murmur is usually heard in the aortic area, even in the absence of aortic stenosis, due to increased stroke volume.

ECG demonstrates left ventricular hypertrophy. Chest radiography reveals cardiomegaly and possibly an enlarged ascending aorta. Echocardiography with Doppler will confirm the diagnosis, define the valve morphology, delineate the aortic root size and left ventricular size and function, and quantify the severity of the regurgitation. Cardiac MRI will provide additional anatomic information regarding the valve and aortic root, as well as left ventricular volume, function, and mass.

Medical treatment for aortic regurgitation consists primarily of vasodilators such as nifedipine or angiotensin-converting enzyme (ACE) inhibitors for afterload reduction.

Surgical valve repair or replacement is indicated for any patient who is symptomatic or who has evidence of impending or existing left ventricular dysfunction (9, 10). In cases where the regurgitation is primarily due to aortic root dilation rather than primary valve leaflet disease, valve-sparing aortic root replacement may be an excellent option. Options for aortic valve repair or replacement are outlined above in the section on aortic valve stenosis.

Sudden death is not common with aortic valve regurgitation alone and, in general, aerobic exercise is well tolerated. Isometric exercise, however, results in a significant increase in afterload and should be discouraged in patients with aortic regurgitation that is more than mild. Pregnancy is generally well tolerated in asymptomatic patients with aortic regurgitation and normal left ventricular function. Pregnancy is accompanied by reduced afterload, which may help compensate for the increased cardiovascular demands.

6.4 Coarctation of the aorta

Coarctation of the aorta is a narrowing or obstruction in the aorta that is usually located in the proximal descending aorta near the aortic insertion of the ductus arteriosus. Constriction of ductal tissue within the aorta may be a factor in the etiology of coarctation. The obstruction may be discrete, with a shelf-like ridge, or diffuse with tubular hypoplasia of the aortic isthmus or the entire aortic arch. In adults, coarctation may be native (untreated or not previously diagnosed) or previously treated by surgery or transcatheter intervention. Coarctation of the aorta may occur as an isolated lesion, but is frequently associated with obstruction of the bicuspid aortic valve or other left heart obstruction. Most cases are sporadic, but genetic factors are implicated in some cases. Coarctation is more common in males (~2:1 male-to-female ratio) (19) and is commonly present in patients with Turner syndrome.

Most adults with coarctation are asymptomatic, presenting with hypertension or a murmur. Particularly if the hypertension is severe, patients may present with headaches, nosebleeds, dizziness, and fatigue. The diagnosis is established by demonstration of a blood pressure differential between the upper and lower extremities. A systolic murmur is frequently heard in the left infraclavicular area and left back. If prominent collateral flow via the intercostal arteries is present, a continuous murmur may be audible. Femoral pulses are generally weak and delayed with respect to the brachial pulses, but may be deceivingly easy to detect if extensive collateral flow is present.

Except in mild cases, ECG demonstrates left ventricular hypertrophy. Chest radiography may be normal, but may demonstrate an indentation in the aortic contour distal to the aortic knob ("3" sign) and/or rib notching (from enlarged intercostal arteries).

Echocardiography with Doppler confirms the diagnosis, quantifies the degree of obstruction, and evaluates for associated cardiac lesions. Imaging of the entire anatomy of the coarctation and surrounding aorta by echocardiographyis frequently difficult, however, and more detailed anatomic definition is obtained by MRI (▶ Fig. 6.5) or CT angiography. Cardiaccatheterization may be done to obtain direct measurements of aortic pressures, to define the anatomy by angiography, and to undertake intervention via balloon angioplasty and/or stent placement.

Despite the relative rarity of symptoms at presentation, untreated coarctation is associated with a poor prognosis, with a mean life expectancy of 35 years (20).

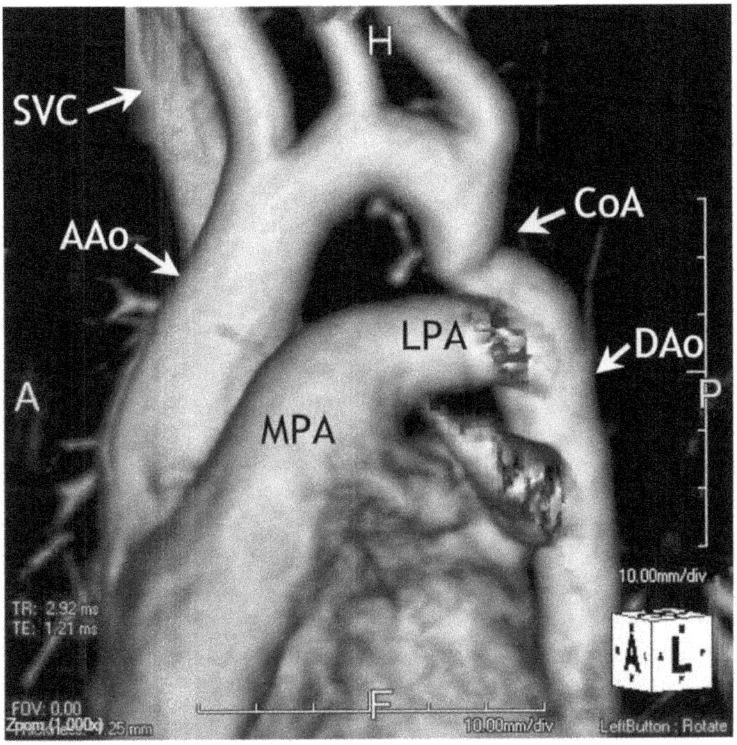

Fig. 6.5: Three-dimensional reconstruction from an MRI scan in a teenager with coarctation of the aorta. MPA, main pulmonary artery; LPA, left pulmonary artery; AAo, ascending aorta; SVC, superior vena cava; CoA, coarctation; DAo, descending aorta.

Complications are mostly related to long-term severe hypertension, and include left ventricular failure, cerebral aneurysms, early coronary artery disease, and dissection or rupture of the aorta. Treatment for coarctation is effective but not curative. Options include surgery by various techniques as well as catheter intervention. Because no treatment renders the aorta completely normal, significant complications may arise even after treatment.

Surgical techniques include resection with end-to-end anastamosis, patch aortoplasty, interposition tube graft, and subclavian flap. Transcatheter techniques include balloon angioplasty and stent placement. Although there is debate regarding which approach is optimal, it is clear that short- and intermediate-term results are generally very good but subsequent complications occur regardless of technique. Recurrent or residual obstruction, anseurysms, dissection, and aortic rupture are not rare. Residual hypertension is common, and its complications (including coronary artery disease, stroke, and heart failure) result in significant long-term morbidity and mortality. The frequently associated aortic valve disease is also important for long-term management and prognosis.

Adults with repaired coarctation require attentive long-term follow-up (10). Periodic imaging of the aorta by MRI or CT angiography is important in the detection of aneurysms or other important changes in anatomy that may herald impending life-threatening complications. Residual hypertension should be monitored closely and aggressively treated. Patients should be monitored closely for symptoms or signs of coronary artery disease and stroke.

Patients with repaired coarctation without residual or recurrent obstruction, aneurysm, or hypertension may participate in athletics, but are advised to avoid exercises with high static components (15). Those with residual hypertension, left ventricular dysfunction or hypertrophy, residual obstruction, or other complications should be advised to participate in only low-intensity exercises, and in particular should avoid isometric exercises. Avoidance of activities which have a risk of significant contact or trauma is also prudent, particularly if there is aortic enlargement or aneurysm. Similarly, women without residual hypertension or obstruction generally tolerate pregnancy well, but untreated patients or those with significant residua are at increased risk of complications (10). Optimal relief of obstruction should be achieved before pregnancy is contemplated, and pregnancy should be followed very closely with careful attention to blood pressure and aortic complications.

6.5 Mitral valve stenosis

Congenital mitral valve stenosis is rare. It is usually associated with other congenital heart disease such as repaired atrioventricular canal or as an element of the Shone complex (multiple left heart obstructions, including coarctation, aortic valve stenosis, subaortic stenosis, and/or mitral valve stenosis) (21). The pathology of congenital mitral stenosis is variable and includes elements of annular hypolasia, papillary muscle and chordae tendineae abnormalities that limit leaflet mobility, incompletely formed commissures, and thickening of valve leaflets. A parachute mitral valve is one which has only one papillary muscle to which all the chordae attach. A mitral arcade ("hammock mitral valve") has an arcade of shortened chordae tendinae that restrict leaflet motion. Another form is the supravalvar mitral ring, in which a fibrous membrane is present on the atrial surface of the valve. Repair of an atrioventricular septal defect frequently involves suturing of the "cleft" in the reconstructed anterior mitral leaflet, and mitral stenosis may result if the orifice size is significantly diminished.

Because it is quite rare for isolated congenital mitral valve stenosis to present as a native disease in adults, most adults with non-rheumatic mitral valve stenosis have mild stenosis or have had surgical procedures for mitral valve dysfunction or other significant congenital heart disease in childhood. The symptoms of mitral stenosis are those of congestive heart failure. Atrial fibrillation is not uncommon in adults with significant mitral stenosis. A diastolic murmur is heard at the apex, and an early diastolic opening snap may be heard. A prominent second heart sound is present if the stenosis is severe with resultant pulmonary hypertension. ECG and chest radiography demonstrate signs of left atrial enlargement. Echocardiography delineates the anatomy of the stenosis, and Doppler evaluation demonstrates high left ventricular inflow velocity. Cardiac catheterization demonstrates elevated left atrial pressure (or pulmonary artery wedge pressure) that is higher than left ventricular diastolic pressure, and pulmonary artery hypertension is present if the mitral stenosis is severe.

Mild mitral stenosis is generally well tolerated, and asymptomatic patients may not require treatment other than observation. For symptomatic patients with moderate or severe stenosis, surgery to repair or replace the mitral valve should be considered. Medical therapy will not relieve the obstruction, but medications that slow the heart rate (e.g., beta-blockers) may improve cardiac performance by lengthening the diastolic filling time. Diuretics may be helpful in alleviating symptoms. Maintenance of sinus rhythm is desirable, and may require medications or ablation (catheter or surgical). Anti-coagulation is important in patients with atrial fibrillation or a markedly enlarged left atrium.

Exercise is usually self-limiting for patients with mitral stenosis. Faster heart rate and increased cardiac output lead to increased left atrial pressure and may lead to pulmonary edema. Sudden death, however, is not common. Pregnancy is high-risk in patients with more than mild mitral stenosis. As with exercise, increased cardiac output with a fixed valve area results in higher left atrial and pulmonary vascular pressures. Exacerbation of symptoms, including onset of atrial fibrillation, may occur. Pregnancy is best deferred until after surgicalrelief of the stenosis is undertaken, if possible.

6.6 Mitral valve regurgitation

6.6.1 Mitral valve prolapse

Although mitral valve prolapse (MVP) is common (reported to be present in ≤15% of the population) (22), most of the individuals with this diagnosis have excellent prognosis and do not develop significant mitral regurgitation. However, a subset of MVP patients is at risk of progressive mitral valve dysfunction. The disorder is associated with connective-tissue abnormalities such as MFS and Ehlers–Danlos syndrome, as well as other inherited disorders such as muscular dystrophy, Grave's disease, and polycystic kidney disease. Due to "myxomatous" changes in the leaflets (overproduction of mucopolysaccharides in the spongiosa layer of valve tissue), the mitral valve leaflets become thickened and redundant, with elongation of the chordae tendineae, resulting in prolapse of one or both leaflets into the left atrium during systole. The resultant suboptimal coaptation of the leaflet edges may lead to regurgitation, which may be progressive.

Although the cause of most symptoms in patients with MVP remains unknown, those with significant regurgitation may develop symptoms of congestive heart failure such as exercise intolerance and dyspnea on exertion. Because the regurgitation is a dynamic process, augmented by factors that decrease left ventricular volume (e.g., hypovolemia, tachycardia, postural hypotension), physical examination findings are best detected just after the patient stands up from a supine or squatting position. A mid-to-late systolic click is heard at the apex, followed by a late systolic murmur. Echocardiography confirms the diagnosis, defines the valve anatomy, and quantifies the regurgitation. Images with the patient in the sitting or standing position may be necessary to definitively demonstrate the prolapse and regurgitation.

For patients with mild regurgitation and normal left ventricular size and function, treatment consists of reassurance and observation. Exercise limitations are not recommended, but avoidance of dehydration/hypovolemia is important. Beta-blockers may be helpful by decreasing the heart rate and increasing left ventricular volume, both of which tend to lessen the degree of regurgitation. For patients with congestive heart failure symptoms or significant left-heart chamber enlargement, surgical repair of the mitral valve is undertaken. Although mitral valve replacement remains an option, techniques for valve repair have developed such that results of repair are generally excellent and durable.

Ventricular arrhythmias are more common in patients with MVP (23), although this appears to be true primarily for those with significant regurgitation and left ventricular dysfunction. Usually these are premature ventricular contractions that are considered to be benign. In patients with thickened valve leaflets and significant regurgitation, however, there is a small increased risk of sudden death. Exercise restrictions are not recommended for most asymptomatic patients with MVP with regurgitation as long as they are in sinus rhythm and their left ventricular size and systolic function are normal. If there is left ventricular enlargement or dysfunction, history of syncope from dysrhythmia, history of documented atrial or ventricular dysrhythmia, or family history of sudden cardiac death associated with MVP, then exercise restrictions are advisable (15).

Pregnancy is generally well tolerated in patients with mitral regurgitation from MVP, unless the regurgitation is severe and there is left ventricular dysfunction. In those with atrial or ventricular dysrhythmia, close observation is advisable.

6.6.2 Postoperative mitral regurgitation

Aside from MVP, the most common setting for mitral regurgitation in adults with congenital heart disease is patients with repaired atrioventricular septal defects (ostium primum atrial defects or complete atrioventricular canal defects). In addition, patients with mitral valve repair for congenital mitral stenosis or resulting from other intracardiac reconstructive surgery may have significant residual or recurrent mitral valve regurgitation. There may also be some degree of concomitant mitral stenosis. Lastly, patients with poor left ventricular function after one or more surgeries for congenital heart disease may develop mitral regurgitation due to left ventricular enlargement, annular dilatation, and papillary muscle dysfunction.

Symptoms are dependent upon the degree of regurgitation and other associated lesions, and include fatigue, dyspnea on exertion, orthopnea, and exercise intolerance. Atrial fibrillation or flutter is not uncommon. Examination reveals lateral displacement of the cardiac impulse and a holosystolic murmur at the apex. Chest readiography demonstrates cardiomegaly with left ventricular and left atrial enlargement, and ECG demonstrates left atrial enlargement and left ventricular hypertrophy. Echocardiography, including transesophageal echocardiography, demonstrates the mechanism and severity of the regurgitation (▶ Fig. 6.6), and defines associated lesions.

Medical treatment for mitral regurgitation consists of afterload reduction, diuretics, and digoxin. Treatment of atrial fibrillation or flutter comprises anti-coagulation and anti-dysrhythmic medications to preserve sinus rhythm or control ventricular rate. Patients with symptoms or significant ventricular enlargement or dysfunction are candidates for surgical valve repair or replacement. Repair is preferable if possible, but frequently the underlying anatomy and mechanism of the regurgitation preclude repair and necessitate replacement. Tissue valves in the mitral position are generally not very durable, therefore mechanical prosthetic valves are usually preferred. Long-term anti-coagulation is required for prosthetic valves in the mitral position.

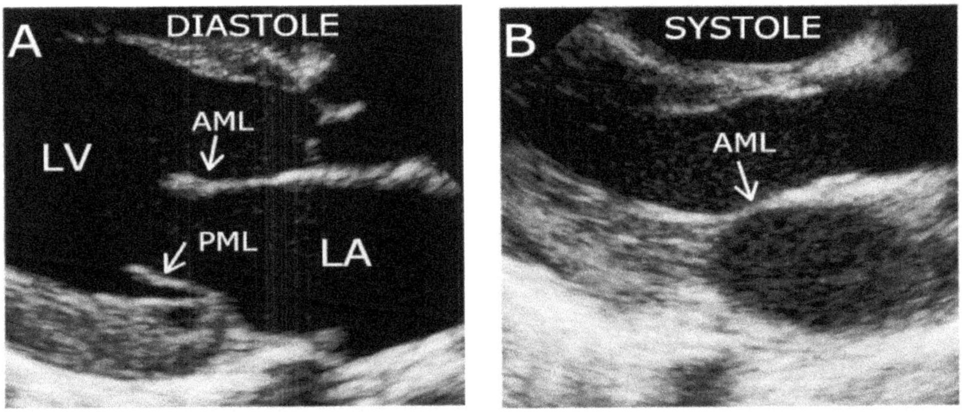

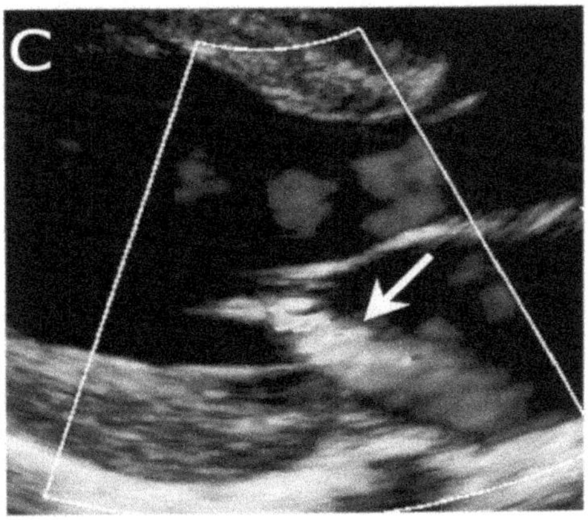

Fig. 6.6: Echocardiography with color Doppler of mitral valve regurgitation. **A:** Open mitral valve in diastole. **B:** Closed mitral valve in systole. **C:** Color flow Doppler of mitral regurgitation jet during systole (arrow). LV, left ventricle; LA, left atrium; AML, anterior mitral leaflet; PML, posterior mitral leaflet.

6.7 Tricuspid stenosis

Congenital tricuspid stenosis is most often associated with right ventricular hypoplasia and right ventricular outflow obstruction or atresia; isolated congenital tricuspid stenosis is extremely rare. In adults, tricuspid stenosis may occur as a consequence of previous valve surgery such as atrioventricular canal repair. Complete atresia of the tricuspid valve is almost always associated with a hypoplastic right ventricle and is a cyanotic condition.

6.8 Tricuspid valve regurgitation

Congenital tricuspid valve regurgitation is rare, and most commonly occurs due to Ebstein's anomaly. Other congenital cardiac malformations that may result in tricuspid regurgitation in adult life include repaired atrioventricular septal defect, congenital tricuspid valve dysplasia (non-Ebstein), VSD with endocarditis, repaired or untreated congenital heart lesions that have lead to right ventricular dilation and dysfunction (such as repaired tetralogy of Fallot or unrepaired ASD), and lesions that cause high right ventricular afterload (such as branch pulmonary artery stenosis or pulmonary hypertension). In the setting of normal PVR and absence of right ventricular outflow tract obstruction, tricuspid regurgitation is generally well-tolerated but eventually may lead to progressive right atrial enlargement with clinical right heart failure and development of atrial arrhythmias.

6.8.1 Ebstein's anomaly of the tricuspid valve

Ebstein's anomaly of the tricuspid valve is rare, accounting for < 1% of congenital heart defects (24). The etiology is not known, although there is an association with fetal lithium exposure in the first trimester. Familial cases have occurred, but most cases are sporadic. The defect involves abnormal attachment of the septal and posterior mural tricuspid valve leaflets, which are displaced towards the apex of the right ventricle. This results in abnormal coaptation of the tricuspid valve leaflets, leading to tricuspid regurgitation. Because of the apical displacement of the leaflet attachments, a portion of the right ventricle is "atrialized" such that it is above the tricuspid valve. In severe cases, there may be right ventricular outflow tract obstruction or even pulmonary atresia. Most patients with Ebstein's anomaly have a patent foramen ovale (PFO) or ASD. Patients with Ebstein's anomaly have an increased incidence of accessory atrioventricular conduction pathways with ventricular pre-excitation. Patients with congenitally corrected transposition of the great arteries ("ventricular inversion") have a relatively high incidence of Ebstein's anomaly; the tricuspid valve is the "systemic" atrioventricular valve in this situation and the physiological impact is that of mitral regurgitation in hearts without ventricular inversion.

Once outside the neonatal period, after the PVR has fallen, patients with Ebstein's anomaly are commonly asymptomatic or minimally symptomatic, even in the presence of significant tricuspid regurgitation. The severity of the valve malformation is highly variable, and those with mild disease may remain asymptomatic. Patients with severe Ebstein's deformity will probably have had surgical valve repair or replacement in childhood, but many reach adult life without having had surgery. Over time, however, right atrial enlargement progresses, and right-to-left shunting across the PFO or ASD may lead to cyanosis. Symptoms may be due to arrhythmia (atrial flutter, atrioventricular re-entry tachycardia, or sudden death) or right heart dysfunction. Patients frequently report fatigue and dyspnea on exertion. Left heart dysfunction is also reported to occur at a surprisingly high frequency for what is generally considered a right heart lesion.

The physical examination findings are dependent upon the severity of the valve deformity and tricuspid regurgitation. Cyanosis and clubbing may be evident. The jugular veins and/or liver may be distended, and the right ventricular impulse may be prominent. A holosystolic murmur is present at the mid, lower left and right sternal borders; the intensity varies according to the severity of the regurgitation. The classic radiographic finding is that of marked right atrial enlargement; pulmonary vascular markings may be diminished. ECG demonstrates right atrial enlargement and ventricular pre-excitation. The definitive diagnosis is made or confirmed by echocardiography with Doppler.

Medical therapy is limited in adults with Ebstein's anomaly other than treatment of arrhythmias with anti-arrhythmic agents. Treatment for Ebstein's anomaly is primarily surgical, and is indicated in patients with cyanosis or symptoms of right heart dysfunction (10). Surgical options include tricuspid valve repair or replacement, ASD or PFO closure, and right atrial placation/reduction. Patients with severe right heart dysfunction may benefit from the presence of an ASD, allowing for improved cardiac output at the expense of cyanosis from a right-to-left shunt. Alternatively, patients with cyanosis from a right-to-left shunt but relatively preserved right heart function may benefit from transcatheter ASD closure alone. Surgical or transcatheter ablation of accessory conduction pathways may also be beneficial.

The prognosis of patients with Ebstein's anomaly is variable according to the severity of the malformation. Severe cases that require surgery in infancy may ultimately require a single ventricle palliation pathway, with eventual bidirectional Glenn, Fontan, or even heart transplant. Mild cases have a good prognosis. With improvement in surgical techniques over the past several years, the prognosis has improved significantly even for those with severe valve abnormality and right heart dysfunction. Due to the risk of arrhythmia and sudden death, restriction from vigorous athletic activities is appropriate for those with more than mild disease. Most patients self-regulate their activities based on symptoms. The risks of arrhythmia, cardiac decompensation, and paradoxical embolism should be weighed carefully for those considering pregnancy.

6.9 Pulmonary stenosis

Pulmonary stenosis is present in ~10% of patients with congenital heart disease, and usually exists as valvular stenosis. Subvalvular and supravalvular pulmonary stenosis may also occur, and pulmonary stenosis may accompany complex congenital heart malformations including tetralogy of Fallot and a double-chambered right ventricle. If a VSD is present (as with tetralogy of Fallot) the patient may be cyanotic. As with most forms of congenital heart disease, genetic factors appear to be involved (although most cases are sporadic). Pulmonary stenosis is common in some genetic syndromes (e.g., Noonan, Alagille, Williams, Leopard).

Pulmonary stenosis is also common in postoperative patients with homograft or valved conduit connections between the right ventricle and pulmonary arteries. This includes patients with repaired tetralogy of Fallot, pulmonary atresia, double outlet right ventricle, and patients who have had a Ross procedure. In contrast to stenotic native pulmonary valves, which do not tend to worsen over time, homograft valves and conduit valves in the pulmonary position develop progressive stenosis and calcification which eventually necessitates repeat valve replacement.

In congenital pulmonary valve stenosis, the pulmonary valve leaflets are usually fused with a conical shape and central opening, although sometimes the leaflets are thickened and "dysplastic" with distinctly defined cusps and commissures. The main pulmonary artery is usually enlarged. The muscular right ventricular infundibulum may be hypertrophied and narrow, causing an element of dynamic subvalvular obstruction. In the absence of a VSD, the physiological impact of pulmonary stenosis is elevation of right ventricular pressure.

Other than patients with critical pulmonary stenosis that present as neonates, pulmonary stenosis is generally discovered at the time of evaluation for a heart murmur in an asymptomatic patient. If the obstruction is severe, symptoms may include exercise intolerance, fatigue, dyspnea on exertion, or syncope. Although this lesion is generally well-tolerated, moderate-to-severe pulmonary stenosis may eventually lead to clinical right heart failure if untreated. Symptoms may be triggered or exacerbated by the onset of atrial dysrhythmia.

Examination findings of pulmonary stenosis include a prominent right ventricular precordial impulse, a systolic ejection murmur at the upper left sternal border radiating to the back, and oftena systolic ejection click. Except in mild cases, where it may be normal, ECG usually demonstrates right ventricular hypertrophy, right axis deviation, and right atrial enlargement. Chest radiography usually shows normal heart size but with a large main pulmonary artery segment, and normal pulmonary vascular markings otherwise. Echocardiography with Doppler confirms the diagnosis and quantifies the degree of obstruction. Cardiac MRI may be useful to help delineate the anatomy of multilevel obstructions (particularly if branch pulmonary artery stenosis is suspected and difficult to image by echocardiography). Cardiac MRI is also helpful in quantifying the degree of pulmonary regurgitation (if present).

Patients with mild pulmonary stenosis have an excellent prognosis and do not require treatment; progression of stenosis to more severe obstruction is not common. However, even if asymptomatic, those with moderate-to-severe stenosis are at risk of late complications, and relief of the obstruction is indicated (10). Most patients with valvular pulmonary stenosis have an excellent result from balloon pulmonary valvuloplasty in the catheterization laboratory.

Some patients, especially those with dysplastic pulmonary valve leaflets and those with significant subvalvular or supravalvular stenosis, do not respond well to valvuloplasty and require surgical valvotomy. In either case, the prognosis is usually excellent even though most patients have mild residual stenosis and some degree of regurgitation. Most will not require subsequent intervention. Those patients with significant residual pulmonary valve regurgitation, however, may eventually benefit from pulmonary valve replacement. In contrast to patients with native pulmonary valve stenosis, those with

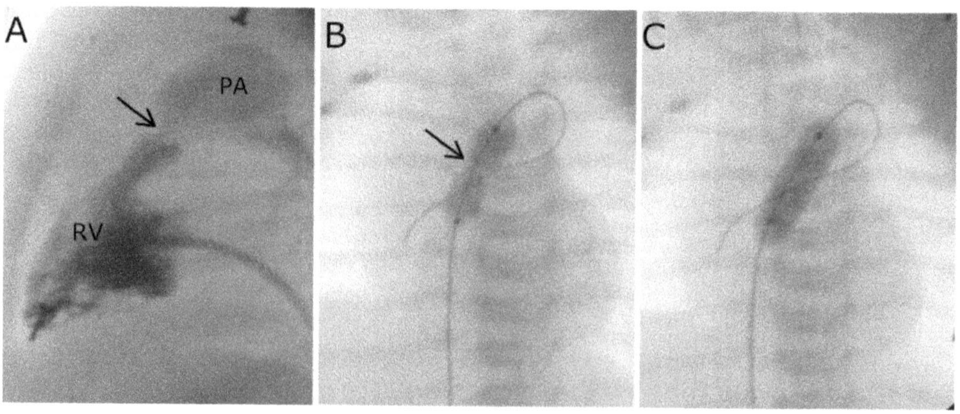

Fig. 6.7: Angiograms of balloon pulmonary valvuloplasty. **A:** Right ventriculogram demonstrating a thickened and stenotic pulmonary valve with a narrow jet of flow through the valve during systole (arrow). **B:** Angioplasty balloon inflating, with a "waist" at the site of the orifice of the stenotic valve (arrow). **C:** Elimination of the waist at full balloon inflation, representing successful tearing of leaflets to open the valve orifice. RV, right ventricle; PA pulmonary artery.

homograft or conduit valves in the pulmonary position develop progressive stenosis over time and eventually repeat valve replacement is to be expected.

Despite the generally excellent prognosis for patients with mild or treated pulmonary stenosis, long-term follow-up is important to assess right ventricular function and to look for possible progression of pulmonary regurgitation. Patients with mild stenosis and normal right ventricular function do not require exercise restrictions. In general, patients with moderate or severe pulmonary stenosis should have catheter or surgical relief of the obstruction before participating in vigorous exercise activities. Patients with right ventricular enlargement or dysfunction, even after relief of obstruction, should not participate in high-intensity exercise activities due to the risk of dysrhythmia or sudden death (15). Pregnancy is generally well tolerated, but ideally should be deferred in women with moderate or severe stenosis until after transcatheter or surgical relief of obstruction. Patients with significant right ventricular dysfunction should be followed closely during pregnancy, and residual stenosis or significant regurgitation should be addressed prior to pregnancy if possible.

6.10 Pulmonary regurgitation

Pulmonary valve regurgitation is a relatively common residual problem in adults with congenital heart disease. Any patient with surgical right ventricular outflow tract reconstruction, such as in tetralogy of Fallot or double outlet right ventricle, is at risk of developing progressive pulmonary valve regurgitation with right ventricular enlargement and dysfunction. Tetralogy of Fallot repairs that involve patch augmentation of the pulmonary valve annulus are particularly prone to subsequent regurgitation. Some patients after pulmonary balloon valvuloplasty will develop progressive pulmonary valve regurgitation, and many homograft or conduit valves in the pulmonary position will develop progressive regurgitation.

Pulmonary valve regurgitation is very well tolerated until right ventricular enlargement and dysfunction develop from the chronic volume overload. Symptoms, which may be precipitated by the onset of atrial or ventricular dysrhythmia, are those of right heart failure and develop late, and are associated with signs of increased central venous pressure such as jugular vein distention and hepatomegaly. The right ventricular impulse is prominent, and the second heart sound is soft or absent. The intensity of the diastolic murmur of pulmonary regurgitation does not necessarily correlate with the degree of regurgitation because the flow is usually low-velocity without any significant pressure gradient between the pulmonary artery and right ventricle during diastole. Chest radiography demonstrates cardiomegaly with enlarged main and proximal branch pulmonary arteries. ECG demonstrates right ventricular hypertrophy typically with concomitant right bundle branch block and right axis deviation. The degree of QRS prolongation may correlate with the degree of right ventricular enlargement.

Echocardiography with Doppler is helpful in determining the degree of regurgitation and right ventricular size and function. Cardiac MRI is used to quantify the size and function of the right ventricle, and defines the anatomy of the valve and pulmonary arteries. Cardiac catheterization is no longer routinely used for diagnostic purposes in this setting, but is undertaken for percutaneous pulmonary valve replacement as well as angioplasty or stent placement if pulmonary artery stenosis is present. Electrophysiology studies may be helpful in those with suspected ventricular or atrial dysrhythmia.

Medical treatment with diuretics and digoxin may be helpful to alleviate symptoms in those with clinical right heart failure. Anti-arrhythmia agents are useful to control dysrhythmias, and catheter ablation may be undertaken to treat some dysrhythmias. Pacemaker therapy may be helpful to treat and prevent certain atrial dysrhythmias, and biventricular pacing may improve right ventricular function in some patients (25). In patients deemed to be at high risk for sudden death from ventricular dysrhythmia, defibrillator systems may be considered. More definitive treatment involves pulmonary valve replacement by surgery or a percutaneous technique. The optimal timing of surgery is before development of right ventricular dysfunction or symptoms but, because many patients with severe pulmonary regurgitation and right ventricular enlargement do extremely well for many years (even decades) before right heart failure develops, determining the indications for pulmonary valve replacement may be challenging. Quantification of right ventricular enlargement and function by cardiac MRI is an objective way to determine the need for pulmonary valve replacement. Patients with significant pulmonary valve regurgitation should be followed periodically to assess for progression in right ventricular enlargement or development of symptoms or signs of right ventricular dysfunction or arrhythmia. Although pulmonary valve replacement has been shown to improve hemodynamic status and degree of right ventricular enlargement, it does not eliminate the risk of arrhythmia and/or sudden death.

Due to the risk of arrhythmia and sudden death, patients with pulmonary regurgitation and moderate or severe right ventricular enlargement, right ventricular dysfunction, concomitant pulmonary stenosis, or history if significant arrhythmia should not participate in athletics or vigorous exercise (15). If the regurgitation is only mild-to-moderate and the right ventricle is normal or only mildly enlarged, and there is no history of dyrhythmia or syncope, then participation in athletics is not restricted. Pregnancy in patients with pulmonary regurgitation is generally well tolerated in the absence of right ventricular dysfunction, dysrhythmia, or other significant associated cardiac problems.

References

1. Mitchell, S. C., Korones, S. B., Berendes, H. W. (1971) Congenital heart disease in 56,109 births. Circulation 43: 323–332.
2. Hoffman, J. I., Christianson, R. (1978) Congenital heart disease in a cohort of 19,502 births with long-term follow-up. Am. J. Cardiol. 42:641–647.
3. Sabet, H. Y., Edwards, W. D., Tazelaar, H. D., Daly, R. C. (1999) Congenitally bicuspid aortic valves: a surgical pathology study of 542 cases (1991 through 1996) and a literature review of 2, 715 additional cases. Mayo Clin. Proc. 74:14–26.
4. Roberts, W. C. (1970) The congenitally bicuspid aortic valve. A study of 85 autopsy cases. Am. J. Cardiol. 26:72–83.
5. Campbell, M. (1968) The natural history of congenital aortic stenosis. Br. Heart J. 30:514–526.
6. Keane, M. G. Wiegers, S. E., Plappert, T., Pochettino, A., Bavaria, J. E., Sutton, M. G., et al. Bicuspid aortic valves are associated with aortic dilatation out of proportion to coexistent valvular lesions. Circulation 102(Suppl. III):35–39.
7. Fenoglio, J. J. Jr., McAllister, H. A. Jr., DeCastro, C. M., Davia, J. E. Cheitlin, M. D., et al. (1977) Congenital bicuspid aortic valve after age 20. Am. J. Cardiol. 39:164–169.
8. Ward, C. (2000) Clinical significance of the bicuspid aortic valve. Heart 83:81–85.

9. Bonow, R. O., Carabello, B., Chatterjee, K., de Leon, A. C., Faxton, D. P., Freed, M. D., et al. (2006) ACC/AHA 2006 guidelines for the management of patients with valvular heart disease: a report of the American College of Cardiology/American Heart Association Task Force on Practice Guidelines (Writing Committee to Develop Guidelines for the Management of Patients With Valvular Heart Disease) Circulation 114:e84–e231.
10. Warnes, C. A., Williams, R. G., Bashore, T. M., Child, J. S., Connolly, H. M., Dearani, J. A. et al. (2008) ACC/AHA 2008 guidelines for the management of adults with congenital heart disease: a report of the American College of Cardiology/American Heart Association Task Force on Practice Guidelines (Writing Committee to Develop Guidelines for the Management of Adults With Congenital Heart Disease). J. Am. Coll. Cardiol. 52:e143–e263.
11. Kelly, T. A., Rothbart, R. M., Cooper, C. M., Kaiser, D. L., Smucker, M. L., Gibson, R. S. (1988) Comparison of outcome of asymptomatic to symptomatic patients older than 20 years of age with valvular aortic stenosis. Am. J. Cardiol. 61:123–130.
12. Pacileo, G., Calabrò, P., Limongelli, G., Russo, M. G., Pisacane, C., Sarubbi, B. et al. (2003) Left ventricular remodeling, mechanics, and tissue characterization in congenital aortic stenosis. J. Am. Soc. Echo. 16:214–220.
13. Vincent, W. R., Buckberg, G. D., Hoffman, J. I. (1974) Left ventricular subendocardial ischemia in severe valvar and supravalvar aortic stenosis. A common mechanism. Circulation 49:326–333.
14. Weidemann, F., Hermann, S., Stork, S., Niemann, M., Frantz, S., Lang, V., et al. (2009) Impact of myocardial fibrosis in patients with symptomatic severe aortic stenosis. Circulation 120: 577–84.
15. Maron, B. J., Zipes, D. P. (2005) 36th Bethesda Conference: eligibility recommendations for competitive athletes with cardiovascular abnormalities. J. Am. Coll. Cardiol. 45:1313–1375.
16. Freedom, R. M., Fowler, R. S., Suncan, W. J. (1981) Rapid evolution from "normal" left ventricular outflow tract to fatal subaortic stenosis in infancy. Br. Heart J. 45:605–609.
17. Brauner, R., Laks, H., Drinkwater, D. C., Shvarts, O., Eghbali, K., Galindo, A. (1997) Benefits of early surgical repair in fixed subaortic stenosis. J. Am. Coll. Cardiol. 30:1835–1842.
18. Gersony, W. M. (2001) Natural history of discrete subvalvar aortic stenosis: management implications. J. Am. Coll. Cardiol. 38:843–845.
19. Fyler, D. C., Buckley, L. P., Hellenbrand, W. E., Cohn, H. E. (1980) Report of the New England regional infant cardiac program. Pediatrics 65:432–436.
20. Campbell, M. (1970) Natural history of coarctation of the aorta. Br. Heart J. 32:633–640.
21. Shone, J. D., Sellers, R. D., Anderson, R. C., Adams, P., Jr., Lillehei, C. W., Edwards, J. E. (1963) The developmental complex of "parachute mitral valve": supravalvular ring of the left atrium, subaortic stenosis and coarctation of the aorta. Am. J. Cardiol. 11:714–725.
22. Levy, D., Savage, D. (1987) Prevalence and clinical features of mitral valve prolapse. Am. Heart J. 113:1281–1290.
23. Devereux, R. B., Kramer-Fox, R., Kligfield, P. (1989) Mitral valve prolapse: causes, clinical manifestations, and management. Ann. Intern. Med. 11:305–317.
24. Corea-Villasenor, A., Ferencz, C., Neill, C. A., Wilson, P. D., Boughman, J. A. (1994) Ebstein's malformation of the tricuspid valve: genetic and environmental factors. TheBaltimore–Washington Infant Study Group. Teratology 50:137–147.
25. Kirsh, J. A., Stephenson, E. A., Redington, A. N. (2006) Recovery of left ventricular systolic function after biventricular resynchronization pacing in a child with repaired tetralogy of Fallot and severe biventricular dysfunction. Circulation 113:e691–e692.

7 Adults with left-to-right cardiac shunts and with shunts treated in childhood

Craig Alexander and Louis I. Bezold

Pediatric cardiac care has advanced over the past decade. Many children born with heart defects have undergone surgery, resulting in improvement of outcome and life expectancy. This review focuses on patients born with left-to-right shunts that survive into adulthood. We believe it is important for the adult Primary Care Physician to realize that increasing numbers of patients with congenital heart defects will enter their practice over the next several decades as improvements in childhood cardiac care continue to be made. The number of cardiologists specifically trained in adult congenital heart disease is not yet adequate to deal with the increasing numbers of patients with these conditions. This requires a concerted effort from cardiologists of adult and pediatric specialties, but perhaps more importantly from the multitude of Primary Care Physicians that will probably be the only physicians many of these patients will ever see. Many adult patients born with left-to-right heart lesions underwent treatment and repair early in childhood, and may not have felt it necessary to continue follow-up with a cardiologist. Many other patients with these defects may have survived to adulthood without diagnosis, and may present to the primary-care provider with new symptoms that finally developed. Primary Care Physicians will most certainly be at the frontlines of caring for these congenital heart defects.

7.1 Introduction

Many advances in pediatric cardiac care have occurred over the past several decades which have improved outcomes and prolonged life in children born with heart defects. These advances have led to an important question: how do we best care for these childhood survivors as they become adults? While this review focuses on patients born with left-to-right shunts that survive into adulthood, whether repaired or not, it is important for the Adult Primary Care Physician to realize that increasing numbers of patients with congenital heart defects will be entering into their practice over the next several decades as improvements in childhood cardiac care continue to be made.

7.2 ASDs

Defects of the atrial septum are relatively common, accounting for ~7% of congenital heart disease, and are the second most common congenital heart lesion presenting in adults (behind bicuspid aortic valve). ASDs vary greatly in size and may occur in several locations within the atrial septum, with the location of the defect generally reflecting the specific abnormality of embryogenesis that led to the anomaly. ASDs can occur in isolation or in association with a multitude of other congenital cardiac anomalies. The functional consequences of an unrepaired ASD are largely related to the size and anatomic location of the defect, and the presence or absence of other cardiac anomalies (1, 2).

The three primary types of ASD discussed in this chapter are secundum ASDs, sinus venosus ASDs and primum ASDs (which are actually a form of endocardial cushion defect). A PFO is also a communication between the right and left atria, but is not technically considered a true ASD because no septal tissue is deficient. PFOs can be clinically significant however, because they represent potential right-to-left shunts which can be associated with a risk of paradoxical embolization.

7.2.1 Secundum ASDs

A secundum ASD is a defect located in the interatrial septum in the region of the fossa ovalis and is the most common type of ASD (70–75% of all ASDs). Secundum ASDs account for ~40% of acyanotic congenital heart defects that survive unrepaired past the age of 40 years. Females outnumber males by approximately 2 to 1. Secundum ASDS most often occur as isolated defects, but may be associated with congenital syndromes, genetic defects or other complex heart disease. Other associations include MVP, partial anomalous pulmonary venous return (rare) and the very rare combination of an ASD with mitral stenosis resulting from rheumatic valvulitis (known as Lutembacher's syndrome) (1).

Anatomy and physiology

Secundum ASDs are usually relatively centrally located in the interatrial septum. They vary in size from < 2–3 mm to > 20 mm, and may be multiple (so-called "fenestrated defects").

In childhood, shunting across a secundum ASD is usually left-to-right, reflective of the relative pressures in the atria (normally left greater than right) and ventricular diastolic compliance (right ventricle more compliant than the thicker-walled left ventricle). The degree of shunting is also obviously dependent on the size of the defect (1, 3, 4). Patients are acyanotic and the volume of blood flow in the pulmonary circulation is greater than that in the systemic circulation (typical pulmonary flow to systemic flow ratio {Qp:Qs} between 2:1 to 5:1). Left-to-right shunting leads to rightheart and pulmonary vascular dilatation. Right ventricular systolic function is generally maintained in childhood but is occasionally decreased in adulthood.

An important long-term factor in the direction and amount of an atrial-level shunt are the diastolic properties of the ventricles, which change over a lifetime and favor increasing left-to-right shunting over time. A previously unrecognized ASD may begin to cause significant symptoms due to this ongoing physiologic process. Pulmonary artery pressure and resistance are usually normal or minimally elevated in secundum ASDs (even in adulthood), but in some cases pulmonary hypertension can develop later in life (5). Even less commonly, the pulmonary resistance and pressure exceeds that of the systemic circulation, resulting in the so-called Eisenmenger syndrome (discussed below). In this physiology, right ventricular failure and right-to-left atrial-level shunting predominate.

Clinical features and natural history

Most small-to-moderate ASDs (including secundum ASDs) do not cause significant symptoms in infancy and childhood. Large ASDs may present with heart failure, recurrent respiratory infections, or failure to thrive as early as the first year or two of life; alternatively even large defects may cause relatively subtle symptoms in many cases in childhood (1, 2).

The diagnosis is usually suspected due to a murmur on physical examination. The murmur is similar to a pulmonary flow murmur or mild pulmonary stenosis, but is distinguished in many cases by a fixed, widely-split S2 (a classic finding in secundum ASDs) and lack of a pulmonic ejection click. A flow rumble due to increased diastolic flow across the tricuspid valve may be audible in large defects. Additional clinical signs of right ventricular volume overload may be evident such as right ventricular heave or lift, a prominent right ventricular impulse, or palpable pulmonary artery pulsations (particularly in the presence of pulmonary hypertension).

Many adults with unrepaired ASDs have a relatively small secundum ASD that has enabled them to progress through childhood without problems. Although many patients report no symptoms, clinical status may improve after correction.

In many patients with uncorrected moderate-to-large ASDs (i.e., Qp:Qs > 2:1), left-to-right shunting increases with age. As a result, the frequency of right heart failure accompanied by shortness of breath, fluid retention, hepatomegaly, and elevated jugular venous pressure increases with advancing age. Most of these adults become symptomatic before age 40 years, but some remain asymptomatic until their 60s or later (1, 6). Common symptoms include atrial arrhythmias, sick-sinus syndrome, exercise intolerance, dyspnea, and fatigue. These findings in an otherwise healthy adult should prompt consideration of a previously unrecognized ASD. Palpitations and atrial arrhythmias, including new-onset atrial fibrillation or flutter, are the most frequent presenting symptom in adults and the prevalence increases with advancing age (from 1% in 18–40 year-olds to 80% in those > 60 years old) and pulmonary artery pressure. Not unexpectedly, patients with atrial fibrillation are at risk for embolic events (1, 5–11).

Although left ventricular failure is uncommon, subtle evidence of left ventricular dysfunction is not. Diastolic function appears to be primarily affected, probably secondary to right ventricular volume overload with resulting secondary left ventricular systolic abnormalities. Systemic hypertension, if present, can exacerbate the hemodynamic changes due to an ASD due to decreased left ventricular compliance, causing an increase in left-to-right shunting.

The pulmonary vasculature can usually handle the increased flow volume due to an ASD without significant rise in pulmonary pressure (≤2.5-times normal flow). Pulmonary vascular injury and hypertension develop in adults with ASDs, and are related to the severity and duration of right heart volume overload.

Moderate-to-severe pulmonary hypertension occurs in < 10% of adults with an ASD (12). The development of severe irreversible pulmonary hypertension with reversal of shunting at the ASD (Eisenmenger syndrome) has fortunately become uncommon due to wide availability of interventions to close these defects. However, ASDs remain a fairly common cause for this syndrome due to their prevalence and sometimes subtle presentation, resulting in delayed diagnosis in adulthood. Eisenmenger syndrome carries a relatively poor prognosis.

Adults with a PFO or ASD with a right-to-left shunt are at risk for stroke due to paradoxical embolization. Right-to-left shunting can occur at rest or with transient increases in right-sided pressure such as with a Valsalva maneuver or coughing, or may be persistent in patients with pulmonary hypertension. PFO is common in patients with cryptogenic stroke (1, 2).

Migraine headaches reportedly occur more frequently in patients with PFO or, less commonly an ASD, possibly due to passage of vasoactive substances such as serotonin into the systemic circulation via right-to-left flow across the atrial septum. Closure of the defect may lead to a reduction in migraine frequency, but appropriate management of PFOs in patients with migraines remains controversial (2).

Diagnostic studies

- **ECG**
  ECG in patients with secundum ASDs typically reveals right axis deviation with an rSr′ patternin the right precordial leads. Right atrial and right ventricular enlargement or hypertrophy may be present to varying degrees. Most adults will show some of these typical findings because they have had a longer period of time to develop signs of right atrial and ventricular enlargement. Very rarely in large secundum ASDs the electrocardiogram has an extreme left axis (similar to primum ASDs).
- **Chest radiography**
  Chest radiographs typically reveal enlargement of the right ventricle and right atrium and possibly dilation of the pulmonary trunk with increased pulmonary vascular markings in significant left-to-right shunts. Tortuous, pruned pulmonary vascular markings with pulmonary oligemia can be seen with pulmonary vascular disease.
- **Echocardiography**
  Two-dimensional (2D) transthoracic echocardiography (TTE) and Doppler echocardiography is the study of choice for the diagnosis of a secundum ASD. Color Doppler imaging can assist in assessing direction and degree of shunting through the ASD. Transesophageal echocardiography (TEE) is useful in adult patients with limited transthoracic acoustic windows and is utilized intraoperatively to assess surgical repair. TEE or intracardiac echocardiography (ICE) is routinely used to assist in transcatheter device closure of secundum ASDs. Use of a laboratory with sonographers and staff experienced in congenital cardiac defects is needed for appropriate evaluation (1).
- **Other imaging methods**
  Cardiac CT and MRI are generally not necessary in evaluation of a secundum ASD, but may be useful if additional malformations are present or echocardiographic acoustic windows are poor.
- **Cardiac catheterization**
  Cardiac catheterization is generally not necessary for diagnostic evaluation of secundum ASDs, and is usually reserved for those circumstances where existing data including TTE and/or TEE is inconsistent or unreliable, in cases where significant pulmonary hypertension is thought to exist, where additional malformations may be present, or if significant coronary artery disease is thought to exist or

requires intervention. Currently, the primary role of cardiac catheterization in the management of secundum ASDs is for trancatheter closure (1, 2).

Management considerations for care of adults with unrepaired secundum ASDs

Many patients with secundum ASDs will survive well into adulthood and often remain relatively asymptomatic until the fourth or fifth decade of life. Atrial arrhythmias and right heart failure eventually develop in unrepaired patients with significant left-to-right shunting (particularly in the 5th–6th decades) and lifespan is shortened. The American College of Cardiology (ACC) and the American Heart Association (AHA) have published excellent guidelines for the care of adults with ASDs (1). Medical treatment includes anti-congestive therapy with digoxin, diuretics and anti-arrhythmics. Patients with pulmonary vascular disease or Eisenmenger syndrome may benefit from pulmonary vasodilator therapy oxygen, diuretics and anti-coagulation with at least aspirin.

Subacute endocarditis (SBE) prophylaxis is not indicated in patients with isolated ASDs of any type, but many authors recommend prophylaxis for 6 months after device or surgical closure. The importance of routine dental care should be stressed to all patients whether they require SBE prophylaxis or not (13).

No specific activity restrictions are needed for most adults with unrepaired secundum ASDs, but the patient should be allowed to self-limit. Intense, isometric physical activities are discouraged in older patients with significant pulmonary hypertension, pulmonary vascular disease or heart failure. Low-resistance isotonic activity may be of benefit in these adults (1, 14).

Definitive treatment for a significant secundum ASD is closure, either surgically or by transcatheter device placement (1). In general, closure should be considered in patients with a Qp:Qs of ≥1.5:1 as evidenced by right atrial and ventricular enlargement in the absence of significant pulmonary vascular disease. Definitive defect closure decreases morbidity and improves life expectancy. The uncommon patient with severe pulmonary hypertension and vascular disease may not be an appropriate candidate for ASD closure, but limited data suggest that even older patients (> 50 years) with moderate-to-severe pulmonary hypertension who undergo surgical repair have better 10-year survival and functional status than those treated medically. For patients who are asymptomatic and have a small ASD (Qp:Qs < 1.5:1), optimal management is controversial because significant differences in outcome from closure *versus* medical treatment are not proven in these patients. Physicians should discuss the risks with these patients and explain the options prior to closure. ASD closure in patients aged > 40 years may not result in the same degree of benefit as seen in younger patients, but is nevertheless likely to improve functional status and survival compared with medical therapy alone (1, 2, 15).

Surgical ASD closure involves cardiopulmonary bypass and consists of patch or primary closure. Surgical risks are those usually associated with cardiopulmonary bypass, anesthesia and thoracic surgery. Long-term results are excellent. Transcatheter device closure for ASDs has become an accepted alternative to surgical closure. A multitude of devices are now availablethat can be delivered with low risk for many secundum ASDs, including relatively large defects. Risks include device embolization, thrombus formation, aortic root perforation, pericardial effusion and arrhythmias with long-term complications of endocarditis, thromboembolism and device strut fracture. Again, long-term results are excellent.

Recent debate has flourished regarding appropriate indications for closure of PFOs or small secundum ASDs in patients with migraine headaches. There appears to be a higher incidence of ASDs or PFOs in patients with migraines (although proof of a direct causal relationship is lacking). Reports of results with closure of the defects vary. Current recommendations call for open discussion of the risks of closure (which remain quite low with continuing advances and with appropriate selection of patients), the understanding that closure may or may not result in resolution of migraine symptoms, and the options for closure (1). Many authors consider closure a justifiable option in those patients with persistent moderate-to-severe migraines in the face of medical treatment who are good candidates for closure whether by interventional device or surgical closure.

Recommendations regarding pregnancy for females with unrepaired secundum ASDs vary depending on the hemodynamics. Small defects typically do not increase the risk of pregnancy from a hemodynamic standpoint and no special precautions are necessary. However, even patients with small shunts are at increased risk of paradoxical emboli by virtue of the atrial-level defect. Patients with left-to-right shunts associated with heart failure can usually tolerate pregnancy, but require close follow-up in a high-risk obstetrical practice because the normal increased intravascular volume load of pregnancy can exacerbate symptoms. Pregnancy is not advisable for patients with pulmonary hypertension or Eisenmenger syndrome due to a high risk of maternal morbidity and mortality. These patients should be appropriately counseled regarding these risks and appropriate contraceptive choices. The recurrence risk for ASD is estimated to be 8–10%. Familial secundum ASD with heart block is an autosomal dominant trait with NKX-2-5 mutations. Although secundum ASDs cannot be reliably diagnosed on fetal echocardiography due to the normal fetal PFO, fetal echocardiography should be considered because there is an increased risk of other congenital heart defects in the fetus whose parent has a secundum ASD (particularly the mother) (1, 2, 16–18).

Whether they have had surgery or not, adult patients should be followed up every 6–12 months by a Pediatric Cardiologist or Adult Cardiologist with expertise in adult congenital heart disease in a center with a multidisciplinary approach.

Management considerations for care of adults with secundum atrial septal defects repaired in childhood

Secundum ASDs with significant left-to-right shunting diagnosed early in life are routinely repaired in childhood (generally between 4 years and 7 years of age). The surgical approach is via a midline sternotomy. Several patients now entering adulthood have been treated via transcatheter device closure. Patients who have had their defects successfully repaired in childhood or adolescence have an excellent long-term outlook and normal life expectancy. Residual lesions and late sequelae occur uncommonly, but include residual atrial level shunting, sinus node dysfunction and atrial arrhythmias. Long-term complications of transcatheter occlusion devices are uncommon, but include endocarditis, thromboembolism and device strut fracture (1, 2).

After successful ASD repair, SBE prophylaxis is not necessary long-term, but good dental hygiene should be stressed (13).

Repaired secundum ASDs with good hemodynamics do not present an increased risk for pregnancy. There is an increased risk of recurrence of congenital heart lesions (not necessarily only ASD) in the fetus whose parent has a congenital heart defect. Fetal echocardiography and counseling should be offered to these families.

Adult patients with complete repair of a secundum ASD in childhood with no residual hemodynamically significant lesions or other issues probably do not need routine cardiology follow-up, but can be seen on an as-needed basis if complications arise.

7.2.2 Sinus venosus atrial septal defect with partial anomalous pulmonary venous return

A second type of ASD that may present in adulthood is the sinus venosus ASD. Sinus venosus ASDs account for ~1% of all congenital heart defects and 10% of ASDs. They are characteristically associated with partial anomalous pulmonary venous drainage of the right upper (most commonly) or lower pulmonary veins to the right atrium. They share many of the physiologic and clinical features of secundum ASDs, essentially being a variable-size left-to-right atrial level shunt. As such, management strategies are very similar (1, 19).

Anatomy and physiology

The sinus venosus ASD gets its name from the embryologic origin of the defect. The sinus venous is the embryologic heart segment which incorporates the vena cavae and ultimately the posterior portions of the right atrium and atrial septum. These defects are located in the superior–posterior septum and continuous with the superior vena cava (SVC; "superior" or "usual" type) or the inferior–posterior septum adjacent to the inferior vena cava (the much less common "inferior" type). Anomalous drainage of the right upper pulmonary vein(s) is associated with the former and right lower pulmonary vein(s) with the latter. Most sinus venosus defects occur in isolation. They do not close spontaneously (19).

The primary physiology of a sinus venosus ASD is left-to-right shunting through the defect resulting in right heart and pulmonary volume overload. This is similar to a secundum ASD with the added feature of increased left-to-right shunting due to the anomalous pulmonary venous drainage. Patients are acyanotic and have increased pulmonary blood flow. Right ventricular systolic function is generally maintained in childhood but is occasionally decreased in adulthood. Changes in ventricular compliance with aging favor increasing left-to-right shunting over time (as discussed above). Systemic hypertension or acquired mitral stenosis can also increase left-to-right shunting. Rarely, pulmonary hypertension can develop later in life, with a decreased or reversed atrial level shunt.

Clinical features and natural history

Like most small-to-moderate ASDs, sinus venosus defects often present in childhood due to a cardiac murmur and/or a fixed-split second heart sound on examination in an otherwise asymptomatic patient. The murmur is similar to a pulmonary flow murmur or mild pulmonary stenosis. Right heart enlargement on ECG or chest radiography may also bring a child to attention. Larger shunts may cause subtle symptoms of easy fatigability or dyspnea with physical activities. A flow rumble due to increased diastolic flow across the tricuspid valve may be audible in large defects.

Many adults with unrepaired sinus venosus ASDs have a relatively small shunt that has gone undetected through childhood. Adults typically are more symptomatic than children and this worsens with time; common signs and symptoms include dyspnea, exercise intolerance, arrhythmias (including atrial fibrillation) and heart failure. These findings in an otherwise healthy adult should prompt consideration of a previously unrecognized ASD.

In many patients with uncorrected moderate-to-large ASDs, left-to-right shunting increases with age. As a result, the frequency of right heart failure accompanied by shortness of breath, fluid retention, hepatomegaly, and elevated jugular venous pressure increases with advancing age. Most such patients become symptomatic before age 40 years, but some remain asymptomatic until their 60s or later. Systemic hypertension, if present, can exacerbate the hemodynamic changes due to an ASD. The risk of stroke due to paradoxical embolism in patients with an ASD is discussed above.

Life expectancy approaches that of the general population with successful repair of sinus venosus defects in the first two decades of life. However, unrepaired ASDs result in a significantly shortened lifespan with a mortality prevalence of ~5% per decade beginning at age 20 years. Cumulative mortality approaches 90% by 60 years of age for untreated patients. Primary causes of mortality are right heart failure, arrhythmias and pulmonary hypertension (1, 2, 19).

Diagnostic studies

- **ECG**
  ECG typically demonstrates P-wave morphology consistent with right atrial enlargement and may show right ventricular hypertrophy. Left axis deviation and a negative P-wave in lead III may be seen. The PR interval may be mildly prolonged and incomplete right bundle branch block (rSR′ in V1) is common.
- **Chest radiography**
  Chest radiography typically demonstrates variable degrees of cardiomegaly with prominence of the right atrium and main pulmonary artery segments and increased pulmonary vascularity. Changes consistent with pulmonary hypertension may be seen.
- **Echocardiography**
  TTE (2D and Doppler) is the diagnostic method of choice for sinus venosus ASDs and can demonstrate the position and size of the defect, relative size and direction of atrial level shunting, and pulmonary venous connections in most patients. Echocardiography can also identify associated anomalies and the degree of right atrial and ventricular volume overload. In older children or adults with poor transthoracic views, TEE may be useful. Intraoperative TEE assists with assessment of surgical repair. Use of a laboratory with sonographers and staff experienced in congenital cardiac defects is needed for appropriate evaluation.
- **Other imaging methods**
  Cardiac magnetic resonance angiography (MRA)/MRI is an excellent modality to completely define the atrial septal anatomy. It is particularly useful in defining pulmonary venous drainage and right ventricular size and function (which can be difficult to visualize well by echocardiography in adults).

- **Cardiac catheterization**
  Catheterization is rarely necessary in the preoperative evaluation of patients with a sinus venosus ASD but may be indicated for (i) further evaluation of known or suspected pulmonary hypertension (including response to pulmonary vasodilators) or (ii) if other associated lesions require invasive hemodynamic study (including exclusion of significant coronary atherosclerosis in adults before surgery). Sinus venosus defects are not amenable to transcatheter closure with currently available devices.

Management considerations for care of adults with unrepaired sinus venosus ASDs

The ACC and the AHA have published excellent guidelines for the management of adults with ASDs (1). Medical management of unrepaired sinus venosus ASD in adults is primarily supportive. Asymptomatic patients require no specific medications or restrictions. Medical treatment of adults with larger left-to-right shunts (Qp:Qs > 1.5–2:1) resulting in heart failure is palliative in anticipation of surgery, including anti-congestive measures such as diuretics and digoxin and anti-arrhythmics as needed. No specific activity restrictions are needed, but the patient should be allowed to self-limit (14). SBE prophylaxis is not indicated in patients with isolated ASDs of any type (except for 6 months after repair). The importance of routine dental care should be stressed to all patients whether they require SBE prophylaxis or not (13).

Compared with patients with secundum ASDs, patients with a sinus venosus defect may be more likely to develop pulmonary hypertension or elevated PVR and to do so at a younger age. They therefore need closer monitoring and may benefit from repair of the defect at a younger age. Patients with pulmonary hypertension not responsive to pulmonary vasodilators may not be appropriate candidates for surgical repair due to the risk of worsening right heart failure after defect closure. They may be need pulmonary vasodilators, oxygen, diuretics and possibly anti-coagulation. Intense physical activities are discouraged in older patients with significant pulmonary hypertension or pulmonary vascular disease.

Surgical repair with cardiopulmonary bypass is the treatment of choice for sinus venosus ASDs and ideally is undertaken by a Congenital Heart Surgeon with experience in adult patients with congenital heart disease (1). The prevalence of surgical mortality is ~1%, although patients aged > 60 years are at greater surgical risk (≤6%). Over 75% of patients are symptomatically improved with surgery; older patients are more likely to have clinical improvement. Surgery is more complicated than secundum ASD repair. The ASD is patch closed and the anomalous right pulmonary vein(s) are baffled or reimplanted via one of several techniques depending on the specific venous anatomy. Potential short- and long-term complications of surgery include vena caval or pulmonary venous stenosis, sinus node dysfunction, pericardial effusion and residual septal defects. The mortality prevalence for patients undergoing repair in childhood is excellent (approaches 0%), but adults undergoing repair may have complications and shortened life expectancy. Transcatheter closure of this type of defect is not possible (1, 2, 19).

Recommendations regarding pregnancy for females with unrepaired sinus venosus ASDs vary depending on the hemodynamics. Small defects typically do not increase the risk of pregnancy from a hemodynamic standpoint, and special precautions are not necessary. However, even patients with small shunts are at increased risk for paradoxical emboli by virtue of the atrial level defect. Patients with left-to-right shunts associated with heart failure can usually tolerate pregnancy, but require close follow-up in a high-risk obstetrical practice because the normal increased intravascular volume load of pregnancy can exacerbate symptoms. Pregnancy is not advisable for patients with pulmonary hypertension or Eisenmenger syndrome due to a high risk of maternal morbidity and mortality (1, 18). These patients should be strongly counseled regarding this risk and appropriate contraceptive choices. As is the case for congenital heart defects in general, there is an increased risk of recurrence of congenital heart lesions (not necessarily only ASD) in the fetus whose parent has a sinus venosus defect (particularly the mother). Sinus venosus defects are detectable on fetal echocardiography and this study should be offered to these families.

Whether they have had surgery or not, adult patients are best followed up every 6–12 months by a Pediatric Cardiologist or Adult Cardiologist with expertise in adult congenital heart disease in a center with a multidisciplinary approach.

Management considerations for care of adults with sinus venosus ASDs repaired in childhood

Sinus venosus defects diagnosed early in life are usually repaired in childhood (generally between 4 years and 7 years of age). Surgery is undertaken via a midline sternotomy. Compared with adults undergoing surgery for a sinus venosus ASD, patients who have had their defects successfully repaired in childhood or adolescence have an excellent long-term outlook and normal life expectancy. In spite of this, late residual lesions and sequelae do occur, but reoperation is rare. Issues to be followed after early repair include residual atrial level shunting, obstruction of systemic or pulmonary venous return, sinus node dysfunction and atrial arrhythmias. Sinus node dysfunction can develop late after repair and may require placement of a permanent pacemaker. Superior vena caval obstruction may complicate or preclude placement of a transvenous pacing system (which is the preferred approach in adults).

Successfully repaired sinus venosus ASDs do not require exercise restrictions (14) or long-term SBE prophylaxis. Good dental hygiene should be stressed to all patients (13).

Repaired sinus venosus ASDs with good hemodynamics do not present an increased risk for pregnancy. There is an increased risk of recurrence of congenital heart lesions (not necessarily only ASD) in the fetus whose parent has a sinus venosus defect (particularly the mother). Fetal echocardiography and counseling should be offered to these families.

As with other types of repaired congenital defects, these patients are optimally followed up and treated by an Adult and/or Pediatric Cardiologist with expertise in adult congenital heart disease in a center with a multidisciplinary team approach. They are typically seen every 6–12 months.

7.2.3 Endocardial cushion (atrioventricular canal) defects

Embryologically, the endocardial cushions of the atrioventricular canal contribute to septation of the crux of the heart and formation of the atrioventricular valves (mitral and tricuspid valves). Defects in this region include the two basic types discussed here: partial and complete atrioventricular canal defects. The so-called "primum ASD" is synonymous with a partial atrioventricular canal defect. Compete atrioventricular canal defects have ASDs and VSDs. Both forms include atrioventricular valve structural and functional anomalies, typically a cleft mitral valve with regurgitation in a primum ASD and more complex anomalies (including a common atrioventricular valve with regurgitation) in complete forms (1, 4).

7.2.4 Primum atrial septal defect (partial atrioventricular canal defect)

Primum ASDs account for 15–20% of all ASDs. They are invariably associated with mitral valve abnormalities, most commonly a cleft anterior leaflet with variable degrees of mitral regurgitation. The tricuspid valve is usually unaffected. The ASD itself involves the most inferior portion of the atrial septum and is usually moderate-to-large in size. Primum ASDs can occur in isolation or in the presence of other complex congenital heart disease. Due to the abnormal position of the left ventricular outflow tract in any atrioventricular canal defect, left ventricular outflow tract obstruction can occur. Primum ASDs do not become smaller with time and never close spontaneously (1, 2, 4).

Physiologically, primum ASDs normally result in a fairly sizable left-to-right shunt; patients are acyanotic with increased pulmonary blood flow. Mitral regurgitation varies but, if it is at least moderate, it results in significantly increased left atrial volume and pressure, thereby increasing the left-to-right shunt. The right atrium and ventricle dilate in compensation for, and commensurate to, the volume load. Significant mitral regurgitation results in left ventricular volume load which typically worsens with age and can lead to left ventricular failure. Right ventricular systolic function is generally maintained in childhood but is occasionally decreased in adulthood. Atrial left-to-right shunting also worsens with age due to the normal progressive decrease in left ventricular compliance in adulthood (especially in the presence of systemic hypertension). Finally, as with other ASDs, pulmonary arterial hypertension and pulmonary vascular disease can develop, primarily after 40 years of age. This physiologic change stresses the right ventricle with an additional pressure load on top of the pre-existing volume overload, often leading to right ventricular failure.

Clinical features and natural history

Although patients born with primum ASDs may go undetected for decades due to subtle findings and lack of symptoms, they are more likely to come to attention than patients with other types of ASD due to the larger left-to-right shunt and mitral regurgitation. Physical examination findings vary depending on the degree and direction of shunting. Patients with the usual left-to-right shunt are acyanotic. A split S2 is common in moderate-to – large left-to-right shunts. In addition to the pulmonary flow murmur common to all ASDs, the holosystolic murmur of mitral regurgitation is generally louder (grade 3–4+) and harsher, and is located in the mitral region with radiation to the left axilla. A tricuspid inflow diastolic rumble and right ventricular lift signifies a large shunt. In older adults with pulmonary hypertension, the S2 narrows and P2 increases in intensity, the pulmonary flow murmur is softer and an right ventricular tap may be felt. Cyanosis suggests atrial shunt reversal associated with severe pulmonary hypertension (Eisenmenger syndrome). Some children or adults are ultimately diagnosed due to an abnormal electrocardiograph or chest radiograph.

If undetected, signs and symptoms may develop gradually over several decades, largely due to right and/or left ventricular failure, atrial arrhythmias, progression of mitral regurgitation and/or development of pulmonary hypertension. Factors for clinical deterioration in adults aged > 40 years with an unrepaired primum ASD include age-related changes in ventricular compliance, an increased incidence of atrial fibrillation and/or flutter, and pulmonary hypertension of at least a moderate degree (1, 2, 4).

Diagnostic studies

- **ECG**
  ECG in partial atrioventricular canal defects characteristically demonstrates leftaxis or extreme left axis deviation, P-wave morphology consistent with right and possibly left atrial enlargement, and incomplete right bundle branch block (rSR′ in V1). First-degree atrioventricular block may be seen as well as findings of right ventricular hypertrophy.
- **Chest radiography**
  Chest radiography typically demonstrates variable degrees of cardiomegaly with prominence of the right atrium and main pulmonary artery segments as well as increased pulmonary vascularity due to left-to right shunting at the atrial level. If mitral regurgitation is significant, the left atrial and left ventricular segments are also prominent.
- **Echocardiography**
  Echocardiography remains the "gold standard" for the diagnosis of primum ASDs with mitral regurgitation. TTE (2D and Doppler) can reliably demonstrate the anatomic and hemodynamic features important to medical and surgical management of this lesion in most patients. TEE may also be useful in older children with poor transthoracic views or in adults. Intraoperative TEE is also routine to assess the adequacy of repair in surgical cases. Use of a laboratory with sonographers and staff experienced in congenital cardiac defects is needed for appropriate evaluation.
- **Other imaging methods**
  Cardiac MRI offers little advantage over echocardiography for anatomic evaluation of primum ASDs in most cases. However, it is useful in assessing other complex associated lesions and for quantifying right ventricular size, volume, and function as needed.
- **Cardiac catheterization**
  Catheterization is rarely necessary in the preoperative evaluation of patients with uncomplicated partial atrioventricular canal defects, but may be indicated for (i) further evaluation of known or suspected pulmonary hypertension, or (ii) if other associated lesions require invasive hemodynamic study (including exclusion of significant coronary atherosclerosis in adults aged > 35–40 years before surgery). Primum ASDs are not amenable to transcatheter closure with currently available devices.

Management considerations for care of adults with unrepaired primum ASDs

The ACC and the AHA have published excellent guidelines for the care of adults with ASDs (1). Medical management of unrepaired primum ASDs in adults is primarily supportive. Asymptomatic patients without significant mitral regurgitation require no specific medications or restrictions. Medical treatment of adults with larger left-to-right shunts (Qp:Qs > 1.5–2:1) resulting in heart failure is palliative in anticipation of surgery, including anti-congestive measures such as diuretics and digoxin and anti-arrhythmics as needed. Afterload reduction with ACE inhibitors or angiotensin receptor blockers (ARBs) may be of benefit in cases with significant mitral regurgitation. No specific activity restrictions are needed, but the patient should be allowed to self-limit. High-intensity sports requiring isometric training (i.e., weightlifting) would be discouraged in patients with mitral regurgitation.

Patients with pulmonary hypertension who are not responsive to pulmonary vasodilators may not be appropriate candidates for surgical repair due to the risk of worsening right heart failure after defect closure. They may be treated with pulmonary vasodilators, oxygen, diuretics and anti-coagulation. Intense physical activities are discouraged in older patients with significant pulmonary hypertension or vascular disease (14). SBE prophylaxis is not indicated in acyanotic patients with unrepaired primum ASDs regardlessof the degree of mitral regurgitation, but good dental care should be stressed. SBE prophylaxis is indicated for 6 months after repair in cyanotic patients and for prosthetic valves (1, 13).

Surgical repair with cardiopulmonary bypass is the treatment of choice for primum ASDs. Surgery is ideally is undertaken by a Congenital Heart Surgeon with experience in adult patients with congenital heart disease. The prevalence of surgical mortality is low (< 1–2%); older patients are at greater surgical risk, but generally have good outcomes with improved survival. Most patients are symptomatically improved with surgery. Surgery includes ASD patch closure and mitral cleft repair; the mitral valve should always be addressed at the time of ASD closure. Potential short- and long-term complications of surgery include residual septal defects, mitral regurgitation or surgicallyinduced mitral stenosis and pericardial effusion. Mitral valve replacement with a prosthetic valve may be needed in patients with residual valve regurgitation or stenosis. The mortality and outcome for patients undergoing repair in childhood is excellent. Adults undergoing repair also do well but may have complications and shortened life expectancy. Best long-term results are expected with repairs before ~25 years of age and with reasonable pulmonary artery pressures (< 40mmHg). Transcatheter closure of this type of defect is not possible (1, 4).

Recommendations regarding pregnancy for females with unrepaired primum ASDs vary depending on the hemodynamics. Patients with small-to-moderate shunts and mild mitral regurgitation tolerate pregnancy relatively well, but require increased follow-up during pregnancy due to the increased blood volume and risk for heart failure. Pregnancy is not advisable if there is evidence of significant pulmonary hypertension. These patients should be strongly counseled regarding this risk and appropriate contraceptive choices. Patients with complete atrioventricular canal defects are at increased risk of paradoxical embolism. As is the case for congenital heart defects in general, there is an increased risk of recurrence of congenital heart lesions of any type in the fetus whose parent has congenital heart disease (particularly the mother). Primum ASDs can be detected on fetal echocardiography; this test and counseling should be offered to these families (1, 18).

Whether they have had surgery or not, adult patients are best followed up by a Pediatric Cardiologist or Adult Cardiologist with expertise in adult congenital heart disease. These patients are typically followed every 6–12 months.

Management considerations for care of adults with primum ASDs repaired in childhood

Primum ASDs and are most appropriately repaired in childhood. There is an excellent long-term outlook and normal life expectancy for these patients after successful intervention. The surgical approach is via a midline sternotomy. Patients with residual ASDs or mitral regurgitation after repair generally also do well, but require monitoring for worsening mitral regurgitation over time. Activity restrictions are not necessary in patients with successful repairs. Intense physical activities are discouraged in older patients with significant pulmonary hypertension or vascular disease (14). SBE prophylaxis for dental or other procedures is not required unless the patient has previously had endocarditis. The importance of routine dental care should be stressed to all patients. Complete atrioventricular block at the time of childhood surgery is fortunately very rare, but some adults may have had pacemakers placed after their repair as a child. Late arrhythmias can also occur (1, 4).

Repaired primum ASDs without hemodynamically significant residual shunts do not present an increased risk for pregnancy. The fetus is at an increased risk for recurrence of congenital heart disease, so fetal echocardiography should be offered. Patients with significant residual mitral regurgitation or septal defects should be followed closely during pregnancy for development of heart failure.

As with other types of repaired congenital defects, these patients are optimally followed and treated by an Adult and/or Pediatric Cardiologist with expertise in adult congenital heart disease in a center with a multidisciplinary team approach. These patients should be routinely seen every year.

7.2.5 Complete atrioventricular canal defect

Complete atrioventricular canal defects consist of a primum ASD and a VSD in the inlet septum, invariably with complex atrioventricular valve anomalies (most commonly a common atrioventricular valve with regurgitation). Complete atrioventricular canal defects can be "balanced" with two good-size ventricles or "unbalanced" with hypoplasia of one or the other ventricles, and are also often associated with left or right ventricular outflow tract obstruction (not discussed here). Patients with complete atrioventricular canal defects of all types generally come to attention in infancy and undergo repair early in life due to a significant left-to-right shunt. Complete atrioventricular canal defects are classically associated with trisomy-21 (1, 4).

Anatomy and physiology

In addition to the typical primum ASD, the VSD is usually large (although in some cases is partially restricted by atrioventricular valve tissue attachments to the ventricular septum). Regurgitation of left and right atrioventricular valves varies from mild to severe, and typically worsens with age. Associated lesions include left or right ventricular outflow tract obstruction, additional septal defects, and coarctation of the aorta.

The typical physiology in uncomplicated complete atrioventricular canal defects is a large left-to-right shunt at the atrial and ventricular levels with pulmonary over-circulation and symptoms of congestive heart failure early in life. If unrepaired, pulmonary vascular disease almost invariably develops, and in adulthood many (if not most) patients ultimately develop Eisenmenger physiology. Patients with trisomy-21 are at greatest risk for developing pulmonary hypertension and vascular disease, some as early as 1–2 years of age.

Clinical features and natural history

Most patients born with complete atrioventricular canal defects become symptomatic in infancy or early childhood due to pulmonary over-circulation. However, some patients survive well into adulthood if the common atrioventricular valve remains competent and the VSD is relatively small. The presence of elevated PVR will typically delay the development of symptoms as it decreases the left-to-right shunt, but may result in the development of pulmonary vascular disease, right heart failure and right-to-left shunting with cyanosis if not addressed early in life. The degree of atrioventricular valve regurgitation worsens with age in adulthood and contributes to the development of symptoms of heart failure. Most patients that do not present early in childhood will usually show some signs of exercise intolerance, shortness of breath, fatigue, or other signs of developing heart failure by the second or third decade of life, and ultimately succumb early to heart failure or pulmonary vascular disease. Reports of survival into the eighth decade without repair have been reported.

Diagnostic studies

- **ECG**
  ECG in complete atrioventricular canal defects characteristically demonstrates extreme left axis deviation (northwest axis), left and/or right atrial atrial enlargement and incomplete right bundle branch block (rSR′ in V1). First-degree atrioventricular block may be seen as well as findings of right and/or left ventricular hypertrophy.
- **Chest radiography**
  Chest radiography typically demonstrates variable degrees of cardiomegaly with prominence of the right and/or left atrium and main pulmonary artery segments as well as increased pulmonary vascularity in patients with significant left-to right shunts and atrioventricular valve regurgitation. Findings consistent with pulmonary vascular disease may predominate later in life.
- **Echocardiography**
  In most younger patients, the anatomy and physiology pertinent to management of complete atrioventricular canal defects and associated lesions can be adequately delineated by 2DTTE and Doppler echocardiography. TEE may provide better anatomic detail in older children and adults with limited acoustic windows. Intraoperative TEE is routinely employed in surgical treatment of complete atrioventricular canal defects to assess the adequacy of repair. Three-dimensional (3D) echocardiography may assist in defining the exact shape and size of the defect and for atrioventricular valve delineation in preparation for surgery. Doppler echocardiography can be used to estimate Qp:Qs, ASD and VSD gradients as well as right ventricular and pulmonary artery pressure. Use of a laboratory with sonographers and staff experienced in congenital cardiac defects is needed for appropriate evaluation.
- **Other imaging methods**
  Cardiac MRI is usually not needed, but can demonstrate the intracardiac anatomy and estimate shunt flow. MRI is not generally superior to echocardiography except in cases of poor echocardiographic acoustic windows.

- **Cardiac catheterization**
  Cardiac catheterization is rarely necessary in the preoperative evaluation of patients with uncomplicated complete atrioventricular canal defects, but may be indicated for (i) further evaluation of known or suspected pulmonary hypertension, or (ii) if other associated lesions require invasive hemodynamic study (including exclusion of significant coronary atherosclerosis in adults aged > 35–40 years before surgery). Complete atrioventricular canal defects are not amenable to transcatheter closure with currently available devices.

Management considerations for care of adults with unrepaired complete atrioventricular canal defects

Patients with complete atrioventricular canal defects generally come to attention in infancy and undergo repair early in life due to a significant left-to-right shunt. Patients who are unrepaired often die before adulthood from congestive heart failure; those who survive usually have pulmonary hypertension with high PVR and vascular disease. Many are inoperable and are cared for medically (as discussed in other sections of this review). The ACC and AHA have published excellent guidelines for the care of adults with ASDs (1). Intense physical activities are discouraged in older patients with significant pulmonary hypertension or vascular disease (14). SBE prophylaxis is not required in patients with left-to-right shunts, but cyanotic patients, patients with residual defects or prosthetic valves require SBE prophylaxis. Good dental care should be stressed (13).

Adults who are fortunate to have a small inlet VSD and who do not have irreversible pulmonary vascular disease can be repaired surgically, ideally by a Congenital Heart Surgeon with expertise in adult congenital heart disease. Surgery consists of patch repair of ASDs and VSDs (via one or two patch techniques) and atrioventricular valvuloplasty. Complications of surgery include residual septal defects, atrioventricular block (may require permanent pacemaker placement), atrioventricular valve regurgitation or stenosis, and pericardial effusion. Long-term issues include the need for late mitral, or less commonly, tricuspid valve replacement. Interestingly, patients with trisomy-21 tend to have atrioventricular valves that are more amenable to repair and are less likely to need subsequent valve replacement.

Recommendations regarding pregnancy for females with unrepaired complete atrioventricular canal defects vary depending on the hemodynamics. Patients with small VSDs behave much like a patient with a primum ASD. These patients do well but require increased vigilance during pregnancy due to the increased blood volume and risk of heart failure. More typically the VSD is large with significant shunting and/or there is evidence of pulmonary hypertension. While patients with moderate left-to-right shunts can tolerate pregnancy, they are at increased risk of heart failure and require close monitoring. Pregnancy is not advisable for patients with pulmonary hypertension or Eisenmenger syndrome due to a high risk of maternal morbidity and mortality. These patients should be appropriately strongly counseled regarding this risk and appropriate contraceptive choices. Due to the cardiac septal defects, all patients with complete atrioventricular canal defects are at increased risk of paradoxical embolism (1, 18). As is the case for congenital heart defects in general, there is an increased risk of recurrence of congenital heart lesions of any type in the fetus whose parent has congenital heart disease (particularly the mother). Complete atrioventricular canal defects are readily detectable on fetal echocardiography, and this test should be offered to these families.

These patients should be routinely followed every 6–12 months by an Adult and/or Pediatric Cardiologist with expertise in adult congenital heart disease, ideally at a center with a multidisciplinary approach.

Management considerations for care of adults with complete atrioventricular canal defects repaired in childhood

Complete atrioventricular canal defects are always hemodynamically significant. They are most appropriately repaired in infancy or childhood. An excellent long-term outlook and relatively normal life expectancy for these patients can be expected after successful intervention. Surgical repair is undertaken via a midline sternotomy.

Patients with atrial and ventricular defects which are completely closed do not require SBE prophylaxis for dental or other procedures. Small residual VSDs after repair are common, but do not require re-intervention in most cases. SBE prophylaxis is required in any patient with a residual defect bordering a patch (because this prevents endothelialization in this area), with a prosthetic valve, or in any patient with a previous episode of endocarditis (13). The importance of routine dental care should be stressed to all patients whether they require SBE prophylaxis or not.

Right bundle branch block identifiable on ECG is fairly common after repair. This is of no significance by itself, but may progress to higher grade or complete heart block if the patient develops subsequent disease of the left bundle branch system (as can occur in adults after myocardial infarction). Complete atrioventricular block at the time of childhood surgery is fortunately rare, but some adults may have had pacemakers placed after their repair as a child. Other residual lesions that may require follow-up after early complete atrioventricular canal surgery include mitral or tricuspid regurgitation or stenosis. Late arrhythmias can also occur.

Repaired complete atrioventricular canal defects with no hemodynamically significant residual shunts or other lesions do not present an increased risk for pregnancy. As is the case for congenital heart defects in general, there is an increased risk of recurrence of congenital heart lesions of any type in the fetus whose parent has congenital heart disease (particularly the mother); fetal echocardiography should be offered to these families.

As with other types of repaired congenital defects, these patients are optimally followed up and treated by an Adult and/or Pediatric Cardiologist with expertise in adult congenital heart disease in a center with a multidisciplinary team approach. These patients should be routinely seen every 6–12 months.

7.2.6 VSDs

VSDs are abnormal openings in the ventricular septum resulting in exchange of blood between the right and left ventricles. The large majority of VSDs are congenital (2–3 cases/1,000 live births), resulting from failure of closure of the normal embryonic connection between the developing ventricles. VSDs can also occur due to trauma or after myocardial infarction. They may be single or multiple, and are often associated with other more complex lesions; VSDs associated with complete atrioventricular canal defects are discussed above. VSDs vary in size from tiny pinholes to very large defects, and can be found in various locations along the interventricular septum. The size of the defect, location with respect to other important structures (such as the aortic valve) and associated lesions are the primary factors in determining the clinical significance of a VSD for a given patient (1).

Anatomy and physiology

VSDs are most commonly classified by location, with many different systems of nomenclature in use (20). Essentially, four characteristic types are usually recognized: atrioventricular septal (or inlet), muscular, perimembranous and outlet. Perimembranous VSDs are the most common (~75% of VSDs) and are frequently associated with other complex defects such as tetralogy of Fallot and transposition of the great arteries. Muscular VSDs account for ~10–15% of all VSDs and are quite variable in size. Perimembranous and muscular defects often become smaller with time or spontaneously close. Outlet defects are relatively unusual (5% of VSDs, but more common in people of Asian descent) but due to their proximity to the aortic valve annulus may be associated with aortic valve cusp prolapse and progressive aortic regurgitation. Aortic regurgitation is (less commonly) also seen in perimembranous VSDs. Atrioventricular septal defects are relatively uncommon (~5–10% of all VSDs) and are associated with primum ASDs and atrioventricular valve abnormalities (discussed above).

The predominant physiology in VSDs is a left-to-right shunt, the magnitude of which is determined by defect size and the relative resistance of the systemic and pulmonary vascular beds. Tiny or small restrictive VSDs are usually hemodynamically insignificant. With moderate-to-large shunts, left heart volume overload and pulmonary over-circulation occur early in life. As with other defects with significant left-to-right shunts, increases in PVR and/or pulmonary vascular disease can develop, potentially progressing to Eisenmenger physiology with shunt reversal and cyanosis (1, 21–23).

Clinical features and natural history

Due to the great variability in size, location and associated lesions, VSDs present in different ways and at different ages.

Small defects usually present in infancy or childhood due to a cardiac murmur in an asymptomatic, thriving child. The murmur of a small VSD is very characteristic: high-pitched, harsh, holosystolic, grade III–VI with a thrill; a smaller defect often equals a louder murmur. The second heart sound is normal and diastole is silent in the absence of aortic regurgitation associated with outlet or perimembranous defects.

Moderate-to-large VSDs resulting in pulmonary over-circulation may present in infancy with tachypnea, tachycardia, diaphoresis, poor-feeding/failure to thrive, hepatomegaly and recurrent respiratory tract infections. These signs of congestive heart failure differ from those seen in adults, who may exhibit more classic findings of congestive heart failure, including edema (pulmonary and peripheral), hepatomegaly and shortness of breath. The murmur of a large left–right ventricular level shunt is lower pitched and may be associated with a loud P2, a diastolic rumble due to increased flow across the mitral valve, and a gallop rhythm.

In the presence of pulmonary hypertension and Eisenmenger syndrome, adults may present with cyanosis, exertional dyspnea, chest pain, syncope, clubbing, hemoptysis, polycythemia and atrial or ventricular arrhythmias. In these patients, the VSD murmur decreases, S2 becomes louder and murmurs of tricuspid and/or pulmonary regurgitation may be heard. Right ventricular lift may also be noted on examination.

The natural history of unrepaired VSDs varies widely. Small defects may close spontaneously; those that do not are usually hemodynamically insignificant. Larger defects can lead to congestive cardiac failure and, if untreated, death in early infancy. A similar spectrum can be seen in adults, with the additional higher risk of developing pulmonary hypertension and pulmonary vascular disease. VSDs are one of the most common lesions that progress to Eisenmenger physiology. The natural history of VSDs may be modified by additional associated congenital or acquired lesions, including right ventricular outflow obstruction (double chamber right ventricle), subaortic membranes and aortic regurgitation or by the development of endocarditis. Adults with unrepaired VSD are also at risk for recurrent respiratory infections and arrhythmias. Independent of the presence or absence of congestive failure or pulmonary vascular disease, adults with moderate-to-large unrepaired VSDs have a shortened life expectancy (1, 21–23).

Diagnostic studies

- **ECG**
  ECG varies according to defect and shunt size. It is normal in small defects. Larger shunts/defects may show left atrial enlargement, left ventricular hypertrophy and possibly biventricular hypertrophy. Pulmonary hypertension is associated with right axis deviation, right atrial enlargement and right or bi-ventricular hypertrophy.
- **Chest radiography**
  The chest film varies according to defect and shunt size. It is usually normal in small defects. Moderate-to-large shunts demonstrate variable degrees of cardiomegaly (primarily left ventricular contour and left atrial enlargement) and increased pulmonary vascular markings. The main pulmonary artery segment may be increased. Interstitial edema is seen in large left-to-right shunts. With the development of pulmonary hypertension and Eisenmenger physiology, the cardiac shadow decreases, but may increase later due to right atrial and ventricular enlargement. The pulmonary vasculature may exhibit changes of distal pruning and proximal dilation and tortuosity.
- **Echocardiography**
  In most younger patients, the anatomy and physiology pertinent to patient care of VSDs and associated lesions can be adequately delineated by 2D TTE and Doppler echocardiography. TEE may provide better anatomic detail in older children and adults with limited acoustic windows. Intraoperative TEE is routinely employed in surgical and transcatheter closure of VSDs to assist in device placement and to assess the adequacy of defect closure. Three-dimensional echocardiography may assist in defining the exact shape and size of the defect. Doppler echocardiography can be used to estimate Qp:Qs, VSD pressure gradients and right-heart pressures. Use of a laboratory with sonographers and staff experienced in congenital cardiac defects is needed for appropriate evaluation.
- **Other imaging methods**
  MRI can demonstrate VSDs and other lesions and estimate shunt flow. However, it is not generally superior to echocardiography except in cases of poor echocardiographic acoustic windows.

- **Cardiac catheterization**
  Cardiac catheterization is less accurate than echocardiography in defining VSD anatomy, but more accurate in determination of shunt magnitude. Catheterization may also be useful in cases of unrepaired VSDs with pulmonary hypertension and potentially significant pulmonary vascular disease. Catheterization may be used to directly determine PVR and architecture as well as the response to oxygen or other pulmonary vasodilators because this may affect operability in some adult patients. Catheterization may also be indicated in patients aged > 35 years to evaluate for coronary artery disease prior to surgical intervention. Some VSDs are amenable to transcatheter device closure.

Management considerations for care of adults with unrepaired VSDs

Management strategies in adults with unrepaired VSDs hinges on several factors, the most basic of which is defect and shunt size. Other factors include defect location, presence of pulmonary hypertension or Eisenmenger syndrome and associated lesions (most of which have usually already been addressed in childhood if significant). Apart from other congenital lesions associated with VSDs, additional acquired cardiac anatomic features can develop, including right or left ventricular outflow obstruction and aortic regurgitation, which may independently require surgical intervention. The ACC and the AHA have published excellent guidelines for the care of adults with ASDs (1).

Tiny or small VSDs without significant left heart volume overload and with normal pulmonary artery pressures are usually clinically silent and require no special intervention or medical therapy (21). One exception is defects that have directly caused distortion and regurgitation of the aortic valve. This is often a progressive problem, so even very small defects causing aortic regurgitation should be surgically closed and the aortic cusps resuspended to protect the valve. No activity or occupational restrictions are necessary for small VSDs (21–23).

Moderate or large defects may have two potential clinical consequences: (i) pulmonary and left heart volume overload with symptoms of congestive heart failure in patients with significant left-to-right shunts or (ii) development of pulmonary hypertension and pulmonary vascular disease with right-to-left shunting and cyanosis in severe cases.

Management of congestive heart failure consists of medical therapy with diuretics, digoxin and afterload reduction with ACE inhibitors or ARBs, and more permanent treatment consisting of closure of the defect. Most defects can be closed surgically utilizing cardiopulmonary bypass with selected defects amenable to placement of transcatheter VSD occlusion devices. Surgery is most appropriately undertaken by a dedicated Congenital Heart Surgeon with experience in adult patients with congenital heart disease. Patients with apical muscular defects which are very challenging surgically probably benefit the most from a transcatheter approach. Both methods of defect closure can be done with a high degree of success and very low morbidity and mortality (1). Atrial dilation predisposes patients to atrial arrhythmias which are generally treated medically. No specific activity restrictions are necessary, although patients should be allowed to self-limit if involved in relatively strenuous sports or occupations (14).

Adults with pulmonary hypertension associated with a VSD typically require further workup. This includes cardiac catheterization to evaluate PVR, perform pulmonary wedge angiography to grade the degree of vascular disease, and evaluation of the reactivity of the pulmonary vascular bed by the response to various pulmonary vasodilators. If PVR is sufficiently low or is reactive to pulmonary vasodilators then surgical or transcatheter closure is possible and recommended. If pulmonary resistance and/or systolic pressure are > 60–70% of systemic values and fixed, patients are usually considered inoperable. However, a select group with borderline pressure data may be able to undergo a technique of fenestrated two-patch closure whereby shunting from right to left can occur if the right ventricular pressure exceeds the left ventricular pressure, but left-to-right flow is blocked by the second patch (which acts as a one-way valve). If inoperable, a trial of pulmonary vasodilator therapy may improve the clinical condition; rarely the hemodynamic status improves sufficientlyfor patients to be considered suitable for defect closure.

Patients with inoperable hemodynamics who develop Eisenmenger syndrome suffer complications such as cyanosis, polycythemia and hyperuricemia (gout). In spite of an increased red blood cell (RBC) mass, they are often iron-deficient, which can be exacerbated by the need for periodic phlebotomy if they are symptomatic due to polycythemia. They are at increased risk for stroke and brain abscesses, and may be hypercoagulable or coagulopathic, putting them at risk of pulmonary hemorrhage. Medical therapy for these patients may include anti-coagulants, diuretics and digoxin in patients with right heart failure. Arrhythmias (atrial and ventricular) become more common with age and in some cases are life-threatening (1, 21–23). Patients with pulmonary hypertension should be limited to relatively low-intensity physical activities and non-manual labor occupations, depending on severity (14).

SBE prophylaxis for unrepaired isolated VSDs in acyanotic patients is no longer recommended by the AHA. However, regular dental checkups and good daily dental care should be stressed (13).

Recommendations regarding pregnancy for females with VSDs vary depending on hemodynamics. Small defects typically do not increase the risk of pregnancy and no special precautions are necessary. Patients with left-to-right shunts associated with heart failure can usually tolerate pregnancy, but require close follow-up because the normal increased volume load of pregnancy can exacerbate symptoms. Pregnancy is not advisable for patients with pulmonary hypertension or Eisenmenger syndrome due to the high risk of maternal morbidity and mortality. These patients should be strongly counseled regarding this risk and appropriate contraceptive choices (1, 18). Pregnant patients or those considering pregnancy should also be counseled that the fetus is at an increased risk of congenital heart disease (not just VSD). Maternal VSD (and less commonly paternal VSD) is an accepted indication for fetal echocardiography, with best images usually obtained ~20–22 weeks' gestation.

If possible, adults with VSDs should be followed up by a Pediatric or Adult Cardiologist with expertise in adult congenital heart disease in a center with a multidisciplinary approach. The usual frequency of follow-up is 1–2 times per year.

Management considerations for care of adults with ventricular septal defects repaired in childhood

VSDs which are recognized early and which are sufficiently large to be hemodynamically significant are most appropriately repaired in infancy or childhood. An excellent long-term outlook and normal life expectancy can be expected for these patients after successful intervention. Surgical repair is via a midline sternotomy.

Patients with defects which are completely closed do not require SBE prophylaxis for dental or other procedures. Small residual VSDs with < 1.5:1 shunts after repair are common, but are of little consequence in most cases and do not require re-intervention (1, 22, 23). No exercise restrictions are necessary (14). SBE prophylaxis is required in any patient with a residual defect bordering a patch (because this prevents endothelialization in this area) or in any patient with a previous episode of endocarditis. The importance of routine dental care should be stressed to all patients whether they require prophylaxis or not (13).

Right bundle branch block identifiable on ECG is fairly common after VSD closure. This is of no significance by itself, but may progress to higher grade or complete heart block if the patient develops subsequent disease of the left bundle branch system (as can occur in adults after myocardial infarction). Complete atrioventricular block at the time of childhood surgery is fortunately rare, but some adults may have had pacemakers placed after their repair as a child. Other residual lesions that may require follow-up after early VSD closure include mitral or tricuspid regurgitation, aortic regurgitation and occasionally tricuspid stenosis. Late arrhythmias can also occur.

Repaired VSDs with no hemodynamically significant residual shunts or other lesions do not present an increased risk for pregnancy. As is the case for congenital heart defects in general, there is an increased risk of recurrence of congenital heart lesions (not necessarily only VSD) in the fetus whose parent has a VSD (particularly the mother). Significant VSDs are readily detectable on fetal echocardiography, although tiny defects may not be visualized. Fetal echocardiography and counseling should be offered to these families.

As with other types of repaired congenital defects, these patients are optimally followed up and treated by an Adult and/or Pediatric Cardiologist with expertise in adult congenital heart disease in a center with a multidisciplinary team approach. Usual frequency of follow-up is 1–2 times per year.

7.2.7 Patent ductus arteriosus

The ductus arteriosus is a fetal structure that allows nutrient-rich blood returning from the placenta to bypass the lungs to be shunted to the developing tissues of the body during intrauterine life. It develops embryologically from the left sixth aortic arch in combination with the left pulmonary artery. The ductus normally closes within hours-to-days after birth, but in some cases remains patent, thus representing a left-to-right shunt between the aorta and pulmonary artery. The PDA is more common in premature infants and infants with congenital rubella syndrome.

Anatomy and physiology

The PDA is a vessel connecting the aorta directly to the main pulmonary artery, and varies in size from tiny to very large. The usual physiology is that of a variable left-to-right shunt. Depending on the size of the defect and PVR, the shunt can be trivial to very large. Larger shunts are associated with left atrial and ventricular dilation. Pulmonary hypertension and pulmonary vascular disease (including Eisenmenger syndrome) can develop in moderate-to-large PDAs (1, 24).

Clinical features and natural history

The PDA is known to cause a machinery-like heart murmur which is continuous (i.e., has systolic and diastolic components). In some cases, a very small PDA is silent and found during echocardiography for unrelated indications; these defects are typically insignificant and do not require therapy. Children and adults with a tiny or small PDA are generally completely asymptomatic. Moderate-to-large defects cause the signs and symptoms of heart failure if the shunt is large, or findings consistent with pulmonary hypertension if the pulmonary resistance is elevated and the shunt reduced. Patients are acyanotic unless the shunt reverses due to Eisenmenger physiology.

The natural history of PDAs varies depending on the size and direction of shunting. Defects still present in adulthood typically do not spontaneously close. Restrictive defects do not cause clinically significant problems in adulthood, nor shorten lifespan in general (although there is an increased lifetime risk of endocarditis). Larger defects may be associated with heart failure or pulmonary hypertension in adulthood, and therefore can result in early death if untreated (1, 24).

Diagnostic studies

- **ECG**
  ECG is normal in small defects. Findings in larger defects vary according to the shunt and presence/absence of pulmonary hypertension (as discussed in other sections of this chapter).
- **Chest radiograph**
  The chest film varies from normal in small defects to variable cardiomegaly with increased pulmonary blood flow in PDAs with larger shunts. Findings consistent with pulmonary hypertension and pulmonary vascular disease are seen in patients with these manifestations.
- **Echocardiography**
  Two-dimensional TTE and Doppler echocardiography are the imaging methods of choice in most patients with PDAs. Doppler echocardiography can be used to estimate Qp:Qs, PDA pressure gradients, and right ventricular and pulmonary artery pressures. TEE is not particularly useful, and in some cases may fail to demonstrate the ductus. Use of a laboratory with sonographers and staff experienced in congenital cardiac defects is needed for appropriate evaluation.
- **Other imaging methods**
  CT and/or MRI/MRA can demonstrate the PDA, aortic arch and pulmonary artery anatomy well. It can be useful in larger patients with poor echocardiographic acoustic windows.
- **Cardiac catheterization**
  Diagnostically, cardiac catheterization is limited to adult patients with significant PDAs where pulmonary hypertension and vascular disease is a concern, or is used to determine shunt magnitude. By far, the primary role of cardiac catheterization is for transcatheter coil or device closure of the PDA (if indicated).

Management considerations for care of adults with an unrepaired PDA

Patent ductus arteriosus is a lesion that is sometimes first diagnosed in adult years. The ACC and the AHA have published excellent guidelines for the care of adults with

ASDs (1). Asymptomatic patients with insignificant left-to-right shunts require no therapy, including no need for SBE prophylaxis, although they are at increased risk for endocarditis compared with the general population (13). Good dental care should be stressed. No precautions are necessary for pregnancy. Medical therapy for symptomatic patients with significant left-to right shunts and heart failure is supportive; definitive treatment is surgical ligation versus transcatheter occlusion with one of several types of coils or devices. The transcatheter approach is appropriate for nearly all patients. SBE prophylaxis is needed only if there is a residual shunt with an intravascular device(13). Individuals who do not have advanced pulmonary vascular disease are usually helped by ductal closure (even as adults). Long-term outcomes are excellent whether surgery or device closure is undertaken. Patients with significant pulmonary vascular disease not responsive to vasodilators in the Catheterization Laboratory may not be candidates for PDA closure. These patients are cared for medically with anti-congestive measures and pulmonary vasodilators. Pregnancy is contraindicated in these patients for reasons noted above (1, 18, 24).

Management considerations for care of adults with a PDA repaired in childhood

Ligation of a PDA was the first surgical treatment available for a congenital heart defect. Many modern-day patients undergoing ductal ligation were premature infants. Typically ligation alone (rather than ligation and division) is carried out due to the friability of ductal tissue in premature babies; a residual PDA due to recanalization of the ductus is possible in these patients. PDA surgery in older infants and children generally includes ligation and division of the ductus. In the early history of PDA surgery, ligation without division was done on some older children and these cases are at risk for having a residual ductus or one that reopens. The typical surgical scar on an adult with ductal surgery in childhood is a left posterolateral incision in the fourth intercostal space. Several patients now entering adult years will have been treated by closure via cardiac catheterization.

In general, PDAs successfully closed in childhood present no clinical issues in adulthood and do not require SBE prophylaxis or follow-up. PDAs closed via a transcatheter approach may have small residual shunts, but these are of little consequence other than a need for SBE prophylaxis as long as the residual defect remains. Occasionally there is mild flow disturbance in the left pulmonary artery or aorta due to the coil or device which requires follow-up. Small residual PDAs or recanalization of the ductus after ligation should also be followed up, but does not require intervention or SBE prophylaxis, although there is an increased lifetime risk of developing endocarditis. Larger residual defects (Qp:Qs ~2:1) can be present and may demonstrate a continuous murmur; an experienced examiner may identify a low-frequency diastolic flow murmur at the apex due to increased flow across the mitral valve. Aneurysm of the PDA is most often found in the very young, very old, or in association with bacterial endocarditis. There may be compression of adjacent structures, and rupture can occur.

There is no need for exercise restrictions. There are no contraindications or special precautions needed for pregnancy in patients with successful PDA closure in childhood (1, 18, 24).

7.2.8 Pulmonary hypertension and Eisenmenger syndrome

In patients with unrepaired congenital heart disease with a systemic-to-pulmonary communication, increased pulmonary blood flow from an initial left-to-right shunt may ultimately lead to the development of pulmonary vascular disease and increased PVR. With time, the shunt may reverse and become right-to-left, causing cyanosis (25, 26). The triad of systemic-to-pulmonary communication, pulmonary vascular disease and cyanosis is known as Eisenmenger syndrome, first described in conjunction with an unrestrictive VSD (27).

The most common defects associated with Eisenmenger syndrome are, in decreasing order of prevalence, VSDs, ASDs and PDAs, but other complex defects such as truncus arteriosus can also lead to this physiology (28). Larger left-to-right shunts and those with higher pulmonary artery pressures have an increased risk (29).

On physical examination, patients with Eisenmenger syndrome demonstrate central cyanosis and clubbing. Differential cyanosis and clubbing of the lower extremities can be seen in PDA. The physical examination may reveal findings consistent with pulmonary hypertension, including a right ventricular impulse and a palpable P2, peripheral edema, hepatomegaly, ascites, and potentially murmurs of tricuspid and/or pulmonic regurgitation.

Patients with Eisenmenger physiology have shortened lifespans. The mean age at death is reported to be in the mid-30s. Patients with complex congenital heart lesions die younger. The clinical course is variable, but most patients succumb to progressive heart failure, sudden cardiac death, or die from major intrapulmonary hemorrhage (28, 30). Predictors of mortality include New York Heart Association (NYHA) functional class, heart failure, history of arrhythmias, and long QTc interval. They are also at risk of pulmonary artery thrombosis and complications of polycythemia.

Recommendations for the evaluation of adults with suspected pulmonary artery hypertension are outlined in the 2008 ACC/AHA guidelines (1) and include pulse oximetry, ECG, chest radiography, CBC, nuclear lung scintigraphy and cardiac imaging (echocardiography, MRI or CT). If the etiology of pulmonary hypertension is not identified, additional recommended testing includes pulmonary function tests, CT pulmonary embolism protocols, and cardiac catheterization (including pulmonary vasodilator responsiveness testing and/or anatomic intervention). Additional evaluation of suspected Eisenmenger physiology includes a detailed medical and surgical history, evaluation of severity of pulmonary hypertension, and review of other secondary complications (1). Lung biopsy is not routinely undertaken in the diagnostic assessment for Eisenmenger syndrome.

Patients with Eisenmenger syndrome should be followed up at least yearly, preferably in a center with expertise in adult congenital heart disease and pulmonary hypertension. Routine evaluation should include functional assessment (such as the 6-min walk test) and review of complications, laboratory studies (CBC, iron studies, creatinine, uric acid) and pulse oximetry (on and off oxygen). Patients should be counseled to avoid high-risk behaviors and situations including pregnancy, dehydration, isometric exercise, and high altitude (1).

Pregnancy is particularly dangerous, with maternal mortality in Eisenmenger syndrome reported to be as high as 30–50%. In addition, there is an increased likelihood of intrauterine growth retardation, prematurity, spontaneous abortion and fetal or perinatal demise (16, 18, 26, 31, 32). Permanent forms of contraception should be considered for patients with Eisenmenger syndrome. Combination (estrogen-containing) oral contraceptives are probably contraindicated due to the risk of thromboembolism and resultant risk of paradoxical embolism. Pregnant patients carrying to term should be collaboratively followed up by a High-risk Obstetrician and Adult Congenital Heart Disease Specialist. It is recommended that these patients be admitted for inpatient pregnancy management beginning at ~20 weeks gestation (18, 26). Recommended delivery approach is controlled vaginal delivery, with narcotic epidural analgesia and vacuum extraction or low forceps. The risk of fetal CHD recurrence is discussed above in other sections.

For patients undergoing surgery or other invasive procedures, pre-procedural hydration and consultation with a Physician with expertise in the care of adults with congenital heart disease is recommended. Meticulous care of intravenous catheters and use of filters to avoid air emboli are indicated. Even minor procedures carry a significant risk of mortality (26).

Although it is probably safe for Eisenmenger patients to travel on pressurized commercial aircraft, supplemental oxygen should be available (efficacy not proven) (33).

Previously, care of patients with Eisenmenger syndrome was primarily conservative. Currently, pulmonary vasodilator therapy has shown promise in improving hemodynamics and QoL in selected patients. The 2008 ACC/AHA guidelines suggest pulmonary vasodilator therapy may improve the QoLof patients with Eisenmenger physiology (1). Short-term survival with medical management is reasonably good. Heart and lung transplantation (or lung transplantation with repair of the cardiac defect) is appropriate in selected severely symptomatic patients and is associated with relatively good outcomes (34).

7.2.9 Future considerations

As medical technology and cardiac care continue to advance, increasing numbers of children born with congenital heart defects will reach adulthood (1, 35). Primary Care Physicians dealing with adults (whether Internal Medicine or Family Physicians) must be aware of this growing segment of their patient population. As discussed in this chapter, many defects causing left-to-right shunts may persist in an asymptomatic fashion into adulthood. Therefore, Adult Primary Care Physicians must be prepared to diagnose and treat these conditions as they may first present in adulthood. The number of cardiologists specifically trained in this area is not yet adequate to deal with the growing amount of patients with these conditions. This requires a concerted effort from cardiologists of adult and pediatric specialties, but perhaps more importantly from the multitude of Primary Care Physicians that will most probably be the only physicians many of these patients will ever see. Many adult patients born with left-to-right heart lesions underwent treatment and repair early in childhood and may have not felt it necessary to continue follow-up with a Cardiologist. Many other patients with these defects may have survived to adulthood without diagnosis, and may present to the primary care provider with new symptoms that finally developed. Primary Care Physicians will most certainly be at the frontlines of caring for these congenital heart defects.

References

1. Warnes, C. A., Williams, R. G., Bashore, T. M., Child, J. S., Connolly, H. M., Dearani, J. A., et al. (2008) ACC/AHA 2008 guidelines for management of adults with congenital heart disease. J. Am. Coll. Cardiol. 52:e143–e263.
2. Wiegers, S. E., St. John Sutton, M. G. Management of atrial septal defect in adults. UptoDateonline textbook. Updated May, 2010. URL: http://www.uptodate.com/contents/management-of-atrial-septal-defects-in-adults.
3. Fuse, S., Tomita, H., Hatakeyama, K., Kubo, N., Abe, N. (2001) Effect of size of a secundum atrial septal defect on shunt volume. Am. J. Cardiol. 88:1447–1450.
4. Vick, G. W. III. (1998) Defects of the atrial septum (including atrioventricular septal defects). In: Garson, A. Jr., Bricker, J. T., Fisher, D. J., Neish, S. R., eds. Science and Practice of Pediatric Cardiology, 2nd ed. Baltimore, USA: Williams Wilkins, p. 1141.
5. Vogel, M., Berger, F., Kramer, A., Alexi-Meskishvili, V., Lange, P. E. (1999)Incidence of secondary pulmonary hypertension in adults with atrial septal or sinus venosus defects. Heart 82:30–33.
6. Konstantinides, S., Geibel, A., Olschewski, M, Gornandt L, Roskamm H, Spillner G, et al. (1995) A comparison of surgical and medical therapy for atrial septal defect in adults. N. Engl. J. Med. 333:469–473.
7. Rostad, H., Sorland, S. (1979) Atrial septal defect of secundum type in patients under 40 years of age. A review of 481 operated cases. Symptoms, signs, treatment and early results. Scand. J. Thorac. Cardiovasc. Surg. 13:123–127.
8. Attie, F., Rosas, M., Granados, N., Zabal, C., Buendia, A., Calderon, J. (2001) Surgical treatment for secundum atrial septal defects in patients > 40 years old. A randomized clinical trial. J. Am. Coll. Cardiol. 38:2035–2042.
9. St. John Sutton, M. G., Tajik, A. J., McGoon, D. C. (1981) Atrial septal defect in patients ages 60 years or older: operative results and long-term postoperative follow-up. Circulation 64:402–409.
10. Horvath, K. A., Burke, R. P., Collins, J. J. Jr, Crohn, L. H. (1992) Surgical treatment of adult atrial septal defect: early and long-term results. J. Am. Coll. Cardiol. 20:1156–1159.
11. Berger, F., Vogel, M., Kramer, A., Alexi-Meskishvili, V., Weng, Y., Lange, P. E., et al. (1999) Incidence of atrial flutter/fibrillation in adults with atrial septal defect before and after surgery. Ann. Thorac. Surg. 68:75–78.
12. Steele, P. M., Fuster, V., Cohen, M., Ritter, D. G., McGoon, D. C. (1987) Isolated atrial septal defect with pulmonary vascular obstructive disease – long-term follow-up and prediction of outcome after surgical correction. Circulation 76:1037–1042.
13. Wilson, W., Taubert, K. A., Gewitz, M., Lockhart, P. B., Baddour, L. M., Levison, M., et al. (2007) Prevention of infective endocarditis. Guidelines from the American Heart Association. A guideline from the American Heart Association Rheumatic Fever, Endocarditis, and Kawasaki Disease Committee, Council on Cardiovascular Disease in the Young, and the Council on Clinical Cardiology, Council on Cardiovascular Surgery and Anesthesia, and the Quality of Care and Outcomes Research Interdisciplinary Working Group. Circulation 116:1736–1754.
14. Graham, T. P., Bricker, J. T., James, F. W., Strong, W. B. (1994) 26th Bestheda Conference: recommendations for determining eligibility for competition in athletes with cardiovascular abnormalities. Task Force 1: Congenital Heart Disease. J. Am. Coll. Cardiol. 24:867–873.
15. Landzberg, M. J. (2001) Closure of atrial septal defects in adult patients: justification of the "tipping point". J. Interv. Cardiol. 14:267–269.
16. Weiss, B. M., Zemp, L., Seifert, B., Hess, O. M. (1998) Outcome of pulmonary vascular disease in pregnancy: a systematic overview from 1978 through 1996. J. Am. Coll. Cardiol. 31:1650–1657.
17. Silversides, C. K., Marelli, A., Beauchesne, L., Dore, A., Kiess, M., Salehian, O., et al. (2010) Canadian Cardiovascular Society 2009 Consensus Conference on the management of adults with congenital heart disease: executive summary. Can. J. Cardiol. 26:143–150.

18. Perloff, J. K., Waksmonski, C. A., Foley, M. R. Pregnancy in women with congenital heart disease: Specific lesions. UpToDate online chapter. Updated May, 2010. URL: http://www.uptodate.com/contents/pregnancy-in-women-with-congenital-heart-disease-general-principles.
19. Satou, G. M., Reemtsen, B. L. Atrial septal defect, Sinus Venosus. Updated Jun 12, 2009. Emedicine online chapter. URL: http://emedicine.medscape.com/article/892151-overview.
20. Jacobs, J. P., Burke, R. P., Quintessenza, J. A., Mavroudis, C. (2000) Congenital heart surgery nomenclature and database project: ventricular septal defect. Ann. Thorac. Surg. 69:S25–S35.
21. Gabriel, H. M., Heger, M., Innerhofer, P., Zehetgruber, M., Mundigler, G., Wimmer, M., et al. (2002) Long-term outcome of patients with ventricular septal defects considered not to require surgical closure during childhood. J. Am. Coll. Cardiol. 39:1066–1071.
22. Kidd, L., Driscoll, D. J., Gersony, W. M., et al. (1993) Second natural history study of congenital heart defects. Results of treatment of patients with ventricular septal defects. Circulation 87:138–151.
23. Prosad, S. (2003) Ventricular septal defects. In: Gatzoulis, M. A., Webb, G. D., Daubeny, P. E., eds. Diagnosis and Management of Adult Congenital Heart Disease. London, UK: Churchhill Livingstone, pp. 171–178.
24. Fisher, R. G., Moodie, D. S., Sterba, R., Gill, C. C. (1986) Patent ductus arteriosus in adults-long-term follow-up: nonsurgical versus surgical treatment. J. Am. Coll. Cardiol. 8:280–284.
25. Wood, P. (1958) The Eisenmenger syndrome or pulmonary hypertension with reversed central shunt. BMJ 2:755–762.
26. Vongpatanasin, W., Brickner, E., Hillis, L. D., Lange, L. A. (1998) The Eisenmenger syndrome in adults. Ann. Intern. Med. 128:745–755.
27. Eisenmenger, V. (1897) Die Angeboren Defect der Kammer scheiderwand des Herzens. Z. Klin. Med. Suppl. 32:1–18. [In German]
28. Saha, A., Balakrishnan, K. G., Jaiswal, P. K., Venkitachalam, C. G., Tharakan, J. T. et al. (1994) Prognosis for patients with Eisenmenger syndrome of various aetiology. Int. J. Cardiol. 45:199–207.
29. Granton, J. T., Rabinovitch, M. (2002) Pulmonary arterial hypertension in congenital heart disease. Cardiol. Clin. 20:441–457.
30. Niwa, K., Perloff, J. K., Kaplan, S., Child, J. S., Miner, P. D. (1999) Eisenmenger syndrome in adults: ventricular septal defect, truncus arteriosus, univentricular heart. J. Am. Coll. Cardiol. 34:223–232.
31. Gleicher, N., Midwall, J., Hochberger, D., Jaffin, H. (1979) Eisenmenger syndrome and pregnancy. Obstet. Gynecol. Surv. 34:721–741.
32. Drenthen, W., Pieper, P. G., Roos-Hesselink, J. W., van Lottum, W. A., Voors, A. A., Mulder, B. J., et al. (2007) Outcome of pregnancy in women with congenital heart disease: a literature review. J. Am. Coll. Cardiol. 49:2303–2311.
33. Broberg, C. S., Uebing, A., Cuomo, L., Thein, S. L., Papadopoulos, M. G., Gatzoulis, M. A. (2007) Adult patients with Eisenmenger syndrome report flying safely on commercial airlines. Heart 93:1599–1603.
34. Waddell, T. K., Bennett, L., Kennedy, R., Todd, T. R., Keshavjee, S. H. (2002) Heart-lung or lung transplantation for Eisenmenger syndrome. J. Heart Lung. Transplant 21:731–737.
35. Pillutla, P., Shetty, K. D., Foster, E. (2009) Mortality associated with adult congenital heart disease: trends in the US population from 1979 to 2005. Am. Heart J. 158:874–879.

8 Transition of pediatric endocrine patients to adult care

Manmohan K. Kamboj, Donald E. Greydanus, Lee A. Bricker and Dilip R. Patel

Most children who are born with or who develop a chronic illness during childhood now survive into the adult years. This can present a considerable challenge to adult clinicians who may not be prepared to care for so-called "pediatric disorders". This review presents concepts of transitioning for three pediatric endocrine disorders: Turner syndrome (TS), congenital adrenal hyperplasia (CAH), and type-1 diabetes mellitus (T1DM). Providers of pediatric care have the responsibility of helping their patients learn to optimize their health. Providers of adult care must be willing to "catch" these older adolescents or young adults and help them deal with the challenges that their disorders present in addition to challenges complicated by adult living. A successful transition has considerable rewards for patients and clinicians at both ends of the age spectrum.

8.1 Introduction

The spectrum of management issues for chronic illnesses has changed over the last several decades. Many chronic or congenital illnesses that were the domain of only Pediatricians have now transitioned to also becoming chronic illnesses in adults. This is seen primarily because of improved care with medical as well as surgical treatment options, which have increased longevity for these individuals. Similar to many of the other chronic disorders discussed in this book, endocrine disorders have seen a similar transition. Many of these disorders began to be recognized only several decades ago, and their treatment plans continue to be optimized.

Therefore, many children/adolescents with these conditions never had the chance to seek adult medical care. However, this has challenged conventional medical teaching systems and physicians taking care of adult patients because they are now confronted with endocrine conditions that these clinicians have never saw before. On the flip side, Pediatricians are now challenged with not only providing adequate medical care but also ensuring smooth transitioning of these patients to adult care. This continues to be a work in progress for healthcare systems and the involved clinicians. Several of the pediatric endocrine conditions that present for adult care at age 18–21 years (varies with different programs and physicians) are listed in ▶Tab. 8.1. TS, CAH, and T1DM are now considered in this light of transition from pediatric- to adult-centered care.

8.2 TS

TS is a relatively common genetic syndrome with an approximate incidence of about 1:2000 live births, although varying incidences have been reported in different settings

Tab. 8.1: Some pediatric endocrine conditions for consideration in adulthood.

- Pituitary disorders
  - Panhypopituitarism
  - Isolated growth hormone deficiency (IGHD)
  - Central hypothyroidism
  - Central diabetes insipidus (DI)
- Thyroid disorders
  - Primary congenital hypothyroidism (CH)
  - Acquired hypothyroidism
  - Graves' disease
  - Cysts, nodules or tumors of the thyroid gland
- Adrenal disorders
  - Congenital adrenal hyperplasia (CAH)
  - Addison's disease
- Parathyroid/vitamin D disorders
  - Osteoporosis/osteomalacia
  - Hypoparathyroidism
  - Hyperparathyroidism
- Disorders of sexual differentiation
- Diabetes mellitus (DM)
  - Type-1 DM (T1DM)
  - Type-2 DM (T2DM)
  - Cystic fibrosis-related DM (CFRD)
- Genetic syndromes
  - Turner syndrome (TS)
  - Klinefelter syndrome (KS)
- Endocrine disorders in cancer survivors

(1–5). The underlying genetic defect is the complete or partial absence of the second "X" chromosome, with or without mosaicism. Some of the common karyotypes seen are listed in ▶ Tab. 8.2 (6). The diagnosis of TS encompasses not only the karyotype but the characteristic phenotype, although there may be a great variation of clinical presentations seen. Some of the common characteristic physical and systemic findings are noted in ▶ Tab. 8.3 (6, 7). However, the two almost constant features seen are short stature and ovarian dysgenesis.

Girls with TS may have multisystem involvement which presents not only diagnostic challenges but also management challenges. The concept of multidisciplinary comprehensive clinics is an ideal arrangement for these patients to provide optimal care. There are multiple disciplines involved: pediatrics, adult medical care, genetics, endocrinology, cardiology, nephrology, reproductive specialties, and psychology. The diagnosis of TS is made with a karyotype in girls with unexplained short stature, delayed puberty, primary amenorrhoea, or with the presence of other clinical features listed in Tab. 8.3. The diagnosis may be made *in utero* on ultrasonography based on any of the

Tab. 8.2: Some common karyotypes seen in Turner syndrome (TS).

Karyotype	Approximate frequency of occurrence
• 45, XO or 45, X	60%
• Mosaic TS ◦ 45, X/46, XX ◦ 45, X/46, XY ◦ 45, X/47, XXX	15%
• TS karyotype with a structurally abnormal "X" chromosome ◦ 46, X, I(Xq) (isochrome Xq) ◦ 46, X, Xp- (partial deletion of XP) ◦ 46, X, r(X) (ring X chromosome)	10%
• TS with mosaicism but with a structurally abnormal X chromosome ◦ 45, X/46, X, I (Xq) ◦ 45, X/46, X, r(X)	10%
• Other rare karyotypes	5%

suspected clinical features followed by amniocentesis. However, the diagnosis may be coincidental with a prenatal karyotype obtained for other reasons (8).

8.2.1 Management considerations

The management of TS is not only multidisciplinary but also age-specific and individualized. Depending on the range of manifestations seen, the therapeutic options may address the presence of specific congenital anomalies. However, short stature and gonadal dysgenesis, being the two almost constant features, will need to be addressed in most girls. The needs of each TS patient understandably will also differ starting from the *in-utero* period: infancy, childhood, adolescence, and into adulthood. The management considerations will need to be varied keeping in mind the specific physical, sexual, and psychosocial needs at each different stage of life. It is also important to assure smooth transition from pediatric care to adult care.

8.2.2 Pediatric issues

Prenatal period: If a diagnosis of TS is made *in utero*, no specific treatment is recommended. However, genetic counseling at this stage is very important to educate parents about TS. The parents may elect to terminate pregnancy at this time or continue with pregnancy, and will need ongoing support and counseling.

Infants and children: It is recommended that a karyotype be repeated after birth to confirm a pre-natal chromosomal diagnosis of TS.

Cardiovascular anomalies: At the diagnosis, all TS girls should be screened for cardiovascular anomalies with imaging studies, and a cardiology consultation should be

Tab. 8.3: Common clinical features of Turner syndrome.

- Short stature
- Gonadal dysgenesis
  - Reproductive issues
  - Delayed or incomplete puberty
  - Primary hypogonadism
  - Primary/secondary amenorrhoea
- Skeletal abnormalities
  - Short neck
  - Short fourth metacarpal
  - Modelung deformity
  - Cubitus valgus
  - Abnormal upper:lower segment ratio
  - Genu valgum
  - High arched palate
  - Scoliosis
  - Micrognathia
  - Nail dysplasia
- Cardiovascular abnormalities
  - Hypertension
  - Coarctation of aorta/aortic valve disease
  - Aortic dissection
- Renal and renovascular abnormalities
  - Horseshoe kidney
  - Abnormal renal vasculature
  - Ureteropelvic obstruction
- Ophthalmologic abnormalities
  - Strabismus
  - Eye deformities
- Otitis media
- Features of lymphatic obstruction
  - Cystic hygroma
  - Webbed neck
  - Widely spaced nipples
  - Edema of hands and feet
- Dermatologic features
  - Multiple pigmented nevi
  - Vitiligo
- Metabolic concerns
  - Hypothyroidism
  - Carbohydrate intolerance
- Reproductive issues
  - Gonadal failure
  - Infertility
  - Amenorrhoea
    - Primary
    - Secondary
- Osteoporosis
- Psychologic issues

obtained. Any major concerns in this regard which need immediate surgical intervention should be addressed appropriately. Baseline electrocardiography and four-limb blood pressures are obtained. MRI of the heart is recommended in addition for older girls and adults. If there is no immediate cardiologic issue, then imaging is recommended every 5–10 years. Re-imaging is also recommended: at the time of transitioning from pediatric to adult care; at the time of new-onset hypertension; or before planning for pregnancy is undertaken (8). If and when there is a degree of defect, then the appropriate plan and follow-up should be decided by the involved cardiologist. Coarctation of aorta and a bicuspid aortic valve are the most common cause of morbidity and mortality in TS. Up to ~26% of TS girls have been reported to have cardiovascular malformations (9).

Renal and renovascular malformations: These conditions occur in a relative greater proportion of TS girls as compared with control populations. There may be renal structure and/or reno-vascular abnormalities that are present in the patient with TS. Horseshoe kidney is seen in ~30% of TS girls (10–14). Thus, the recommendations for girls with TS include a renal ultrasound at the diagnosis and then subsequent nephrology consultation if required. If there is a urinary tract infection (UTI), then complete work-up and imaging should be undertaken because ureteropelvic obstruction may be the underlying cause. All these abnormalities, if present, will need to be addressed appropriately.

Cardiovascular issues in adulthood: Approximately 50% of TS young adults have hypertension which should be carefully looked for and aggressively managed. Besides a higher risk of congenital heart disease there is also a high risk of coronary artery disease and atherosclerosis. Thus, monitoring of blood pressure as well as follow-up with a cardiologist and echocardiography as indicated (every 2–5 years) is recommended (15–17). TS women with underlying renovascular disease are predisposed to hypertension. There may be a higher risk of UTI due to underlying renal collecting system abnormalities causing obstruction. These TS patients may need closer monitoring and screening for UTIs.

Short stature: Short stature is almost a constant feature of TS girls (along with ovarian dysgenesis). TS girls are, on average, 20 cm or 8 inches shorter than their mid-parental height; however, they are not growth hormone (GH)-deficient (18). All the other clinical concerns in TS girls will need to be addressed on an ongoing basis from infancy through childhood to adulthood. However, short-stature issues understandably will be a concern only for the Pediatric Endocrinologist, and is a concern that adult caretakers do not have to address.

Current recommendations include the use of recombinant human growth hormone (rhGH) for maximizing the final adult height in TS girls (8, 19). GH stimulation testing is routinely not indicated in these girls. Longitudinal follow-up of linear growth in TS girls reveals that most of them fall below the 5th percentile by 5 years of age. It is recommended that rhGH be started as soon as the height falls below the 5th percentile (8). If rhGH is used as recommended and in a timely manner, it is possible for TS girls to attain their normal height (20). GH therapy in the USA is approved by the US Food and Drug Administration (FDA) at 0.375 mg/kg/week given daily and subcutaneously. This dose can be modified based on insulin growth factor-1 (IGF1) levels and the growth response (8). TS girls should be followed up by a Pediatric Endocrinologist every 3–6 months for rate of growth, scoliosis, and general examination depending on age. GH therapy needs to be stopped at completion of linear growth. GH therapy is not needed in adult TS women because they are not GH-deficient.

Ovarian dysgenesis: This is the second most common feature seen in TS girls next only to short stature. In contrast to short stature, the issues resulting from ovarian dysgenesis present varying clinical features requiring varying treatment and management options over the different age periods. There is no effect of the ovarian dysgenesis in the prenatal period, on the infant, and in early childhood, i.e., until the peri-pubertal period. Therefore, no management issues arise during these ages with regards to ovarian dysgenesis.

Depending primarily on the particular karyotype, issues with pubertal development may arise in the normally expected pubertal period. These may range from the following: delayed puberty with no onset of thelarche; incomplete pubertal progression where thelarche was initiated but did not progress as normally expected; primary amenorrhoea with normal thelarche but no menstrual periods; or secondary amenorrhoeawhere menarche and some menstrual period cycling was initiated but then stopped. In young adult TS women, ongoing concerns about adequate hormone replacement for continued menstrual cycling and reproductive issues arise. In the older adult, hormonal therapy concerns continue (as in post-menopausal women).

Understandably, with different presentations and different expectations, the means of hormone replacement will differ. About one-third of TS girls undergo spontaneous pubertal development whereas 2–5% may even be able to become pregnant; however, ultimately > 90% of TS girls and women will have gonadal failure (21–23). Estrogen replacement therapy is used for the induction and progression of pubertal development. Progestins are then added after adequate estrogenization has been achieved to obtain normal menstrual cycling. The aim of choosing the dose and timing of replacement hormone therapy is to try to mimic normal pubertal development as closely as possible while also ensuring adequate linear growth.

The hormone treatment plan discussed here is primarily from the Turner Syndrome Consensus Study Group (8). Unlike previously practiced, the current recommendations note that estrogen replacement should be initiated at about 12–13 years of age in TS girls if no spontaneous development is seen. Elevated follicle-stimulation hormone (FSH) levels should be documented prior to hormone initiation to confirm primary gonadal failure. Estrogen replacement is initiated at very low doses of about 1/10 to 1/8 of the normal adult dose. Various formulations may be used (▶ Tab. 8.4). Estrogen dose is gradually and progressively increased to adult dose levels over ~2 years. Progestin therapy is then begun after adequate estrogenization as well as breast and uterine development has occurred for adequate menstrual cycling and to prevent endometrial hyperplasia.

Ovarian dysgenesis in adulthood: After pubertal development and menstrual cycles have been initiated, it is important for TS adolescents to understand the importance of ongoing hormone replacement. At this time different methods may be used: estrogen patch with intermittent progestin; oral estrogen with separate intermittent progestin; or facilitating therapy with combination estrogen/progestin preparations. Estrogen replacement (see Tab. 8.4) is usually required until the time of normal menopause to maintain feminization and to prevent osteoporosis (and may be needed even beyond that time period depending on individual requirements) (8).

The other important concerns related to ovarian dysgenesis that are important for TS young adult women are reproduction and fertility. Most TS women are infertile and it is best to start this discussion earlier on in adulthood (or even late adolescence). However, as for all non-TS adolescent girls, it is important to educate these girls about prevention of unwanted pregnancies and sexually transmitted diseases. Women with functional ovaries may need to understand not to unduly postpone pregnancy for risk of early ovarian failure; or to look into cryopreservation of ovarian tissue or ova for future use. However, it is also important for them to realize the greater risk of chromosomal

Tab. 8.4: Estrogen replacement in Turner syndrome.

Options for estrogen replacement	Route	Initial daily dose	Adult daily dose
Estrogen patch	Transdermal	6.25 μg	100–200 μg
Micronised estradiol	Oral	0.25 mg	2–4 mg
Ethinyl estradiol	Oral	-	20 μg
Conjugated equine estrogens (CEE)	Oral	-	1.25–2.5 mg
Estradiol cypionate	Injectable	-	2.5 mg monthly

abnormalities and risk to themselves because of cardiovascular complications. TS girls with pre-existent cardiovascular involvement are best advised against pregnancy.

Even women without apparent cardiovascular concerns need to have extensive pre-conception work-up and close follow-up in pregnancy. This is best addressed by their Cardiologist in conjunction with High-risk Obstetricians. Women without functional ovaries may need donor eggs and require hormone replacement preparation to assure adequate uterine development for carrying through with pregnancy. Research work is ongoing with respect to exploring options for cryopreservation of ovarian tissue/follicles from TS girls in their younger years when they may have more functional ova (24).

Autoimmune issues in TS: TS girls have a higher incidence of autoimmune concerns. Autoimmune thyroid disease (AITD) is seen in ~30% of girls with TS. The anti-thyroid antibodies are present in even a higher number (≤50%) of patients (25). AITD may manifest as early as 4 years of age, so annual screening is recommended in TS girls from this age (25, 26). Celiac disease may also be seen in ~5% of TS girls. Screening with tissue transglutaminase immunoglobulin (Ig)A antibodies is recommended starting also at ~4 years (27). The follow-up for both of these entities should continue on an ongoing basis not only in childhood and adolescence but into adulthood. Appropriate treatment options should be undertaken as needed for hypothyroidism, hyperthyroidism and/or celiac disease.

Psychological and educational issues: Girls with TS are predisposed to a higher risk of cognitive, social, and behavioral issues. Psycho-educational evaluations are recommended at school entry and then during the early school years as needed. If difficulties are noted, necessary referral for appropriate testing and treatment needs to be made. Further discussion on the topic is beyond the discussion of this review. These issues may need to be discussed with age-specific strategies to address age-related concerns. Other issues confronted in TS girls include those listed below.

- Predisposition to keloid formation
- Higher risk of hearing deficits (which may also be conductive with superimposed sensori-neural hearing loss). Hence, all TS women should have an audiologic evaluation every 2–3 years.
- Higher risk of hyperinsulinemia, insulin resistance, hyperlipidemia, dyslipidemia, obesity, prediabetes, type-2 diabetes mellitus (T2DM), and even frank metabolic syndrome. Therefore, TS young adults should be screened annually with blood sugar and lipid profiles, thyroid function test, and liver function (28–30). Adults should be also monitored for hypertension and aortic enlargement. Cardiovascular effects during pregnancy should be considered along with overall bone health during the adult years (30).

8.3 CAH

CAH comprises a group of enzymatic endocrine disorders due to partial or complete deficiency of one of enzymes in the steroid hormone pathway. There are multiple enzymes in this pathway, but > 90% of cases of CAH are due to a defect in the 21-hyroxylase enzyme, which is encoded by the CYP21A2 gene. This enzyme is important for the conversion of 17-hydroxyprogesterone to 11-deoxycortisol. CAH also presents a pertinent chronic pediatric endocrine disorder which needs appropriate transition and subsequent management in adulthood. This is especially important for individuals with severe deficiency, in which case inadequate care may be life-threatening. For the purposes of discussion of this chapter, the term CAH will be used to refer to CAH due to 21-hydroxylase deficiency. The other enzymatic defects causing CAH will not be discussed further. The incidence of CAH (21-hydroxylase) is about 1:15.000 live births, but wide ethnic variations have been noted (31, 32). CAH is an autosomal recessive condition. There is also some genotype–phenotype correlation although it is not always possible to predict the phenotype from a genetic study or *vice versa* (33, 34). 21-hydroxylase CAH may be of classified into three main types based on presentation and severity.

- The classic or severe form of CAH is characterized by severe deficiency or absence of 21-hydroxylase enzyme. These children present with severe decompensation in the neonatal period with adrenal insufficiency and salt-losing crisis, and additionally in girls with a range of ambiguous genitalia.
- The virilizing form of CAH involves infants and toddlers who may present with virilization but no adrenal insufficiency.
- The non-classic form of CAH presents later in life. These patients may present at different ages with varied expression of virilization, including premature adrenarche and advanced skeletal maturation, or in adolescents and adults with hirsutism, menstrual irregularities and essentially a polycystic ovarian syndrome-like picture. Many of the patients may remain asymptomatic.

The 21-hydroxylase deficiency results in interruption of the adrenal steroid pathway and prevents conversion of 17-OH progesterone to 11-deoxycortisol and progesterone to deoxycorticosterone. This results in decreased secretion of cortisol and aldosterone and therefore an increase in adrenocorticotropic hormone(ACTH) secretion. This results in deficiency of cortisol and aldosterone, causing salt wasting but increased androgens because of diversion of precursors in the adrenal hormone pathway towards androgen synthesis, leading to virilization. All these findings are less severe in non-classic CAH because of partial enzyme activity being present.

8.3.1 Diagnostic considerations

The diagnosis of 21-hydroxylase deficiency CAH has been greatly facilitated by inclusion into the newborn screening (NBS) program. All 50 states in the USA include this in their NBS as of July 2008. A dried spot of blood is tested for 17-hydroxy progesterone. Many states have developed reference standards based on birth weight and/or gestation (35–38). This NBS for CAH has prevented a lot of morbidity and mortality in salt-wasting neonates (especially males). Female neonates with the disorder are generally brought to medical attention at birth with ambiguous genitalia.

Laboratory findings for CAH include elevated levels of 17-hydroxy progesterone. Most neonates will definitely have values well over 3, 500 mg/dL (38). A high level on NBS should be confirmed with serum 17-hydroxy progesterone. A complete ACTH (cosyntropin) stimulation test should also be obtained as per standard protocols in which other precursors of the adrenal pathway are measured along with cortisol levels before and after stimulation with cosyntropin (using the standard 250 μg dose). The biochemical levels of these intermediate hormones are overall much lower in non-classic forms of CAH than in classic CAH cases. Genetic testing is now quite widely available for confirmation of the mutant CYP21A2 gene.

Over the last several years, reliable prenatal diagnosis and prenatal treatment of mothers with affected fetuses has been developed and are in use. Prenatal diagnosis should be undertaken if there is a sibling already diagnosed with the condition, or ifboth parents are known to be heterozygous for the mutation. Molecular analyses of fetal CYP21A2 genes in amniotic fluid or in choronic villus sampling are the preferred tests. Other options for testing include amniotic fluid 17-hydroxyproesterone or human leukocyte antigen (HLA) typing in fetal cells (39, 40).

8.3.2 Therapeutic management of CAH

Management of CAH may be discussed under three age-group periods: neonate, childhood and adult.

Management in neonates: A newborn infant with ambiguous genitalia is a very high index of suspicion for CAH. Every newborn with ambiguous genitalia or suspected CAH should be seen by a Pediatric Endocrinologist. 21-hydroxylase deficiency CAH causes virilization in the female neonate whereas no significant ambiguity is seen in the male newborn. The female external genitalia undergo virilization because of exposure to high levels of androgen *in utero*. These infants are typically brought to medical attention at birth and adequately tested and treated. Conversely, the male infant presents with a normal phenotype but if he has classic CAH will present with salt-wasting crisis, which in the past was a cause of high mortality. The ambiguous genitalia in a newborn are an endocrine psychosocial emergency. Appropriate diagnostic testing as noted above should be done to rule out CAH. The newborn is carefully monitored for signs of cortisol deficiency and salt wasting until definitive results are obtained. Females neonates will need extensive reconstructive surgery, usually clitroplasty and vaginoplasty, which should be undertaken only by Pediatric Surgeons or Urologists with expertise in the field (41, 42).

Adrenal crisis with salt wasting is an emergency requiring immediate medical evaluation and treatment. Hypocortisolemia results in hypotension, dehydration, hyponatremia, hypoglycemia, and hyperkalemia requiring intravenous fluid resuscitation with 5% dextrose and normal saline. High-dose hydrocortisone needs to be administered in this phase of acute adrenal crisis. After adequate blood samples are drawn for measurement of corticosteroid hormones, these newborns usually need hydrocortisone (50–100 mg/m^2) followed by the same dose divided every 4 h daily until the baby is clinically stable. Once clinically stable, intravenous hydrocortisone can be switched to oral hydrocortisone at normal physiological doses generally between 12–18 mg/m^2 per day preferably given every 8 h (42). Additional salt supplementation is generally needed in these infants.

Management in children and adolescents: Glucocorticoid replacement continues in children with classic CAH-CYP21A2 deficiency with hydrocortisone at 12–18 mg/m^2 per day. At these physiologic replacement doses of hydrocortisone, mineralocorticoid replacement is also necessary. Mineralocorticoid replacement is accomplished with fludrocortisone, generally in doses of 0.05–0.2 mg per day (42).

Non-classic CAH children generally do not require hydrocortisone or mineralocorticoid replacement (although replacement may be needed in some cases).

Stress dosing of hydrocortisone in oral and injectable form needs to be discussed in detail with the parents of these children. The importance of stress dosing in cases of stress, illness or surgery needs to be emphasized. These children should be given an emergency stress dosing sheet for documentation during periods of emergency and visits to the Emergency Room.

Clinic follow-up: Patients with CAH are followed up by Pediatric Endocrinologists every 3–4 months. Adrenal hormones and overall energy level are used to titrate replacement doses of hydrocortisone. Plasma renin activity and serum electrolytes may be used to titrate the mineralocorticoid dose. Every patient with CAH should have a medic alert on them for cases of emergency (42). The aim of replacement therapy and adequate dose titration is to (i) achieve normal growth and development, (ii) achieve normal final adult height and (iii) prevent episodes of adrenal crisis. This must be done while preventing the adverse effects of chronic glucocorticoid therapy. Overtreatment may result in growth retardation or Cushing's syndrome signs. Because of the importance of adequate therapy in these children and adolescents, smooth transition of CAH adolescents into adult medical care is crucial.

8.3.3 Management in adults

The last 50 years of CAH treatment with glucocorticoids have witnessed considerable understanding of the treatment of children and adolescents, and knowledge of caring for adults with CAH is now emerging. Adults with CAH need continued monitoring of hormonal treatment (i.e., glucocorticoid and mineralocorticoid) based on laboratory testing and compliance with prescribed medications (43). Clinicians continue to look at bone density, cardiovascular risk factors, and catecholamine deficiency. A multidisciplinary-team approach can be useful to provide specialized pregnancy care, psychosexual counseling, and gynecologic surgery (43). Adult men with CAH are noted to be lost to follow-up. This can be problematic because they will not receive recommended monitoring for hypogonadism because of the effects of adrenal rests or suppression of gonadotrophins, leading to a high risk of oligospermia (43).

8.4 DM

DM is a chronic endocrine disorder which also requires smooth transition from pediatric care to adult care. The management of DM becomes very important on an ongoing basis because multiple studies have demonstrated the direct relationship of the level of DM control with the occurrence of chronic complications. The importance of a "team approach" in the management of chronic illnesses cannot be exemplified in pediatric care more than in DM management. DM is a state of absolute or relative insulin deficiency, and can be classified into groups primarily based on underlying etiology (▶ Tab. 8.5). Presently, it is believed that there are environmental influences superimposed on a genetic predisposition which are responsible for overt expression of the disease. For the purpose of this chapter, T1DM will be discussed in further

Tab. 8.5: Types of diabetes mellitus (DM).

I. Type-1 diabetes mellitus (T1DM)
- Also known as insulin-dependent diabetes mellitus (IDDM)
- Juvenile diabetes mellitus (JDM)

II. Type-2 diabetes mellitus (T2DM)
- Non-insulin-dependentdiabetesmellitus (NIDDM)
- Maturity-onsetdiabetesmellitus
- Adult-onsetdiabetes

III. Maturity-onset diabetes mellitus in youth (MODY)

IV. Gestational diabetes mellitus (GDM)

V. Secondary diabetes mellitus
- Cystic fibrosis-related diabetes (CFRD)
- Lipoatrophic diabetes mellitus – due to genetic defects of insulin action
- Diabetes mellitus seen in relation with other endocrine conditions
  - Cushing's syndrome
  - Acromegaly
  - Glucagonoma
  - Pheochromocytoma
- Drug-induced
  - Glucocorticoids
- DM in association with syndromic conditions
  - Prader–Willi syndrome
  - Turner syndrome
  - Klinefelter syndrome
  - Wolfram syndrome

detail because it is a prototypic childhood chronic condition requiring intensive care as well as management in childhood and adolescence followed by smooth transition to adult care.

8.4.1 Incidence and prevalence of T1DM

T1DM is one of the most common chronic illnesses in the pediatric population. The frequency of occurrence of T1DM is 1 in 360 adolescents at 16 years of age, and this incidence declines after the age of 20 years. Only 5–10% of all patients with DM in the USA have T1DM, and ~150.000 people under the age of 20 years have T1DM. About two-thirds of newly diagnosed cases of DM who are < 19 years of age have T1DM (44–48). The incidence of T1DM also varies with ethnicity, with a lower incidence in African–American, American–Indians, Asian–Americans, and Hispanics as compared with that in Caucasians. There is a higher incidence in family members with similar genetic/HLA composition. The age at presentation shows two age groups for peak incidence: 4–6 years of age, and 10–14 years of age (49–51). There is no specific sex difference associated with the incidence of DM (52).

8.4.2 Clinical considerations

The onset of T1 DM may be varied. It may be acute in the decompensated form in diabetic ketoacidosis (DKA); a more classic presentation with polyuria, polydipsia and weight loss; or a very subtle pre-clinical presentation when DM may be diagnosed incidentally on a urine test or blood test ordered for entirely different reasons. The distribution of the occurrence of the initial presentation is quite similar, with about one-third of the new-onset DM cases presenting with each of these clinical scenarios. Children and adolescents presenting in DKA may be quite ill with nausea, vomiting, abdominal pain, Kussmaul breathing, ketotic breath, and even with altered sensorium or frank coma. These patients will require initial intravenous management in the intensive care unit (ICU) with close monitoring of vital signs, fluid balance, and laboratory parameters. High blood glucose, high glucose and ketones in the urine, and an acidic pH are diagnostic. Electrolyte panel may reveal hyponatremia and acidosis.

These are the children presenting to the Emergency Room. They require immediate intensive care in the Emergency Roomand admission to the pediatric ICU. Typically, children present to the Pediatrician or Family Physician because parents have noticed increased frequency of urination. Sometimes there may be nocturia in children who have been otherwise controlled for a long time, as well as increased thirst. Parents may also notice weight loss over a few weeks. These children/adolescents are not sufficiently decompensated to be sick otherwise. When seen by the Primary Care Physician with a high index of suspicion, urinalysis generally reveals glucose in the urine. A subsequent blood glucose check on a glucose testing meter reveals a high blood glucose level in the range for DM.

The subtle or very early presentation is almost a coincidental diagnosis. Either there is a close family member or sibling with DM; a blood sugar test is done first because there is facility to do it at home. The results reveal blood sugar either in the range of impaired glucose tolerance or in the low DM range. The alarmed parents bring the child to then be seen at their Pediatrician's office for further work-up. Sometimes a urinalysis done just for a routine visit or physical at the Primary Care Physician's office may reveal glucose, thereby bringing up the suspicion of DM.

8.4.3 Diagnostic considerations

Aside from the details of history and examination mentioned above, further confirmation of DM needs to be undertaken. Once the diagnosis of DM is established, the underlying type of DM will need to be differentiated so as to optimize therapeutic options. According to the American Diabetes Association (ADA), the diagnostic criteria for diagnosis of DM are:

- A fasting plasma glucose = 126 mg/dL
- A post-prandial plasma glucose = 200 mg/dL
- Glycated hemoglobin (HgbA1c) = 6.5%

Impaired glucose tolerance or pre-DM refers to a fasting plasma glucose of 100–125 mg/dL and post-prandial plasma glucose of 140–199 mg/dL. The plasma glucose must be repeated on a separate day for confirmation unless the level is unequivocally diagnostic. HgbA1c measures the percentage hemoglobin bound to glucose in a non-enzymatic reaction and gives a reflection of the mean blood sugar levels over the prior 3 months

Tab. 8.6: Differences between type-1 and type-2 diabetes mellitus.

	T1DM	T2DM
Age	Bimodal peak: 4–6 years, 10–14 years	After onset of puberty
Body habitus	Not overweight Recent weight loss	Generally overweight
Family history	<5% family members may have h/o T1DM	≥90% have exposure to family members with poorly controlled T2DM, obesity and complications setting up a wrong image
Insulin resistance	Less likely	Likely to have acanthosis nigricans, hypertension, dyslipidemia, and polycystic ovary syndrome
Autoimmunity	Likely to have positive autoantibodies to islet cells, glutamic acid decarboxylase (GAD), insulin, tyrosine phosphatase (IA2)	Less likely to have autoantibodies
Socioeconomic status	No specific difference	More likely in the lower socioeconomic status family distribution (same as obesity)
Lifestyle modifications	Not too many lifestyle modifications required	Extensive modifications in lifestyle are key to successful treatment and management
Technological advancements	Instrumental in improving diabetes care with newer types of insulin and insulin delivery devices	Many of the technological advances are responsible for a poorer lifestyle and causation of T2DM and obesity
Treatment options	Only insulin	Insulin sensitizers and insulin later in the course of illness

relating to the lifespan of a RBC. HgbA1c has been recently recommended to be used as a diagnostic measure by an international consensus statement, and has been endorsed by the ADA. However, appropriate precautions must be exercised for the interpretation of results (53). Once the diagnosis of DM is established, it is necessary to differentiate between T1DM and T2DM in patients where this differentiation may not be as obvious. Some of the differentiating features between T1DM and T2DM are listed in ▶Tab. 8.6.

8.4.4 Management considerations

Management of T1DM is dependentupon the initial presentation. Insulin is the only specific therapeutic agent for the treatment of T1DM. However, successful management of T1DM in children and adolescents involves not only adequate insulin management but also comprehensive management strategies, as listed below.

- Individualized treatment options for each child/adolescent in relation to the whole family dynamics.

- The child's age, maturity, and developmental level are important considerations in addition to the level of family involvement, interest, and dedication to implementation of management plan.
- The overall aim is to set realistic glycemic goals which can be practically followed to achieve a good balance between maintaining the strictest glycemic control, to minimize risk of long-term complications while avoiding short term complications, mainly hypoglycemia.

There are two main phases of management of new-onset T1DM: initial immediate management and the long-term ongoing treatment plan.

Initial management depends on the initial presentation for DKA. Intensive-care management involving intravenous fluids and continuous intravenous insulin is initiated to rehydrate the patient and improve hyperglycemia acidosis, hyponatremia, hypokalemia, and possibly hypophosphatemia. Close monitoring of intake and output, urine dipsticks for glucose, ketones, and specific gravity and electrolytes are necessary along with hourly blood glucose monitoring. The aim is to treat dehydration and achieve euglycemia while taking care to prevent untoward complications such as cerebral edema.

As the DKA resolves and symptoms improve, the insulin regimen is transitioned from intravenous to subcutaneous insulin along with gradual oral intake. If the child or adolescent has a classic presentation and is not sick, then the subcutaneous insulin regimen may be instituted directly. Ongoing management is generally standard for T1DM irrespective of the initial presentation. Depending on specific clinical and hospital setups, outpatient or inpatient initiation of treatment and DM education may be undertaken.

Learning of survival skills is the start of DM education. DM educators and DM nurses educate the child/adolescent and their families about the basic technical skills required to start testing blood glucose and insulin administration. They learn to use their glucose testing meters, to "poke" themselves to test, learn techniques for drawing up insulin, and injection techniques. Depending on each situation and patient capabilities, decisions are made regarding their initial use of insulin vial/syringe or insulin pen, and the particular glucose testing meter they will be using. Blood glucose log sheets are used to keep a record of self-monitored blood glucose (SMBG) levels, insulin given, carbohydrate consumed, and any other special or unusual circumstances noted. For the initial few weeks and then as needed later on, this is very useful to monitor, evaluate, discuss, and make appropriate changes to the insulin regimen (preferably via phone contact) on a daily basis. This opportunity is also used to educate further and address questions or concerns.

8.4.5 Team approach

There are many important components to DM management in the pediatric arena. It is all encompassed, however, under the umbrella term of "comprehensive team approach". This process starts off, more or less at the time of the diagnosis and then continues on into routine outpatient follow-up care. The "team" covers most of the components of comprehensive care, and family/parents are a part of this team. The role of team members varies according to their expertise and serves to assure comprehensive care. The best results can be expected if there is open communication between the child/adolescent with DM, participating family members, and clinic team members.

Clinic team members must have open communication among the multiple members so that the family and patient do not get mixed messages regarding their care. Ideally, the team should include a Diabetes Nurse, Diabetes Educator, Nutritionist, Medical Social Worker, Psychologist and Pediatric Endocrinologist. The Primary Care Physician is an important peripheral part of the team, and it is important that the line of communication also remains open between them and the Diabetes Care Team. Each member of the team addresses specific components affecting DM management.

8.4.6 Main components of DM management

Overall, the main challenge in DM management seems to be the chronicity of the condition as well as the treatment methods, more specifically poking for blood sugar testing and poking for insulin injections. Newer options are becoming popular which decrease the number of pokes required for testing and injections. However, until they become the mainstream standard of care, the challenge continues.

Blood glucose testing

Close testing of self-monitored blood glucose (SMBG) is essential to optimize glycemic control as well as to prevent episodes of severe hypoglycemia (54–56). According to ADA recommendations, SMBG testing should be done at least four times a day. In the pediatric population, however, the testing may end up being much more than that for several reasons, including: fear of severe hypoglycemia; failure of recognition of hypoglycemia or hyperglycemia with clinical signs only; and puberty as well as growth affecting relatively rapid requirements of insulin doses. For intensive-therapy regimens, SMBG testing is required before meals to be able to bolus appropriately.

Newer glucose testing meters and lancet devices have facilitated testing, and some meters require only 0.3–1 μL of blood for testing. Continuous glucose monitoring devices (CGMDs) have also become available. These devices utilize interstitial fluid for glucose testing via electrodes placed in the interstitial space or subcutaneous space. New-generation CGMDs are more accurate and provide real-time blood glucose values. Some of these devices are approved for use in children but remain expensive and therefore not in mainstream use. Once available for use in routine testing they will take away some of the "pain" from testing SMBG.

Insulin preparations and insulin requirements

The mainstay of treatment of T1DM is insulin. Insulin administered exogenously is used to replace missing endogenous insulin. The secretion, action, and factors affecting its function are quite complex and difficult to replicate. Therefore, in day-to-day T1DM management, the three main factors that are considered are blood glucose levels, carbohydrates eaten, and significant physical activity. After estimation of the insulin dose, further "fine-tuning" to achieve adequate glycemic control is done by SMBG. Appropriate dose changes are made based on patterns of blood glucose levels observed. Variouspreparations of insulin and insulindelivery devices are available. The choice of a particular regimen should be individualized to offer the treatment option to best fit the understanding, capabilities, and lifestyle of the family. This tends to assure better compliance. There are three broad categories of insulin types primarily based on their duration of action, as listed below.

- Long-acting insulin preparations have a long duration of action and are generally given once a day. They serve to provide the basal insulin level. Two main insulin types in this category are insulin glargine and insulin detemir. They are used in combination insulin regimens along with rapid-acting preparations.
- Intermediate-acting insulin preparation includes neutral protamine Hagedorn (NPH) insulin generally given twice a day. It has a variable duration of action of ~8–16 h.
- Short-acting insulin preparations primarily include regular insulin with a duration of action of ~4–6 h.
- Rapid-acting insulin preparations have a rapid onset of action of 5–15 min and duration of action of ~2–3 h. In combination regimens, the rapid-acting insulin is used for pre-meal and correction boluses. These preparations and regular insulin are used in insulin pumps and insulin drips. These include insulin lispro, aspart, and glulisine.

Insulin delivery devices

According to individual patient/family preference, an appropriate choice of insulin delivery devices may be used. These include traditional insulin syringes or the newer and more convenient insulin pens. Insulin vials and syringes allow for mixing of insulin as previously used (e.g., mixing of NPH and regular insulin). However, glargine is not currently recommended to be mixed with any other insulin. Insulin pens are available for rapid-acting and long-acting insulin types. They offer more attractive, convenient, and easy portability options than syringes, and replace the need to draw-up insulin; instead, the amount of insulin dose required is "dialed-up". Insulin pumps are other options available for the technically gifted. They offer multiple options to facilitate intensive management, and offer more flexibility with meals and schedules besides eliminating a poke for each insulin shot.

Insulin pumps primarily use only rapid-acting insulin preparations. Management of the insulin pump is often referred to as "continuous subcutaneous insulin infusion" (CSII). The popularity of the insulin pump is increasing. The ADA recommends consideration of pump usefor insulin therapy to address concerns relating to recurrent hypoglycemia, widely ranging blood glucose levels, inadequate control of DM, flexibility in lifestyle being required for good metabolic control, microvascular complications, and/or risk factors for macrovascular complications. Also, pumps may be considered for further individualization of DM management for athletes, pregnant adolescents, or young children and infants who may all benefit from the flexibility offered (57). The overall concept of the insulin pump is to supply a continuous dose of insulin and supplement with extra insulin bolusing for carbohydrate intake. However, it is very important that the child/adolescent and family realize the full implications of using with the insulin pump.

There are multiple combination regimens of insulin that may be utilized without the use of an insulin pump: insulin pens or syringes can be used instead. The preferred regimen generally referred to as the "intensive flexible regimen" utilizes the physiologic concept of having basal insulin which is supplemented with bolus insulin for carbohydrate intake. Primarily, a long-acting insulin preparation is used to provide the basal insulin, and generally comprises ~50% of the total daily insulin (TDI) requirement. This is then supplemented with bolus insulin using the rapid-acting insulin preparations mentioned above (which account for the other ~50% of the TDI).

The conventional insulin regimen involves an intermediate-acting insulin preparation along with a rapid-acting insulin preparation, and is given 2–3 times a day. Most commonly this is NPH combined with a rapid-acting insulin preparation before breakfast, a rapid-acting insulin preparation for dinner, and NPH at bedtime. Although seemingly easier, this regimen is more rigid as far as meal times and meal content are concerned. Two main types of insulin regimens are noted in ▶ Tab. 8.7. Control studies have shown an improvement in DM control with use of intensive insulin regimens versus conventional insulin regimens (58, 59).

Dose of insulin: The TDI requirement is 0.5–1.0 units/kg. Pre-pubertal children, younger children, and children presenting early in the course of the disease require the lower end of the dose range as compared with older pubertal adolescents or adolescents presenting in DKA.

Clinic follow-up: The ADA recommends follow-up of children and adolescents with T1DM in outpatient clinic every 3 months. The team approach alluded to above should preferably be in place at each of these visits. Complete evaluation of the status of glycemic control, overall health, and illness issues are discussed. A complete physical examination is done, and this opportunity is also resourceful for providing DM education. ▶ Tab. 8.8 lists the parameters to be followed at these follow-up visits. The ADA recommends age-specific HgbA1c (as listed in ▶ Tab. 8.9). The common laboratory tests that are done at the time of the visit are listed in ▶ Tab. 8.10.

Transition of care to adults

Transition of older adolescents to adult medical care should be a gradual and well-planned process. Different institutions have varying protocols to ensure smooth transitioning. However, this recommended transition may not be as efficiently undertaken as desired in many clinical settings. It is the responsibility of the Pediatric Team to make the adolescent comfortable and prepared to move onto adult medical/diabetes care. It can be a very challenging situation for many young adults. adult physicians/Endocrinologists will continue the intensive management strategies that many of these individuals should hopefully be already quite comfortable with. The Adult Endocrinologist can focus on the risk of long-term complications as well as management of pregnancy with DM in this now adult patient with DM.

With adolescence come increasingly complex demands associated with rapid growth in height and muscle, puberty and sexual development, and the common urges of the adolescent patient towards varying degrees of rebelliousness. It is into this often uncertain *milieu* that efforts to transition the young patient to adult care must be introduced. Many pediatric patients with DM have proved able (with support) to manage their disease. However, the goal at this critical transitional juncture is to equip the young patient with the skills to become totally independent and capable of effective self-selection of insulin doses, of sound dietary as well as lifestyle choices, and to organize support mechanisms as needed to be an independent adult.

Tab. 8.7: Examples of combination insulin regimens.

- Intensive flexible insulin regimen
  - Type of insulin
    - Long-acting insulin – one the following:
      - Glargine
      - Detemir

      +
    - Rapid acting insulin – one of the following:
      - Lispro
      - Aspart
      - Glulisine
  - Dose of insulin
    - Long-acting insulin
      - About 50% of total daily insulin (TDI) dose
    - Rapid-acting insulin
      - Correction factor (CF)
        - Using rule of 1800 (1800 ÷ TDI)
      - Insulin:Carbohydrate ratio
        - CF ÷ 3
  - This regimen is more flexible with regards to meal timing as well as carbohydrate content
- Conventional regimen
  - Type of insulin
      - Intermediate acting insulin
      - NPH

      +
    - Rapid-acting insulin – one the following:
      - Lispro
      - Aspart
      - Glulisine
  - Dose of insulin
    - Calculate TDI dose
      - 2/3 of TDI at breakfast
        - 2/3 intermediate-acting insulin
        - 1/3 rapid-acting insulin
      - 1/3 of TDI in evening
        - 1/3 rapid acting insulin at dinner
        - 2/3 intermediate acting at bedtime
  - Usually the lunchtime insulin is not required
  - More rigid with meal timing and carbohydrate content

Quite unlike nearly every other known medical condition, DM in an independently living adult patient is a wholly unique problem. Successful management demands all of the patient's intelligence as well as his/her full willingness to be the principal player on his/her management team. Significant deficit in the patient's intellectual grasp of the nuances of the dosing and management of insulin, or of keen interest in participating actively in all decision-making processes, will almost inevitably result in wider

Tab. 8.8: Information obtained at clinic visit upon intake.

- Present insulin regimen being used
  - Insulin pump:
    - Basal rates
    - Insulin:carbohydrate ratio
    - Correction factor
  - Multiple daily injection insulin regimen
    - Type of insulin
      - Long-acting insulin
      - Short-acting insulin
      - Any other insulin being used
    - Dose of insulin
      - Dose of long-acting insulin
      - Insulin:carbohydrate ratio
      - Correction factor
- Supplies being used
  - Type of glucose testing meter
  - Types of syringes
  - Types of insulin pens
- Mean readings of blood sugar values
  - At breakfast
  - At lunch
  - At dinner
  - At bedtime
  - Overnight
- Episodes of illness since last visit
  - What was the illness
  - DKA or not
  - When
  - Mode of treatment
- Information about nutrition
  - Carbohydrate intake
  - Adherence to dietary recommendations
  - Exercise/activity
    - Type of exercise
    - Frequency
    - Effect of exercise on blood sugar:
      - Normal
      - Hypoglycemia
      - Hyperglycemia

glucose fluctuations, more hypoglycemia, and more rapid advance of complications due to DM.

The successful transition to adult care therefore entails the "handing off" of the responsibility of the lion's share of day-to-day management from members of the Pediatric/Adolescent Team to the patient. As an emerging adult, the patient must learn to become knowledgeable in estimating meal content and in making his/her own informed decisions about dosing and timing of insulin(s), and in clearly assuming command of the Pediatric/Adolescent Team.

As well as possessing good intelligence and organizational ability, the new adult patient with DM must possess the motivation, and resistance to "DM burnout" to assume that command. This means that the patient largely takes over the activities listed below.

Tab. 8.9: Age-specific HgbA1c goal recommendations as per ADA.

Age (years)	HgbA1c (%)
<6	7.5–8.5
6–12	≤8
>12	≤7.5

Dietary selection

- Selecting meals that avoid excessive calories or that could result in unacceptably high glucose excursions, and which are "heart healthy."
- Timing of meals.
- Estimating carbohydrate content or other properties of meals for calculating prandial insulin dosing.

Regular and frequent measurements of blood glucose

- Knowledge of, and keen focus on, desired goal blood glucose values (fasting and post-prandial.
- Ability and willingness to change basal dosing or basal pump infusion rates, without consultation, based on blood glucose data.
- Ability and willingness to re-calculate prandial insulin doses or boluses based on appropriately timed, and adequate numbers of, determinations of post-prandial glucose values, without consultation.
- Ability and willingness to obtain pre-prandial glucose values for purposes of correcting calculated prandial insulin doses or boluses, without consultation.

Personal oversight of the ancillary aspects of care

- Assuring adequate and regular exercise.
- Assuring adequate and regular sleep.
- Absolute and total avoidance of smoking and rare use of alcohol.
- Attention to foot care and to daily self-examination of feet.
- Attention to dental hygiene and examinations.
- Attention to eye care, with regular retinal examinations.
- Attention to general medical examinations by Adult Primary Care Physician or Adult Endocrinologist.
- Selection of a peer group whose members are sympathetic and helpful to the young patient (especially at times such as departure for college).
- Willingness to adopt wearing of appropriate bracelet or necklace indicating the existence of insulin-requiring DM.

Until an excellent closed-loop pump becomes available, the complexities of blood glucose management and other aspects of DM care must be the responsibility of the patient transitioning to adult care. Physicians, patients, family, and peers need

Tab. 8.10: Laboratory tests in the Pediatric Diabetes Outpatient Follow-up Clinic.

- At 3-month visit
  - Hemoglobin A1C
  - Urine dipstick for glucose, ketones, and protein
  - Random blood glucose
- Annual Labwork
  - Lipid profile
  - Free T4 and TSH
  - Anti-endomysial antibodies
  - Further testing if required

to understand that a well-informed, motivated young patient is much more likely to succeed over time in taming the illness than is a patient without such attributes.

Insouciance is, in and of itself, a major and potentially deadly risk factor. A patient's systemic inability and or unwillingness to organize and grasp the vicissitudes of self-management is likely to impact tremendously and adversely affect short- and long-term outcome. Furthermore, the risks associated with fixed, Physician-assigned insulin doses and "sliding scales" may be great. Major efforts need to be directed at educating the adolescent patient with DM emerging into adulthood. The Pediatrician, Internist, and Diabetes Educator, along with solid support from family and peers, are crucial ingredients in the process of handing management over to the new, pre-eminent caregiver: the patient who is cognizant of correct care. This is the *sine qua non* in a successful transition of the pediatric patient with DM to an adult patient with DM. The young adult patient who is apolaustic toward life and not serious about optimal self-regulation of his/her DM care will find potentially rapid deterioration of health in the adult independent years. Hopefully, excellent healthcare at both ends of the treatment spectrum and a smooth transition of care will minimize such an egregious outcome.

8.5 Conclusions

The transition of patients with endocrine and other chronic illnesses from the pediatric healthcare model to the adult healthcare model should be a smooth and successful journey and not a perplexing paradox (60–67). Transitioning of care should not be an arcane sesquipedalian term with no meaning for clinicians who feel they are unable to provide this complex care because of limited training in their residency or fellowship programs. This chapter offered reflections on this journey for three endocrine disorders: TS (68), CAH (69–76), and T1DM (77). The goal of this handoff is to present a stable older adolescent or young adult who is cognizant of his/her condition and who is willing to optimize health with the advice of an adult caregiver who is cognizant of the special issues this condition may present in the adult years of life. It can be a daunting challenge, but transitioning of healthcare remains a critical part of practice for those who have the privilege of being healers and clinicians to the child, adolescent, and adult in the 21st century.

> "You have powers you never dreamed of. You can do things you never thought you could do. There are no limitations in what you can do except the limitations of your own mind."
> Darwin P. Kingsley

References

1. Hook, E. B., Hamerton, J. L. (1977) The frequency of chromosome abnormalities detected in consecutive newborn studies – differences between studies: results by sex and severity of phenotypic involvement. In: Hooke, B., Porter, I. H., eds. Population Cytogenetics. New York, USA: Acad Press, p. 63.
2. Hook, E. B., Warburton, D. (1983) The distribution of chromosomal genotypes associated with Turner's syndrome: livebirth prevalence rates and evidence for diminished fetal mortality and

severity in genotypes associated with structural X abnormalities or mosaicism. Hum. Genet. 64:24–27.

3. Jacob, P. A., Betts, P. R., Cockwell, A. E., Crolla, J. A., Mackenzie, M. J., Robinson, D. O. et al. (1990) A cytogenetic and molecular reappraisal of a series of patients with Turner's syndrome. Ann. Hum. Genet. 54(Pt. 3):209–223.
4. Hall, J. G., Sybert, V. P., Williamson, R. A., Fisher, N. L., Reed, S. D. (1982) Turner's syndrome – clinical genetics conference, children's orthopedic hospital and medical center, Seattle, and University of Washington (Specialty Conference). West. J. Med. 137:32–44.
5. Nielsen, J., Wohlert, M. (1991) Chromosome abnormalities found amount 34, 910 newborn children: results from a 13-year incidence study in Arhus, Denmark. Hum. Genet. 87: 81–83.
6. Saenger, P. (2008) Turner syndrome. In: Sperling, M. A., ed. Pediatric Endocrinology, 3rd ed. Philadelphia, USA: Saunders Elsevier, pp. 610–661.
7. Saenger, P. (2010) Clinical manifestations and diagnosis of turner syndrome (gonadal dysgenesis). UpToDate 2010 May. URL: http://www.uptodate.com/contents/clinical-manifestations-and-diagnosis-of-turner-syndrome-gonadal-dysgenesis.
8. Bondy, C. A. (2007) Turner Syndrome Study Group. Care of girls with Turner syndrome: a guideline of the Turner Syndrome Study Group. J. Clin. Endocrinol. Metab. 92:10–25.
9. Gotzsche, C. O., Krag-Olsen, B., Nielsen, J., Sorensen, K. E., Kristensen, B. O. (1994) Prevalence of cardiovascular malformations and association with karyotypes in Turner's syndrome. Arch. Dis. Child. 71:433–436.
10. Sas, T. C., de Muinck Keizer-Schrama, S. M., Stijnen, T., Jansen, M., Otten, B. J., Hoorweg-Nijman, J. J., et al. (1999) Normalization of height in girls with Turner syndrome after long-term growth hormone treatment: results of a randomized dose-response trial. J. Clin. Endocrinol. Metab. 84:4607–4612.
11. Kaneko, N., Kawagoe, S., Hiroi, M. (1990) Turner's syndrome – review of the literature with reference to a successful pregnancy outcome. Gynecol. Obstet. Invest. 29:81–87.
12. Press, F., Shapiro, H. M., Cowell, C. A., Oliver, G. D. (1995) Outcome of ovum donation in Turner's syndrome patients. Fertil. Steril. 64:995–998.
13. Chang, P., Tsau, Y. K., Tsai, W. Y., Tsai, W. S., Hou, J. W., Hsiao, P. H. et al. (2000) Renal malformations in children with Turner's syndrome. J. Formos. Med. Assoc. 99:796–798.
14. Flynn, M. T., Ekstrom, L., De Arce, M., Costigan, C., Hoey, H. M. (1996) Prevalence of renal malformation in Turner syndrome. Pediatr. Nephrol. 10:498–500.
15. Gravholt, C. H., Naeraa, R. W., Nyholm, B., Gerdes, L. U., Christiansen, E., Schmitz, O. et al. (1998) Glucose metabolism, lipid metabolism, and cardiovascular risk factors in adult Turner's syndrome. The impact of sex hormone replacement. Diabetes Care 21:1062–1070.
16. Nathwani, N. C., Unwin, R., Brook, C. G., Hindmarsh, P. C. (2000) Blood pressure and Turner syndrome. Clin. Endocrinol. (Oxf.) 52:363–370.
17. Landin-Wilhelmsen, K., Bryman, I., Wilhemsen, L. (2001) Cardiac malformations and hypertension, but not metabolic risk factors, are common in Turner syndrome. J. Clin. Endocrinol. Metab. 86:4166–4170.
18. Stahnke, N., Keller, E., Landy, H., Serono Study Group. (2002) Favorable final height outcome in girls with Ullrich–Turner syndrome treated with low-dose growth hormone together with oxandroloen despite starting treatment after 10 years of age. J. Pediatr. Endocrinol. Metab. 15:129–138.
19. Saenger, P. Management of turner syndrome (gonadal dysgenesis). UpToDate 2010 May. URL: http://www.uptodate.com/contents/management-of-turner-syndrome-gonadal-dysgenesis.
20. Gunther, D. F., Eugster, E., Zagar, A. J., Bryant, C. G., Davenport, M. L., Quigley, C. A. (2004) Ascertainment bias in Turner syndrome: new insights from girls who were diagnosed incidentally in prenatal life. Pediatrics 114:640–644.
21. Boechat, M. I., Westra, S. J., Lippe, B. (1996) Normal US appearance of ovaries and uterus in four patients with Turner's syndrome and 45, X karyotype. Pediatr. Radiol. 26:37–39.

22. Pasquino, A. M., Passeri, F., Pucarelli, I., Segni, M., Municchi, G., Italian Study Group for Turner's Syndrome. (1997) Spontaneous pubertal development in Turner's syndrome. J. Clin. Endocrinol. Metab. 82:1810–1813.
23. Hovatta, O. (1999) Pregnancies in women with Turner's syndrome. (1999) Ann. Med. 31:106–110.
24. Hreinsson, J. G., Otala, M., Fridstrom, M., Borgstrom, B., Rasmussen, C., Lundqvist, M. et al. (2002) Follicles are found in the ovaries of adolescent girls with Turner's syndrome. J. Clin. Endocrinol. Metab. 87:3618–3623.
25. Livadas, S., Xekouki, P., Fouka, F., Kanaka-Gantenbein, C., Kaloumenou, I., Mavrou, A. et al. (2005) Prevalence of thyroid dysfunction in Turner's syndrome: a long-term follow-up study and brief literature review. Thyroid 15:1061–1066.
26. El-Mansoury, M., Bryman, I., Berntorp, K., Hanson, C., Wilhelmsen, L., Landin-Wilhelmsen, K. (2005) Hypothyroidism is common in Turner syndrome: results of a five-year follow-up. J. Clin. Endocrinol. Metab. 90:2131–2135.
27. Bonamico, M., Pasquino, A. M., Mariani, P., Danesi, H. M., Culasso, F., Mazzanti, L., et al. (2002) Prevalence and clinical picture of celiac disease in Turner syndrome. J. Clin. Endocrinol. Metab. 87:5495–5498.
28. Maraschio, P., Tupler, R., Barbierato, L., Dainotti, E., Larizza, D., Bernardi, F., et al. (1996) An analysis of Xq deletions. Hum. Genet. 97:375–381.
29. Miyabara, S., Nakayama, M., Suzumori, K., Yonemitsu, N., Sugihara, H. (1997) Developmental analysis of cardiovascular system of 45, X fetuses with cystic hygroma. Am. J. Med. Genet. 68:135–141.
30. Bondy, C. A. (2007) Care of girls and women with Turner syndrome: a guideline of the Turner Syndrome Study Group. J. Clin. Endocrinol. Metabol. 92:110–125.
31. Merke, D. P. Genetics and clinical presentation of classic congenital adrenal hyperplasia due to 21-hydroxylase deficiency. UpToDate 2010 May. URL: http://www.uptodate.com/contents/genetics-and-clinical-presentation-of-classic-congenital-adrenal-hyperplasia-due-to-21-hydroxylase-deficiency.
32. Therrell, B. L. (2001) Newborn screening for congenital adrenal hyperplasia. Endocrinol. Metab. Clin. North. Am. 30:15–30.
33. Speiser, P. W., White, P. C. (2003) Congenital adrenal hyperplasia. N. Engl. J. Med. 349:776–788.
34. Ferenczi, A., Garami, M., Kiss, E., Pek, M., Sasvari-Szekely, M., Barta, C. et al. (1999) Screening for mutations of 21-hydroxylase gene in Hungarian patients with congenital adrenal hyperplasia. J. Clin. Endocrinol. Metab. 84:2369–2372.
35. Merke DP. Diagnosis of classic congenital adrenal hyperplasia due to 21-hydroxylase deficiency. UpToDate 2010 May. URL: http://www.uptodate.com/contents/diagnosis-of-classic-congenital-adrenal-hyperplasia-due-to-21-hydroxylase-deficiency.
36. Olgemoller, B., Roscher, A. A., Liebl, B., Fingerhut, R. (2003) Screening for congenital adrenal hyperplasia: adjustment of 17-hydroxyprogesterone cut-off values to both age and birth weight markedly improves the predictive value. J. Clin. Endocrinol. Metab. 88:5790–5794.
37. van der Kamp, H. J., Oudshoorn, C. G., Elvers, B. H., van Baarle, M., Otten, B. J., Wit, J. et al. (2005) Cutoff levels of 17-alpha-hydroxyprogesterone in neonatal screening for congenital adrenal hyperplasia should be based on gestational age rather than on birth weight. J. Clin. Endocrinol. Metab. 90:3904–3907.
38. Witchel, S. F., Nayak, S., Suda-Hartman, M., Lee, P. A. (1997) Newborn screening for 21-hydroxylase deficiency: results of CYP21 molecular genetic analysis. J. Pediatr. 131:328–331.
39. Miller, W. L., Levine, L. S. (1987) Molecular and clinical advances in congenital adrenal hyperplasia. J. Pediatr. 111:1–13.
40. White, P. C., Speiser, P. W. (2000) Congenital adrenal hyperplasia due to 21-hydroxylase deficiency. Endocr. Rev. 21:245–291. Erratum in: Endocr. Rev. 21:550.
41. Merke, D. P. Treatment of classic congenital adrenal hyperplasia due to 21-hydroxylase deficiency in infants and children. UpToDate 2010 May. URL: http://www.uptodate.com/

contents/treatment-of-classic-congenital-adrenal-hyperplasia-due-to-21-hydroxylase-deficiency-in-infants-and-children.
42. Joint LWPES/ESPE CAH Working Group. (2002) Consensus statement on 21-hydroxylase deficiency from the Lawson Wilkins Pediatric Endocrine Society and the European Society for Paediatric Endocrinology. J. Clin. Endrinol. Metab. 87:4048–4053.
43. Ogilvie, C. M., Crouch, N. S., Rumsby, G. et al (2006) Congenital adrenal hyperplasia in adults: a review of medical, surgical, and psychological issues. Clin. Endocrinol. 64:2–11.
44. Levitsky, L. L., Misra, M. Epidemiology, presentation, and diagnosis of type 1 diabetes mellitus in children and adolescents. UpToDate 2010 May. URL: http://www.uptodate.com/contents/epidemiology-presentation-and-diagnosis-of-type-1-diabetes-mellitus-in-children-and-adolescents.
45. Lipton, R. B., Drum, M., Burnet, D., Rich, B., Cooper, A., Baumann, et al. (2005) Obesity at the onset of diabetes in an ethnically diverse population of children: what does it mean for epidemiologists and clinicians? Pediatrics 115:e553–e560.
46. Fagot-Campagna, A., Pettitt, D. J., Engelgau, M. M., Burrows, N. R., Geiss, L. S., Valdez, R., et al. (2000) Type 2 diabetes among North American children and adolescents: an epidemiologic review and a public health perspective. J. Pediatr. 136:664–672.
47. Duncan, G. E. (2006) Prevalance of diabetes and impaired fasting glucose levels amont US adolescents: National Health and Nutrition Examination Survey, 1999–2002. Arch. Pediatr. Adolesc. Med. 160:523–528.
48. Liese, A. D., D'Agostino, R. B. Jr., Hamman, R. F., Kilgo, P. D., Lawrence, J. M., Liu, L. L., et al. (2006) The burden of diabetes mellitus among US youth: prevalence estimates from the SEARCH for Diabetes in Youth Study. Pediatrics 118:1510–1518.
49. Felner, E. I., Klitz, W., Ham, M., Lazaro, A. M., Stastny, P., Dupont, B. et al. (2005) Genetic interaction among three genomic regions creates distinct contributions to early- and late-onset type 1 diabetes mellitus. Pediatr. Diabetes. 6:213–220.
50. Durruty, P., Ruiz, F., Garcia de los Rios, M. (1979) Age at diagnosis and seasonal variation in the onset of insulin-dependent diabetes in Chile (Southern hemisphere). Diabetologia 17:357–360.
51. Elamin, A., Omer, M. I., Zein, K., Tuvemo, T. (1992) Epidemiology of childhood type I diabetes in Sudan, 1987–1990. Diabetes Care 15:1556–1559.
52. Dabelea, D., Bell, R. A., D'Agostino, R. B. Jr., Imperatore, G., Johansen, J. M., Linder, B. et al. (2007) Incidence of diabetes in youth in the United States. JAMA 297:2716–2724.
53. American Diabetes Association. (2010) Standards of medical care in diabetes – 2010. Diabetes Care 33(Suppl. 1):S11–S61.
54. Levitsky, L., Misra, M. Management of type 1 diabetes mellitus in children and adolescents. UpToDate 2010 May. URL: http://www.uptodate.com/contents/topic.do?topicKey=PEDS/5817.
55. Anderson, B., Ho, J., Brackett, J., Finkelstein, D., Laffel, L. (1997) Parental involvement in diabetes management tasks: relationships to blood glucose monitoring adherence and metabolic control in young adolescents with insulin-dependent diabetes mellitus. J. Pediatr. 130:257–265.
56. Haller, M. J., Stalvey, M. S., Silverstein, J. H. (2004) Predictors of control of diabetes: monitoring may be the key. J. Pediatr. 144:660–661.
57. Phillip, M., Battelino, T., Rodriguez, H., Danne, T., Kaufman, F. (2007) Use of insulin pump therapy in the pediatric age-group: consensus statement from the European Society for Paediatric Endocinology, the Lawson Wilkins Pediatric Endocrine Society, and the International Society for Pediatric and Adolescent Diabetes, endorsed by the American Diabetes Association and the European Association for the Study of Diabetes. Diabetes Care 30:1653–1662.
58. Murphy, N. P., Keane Sm Ong, K. K., Ford-Adams, M., Edge, J. A., Acerini, C. L., Dunger, D. B. (2003) Randomized cross-over trial of insulin glargine plus lispro or NPH insulin plus regular human insulin in adolescents with type 1 diabetes on intensive insulin regimens. Diabetes Care 26:799–804.

59. Diabetes Control and Complications Trial Research Group. (1994) Effect of intensive diabetes treatment on the development and progression of long-term complications in adolescents with insulin-dependent diabetes mellitus: Diabetes control and complications trial. J. Pediatr. 125:177–188.
60. Duke, N. N., Scal, P. B. (2009) Adult care transitioning for adolescents with special health needs: A pivotal role for family centered care. Matern. Child Health J.
61. Rapley, P., Davidson, P. M. (2010) Enough of the problem: a review of time for health care transition solutions for young adults with a chronic illness. J. Clin. Nutr. 19(3–4):313–323.
62. Okumura, M. J., Kerr, E. A., Cabana, M. D., et al. (2010) Physician views on barriers to primary care for young adults with childhood-onset chronic disease. Pediatrics 125:e748–e754.
63. Berkowitz, S. (2009) Transitioning adolescents to adult care: putting theory into practice. Minn. Med. 92:42–44.
64. Peter, N. G., Forke, C. M., Ginsburg, K. R., et al. (2009) Transition from pediatric to adult care: Internists' perspectives. Pediatrics 123:417–423.
65. Tuchman, L. K., Slap, G. B., Britto, M. T. (2008) Transition to adult care: experiences and expectations of adolescents with a chronic illness. Child Care Health Dev. 34:557–563.
66. Harden, P. N., Nadine, P. (2006) Pediatric to adult transition: a personal experience. Prog. Transplant 16:324–328.
67. Betz, C. L. (2004) Adolescents in transition of adult care: why the concern? Nurs. Clin. North Am. 39:681–713.
68. Rubin, K. (2003) Transitioning the patient with Turner's syndrome from pediatric to adult care. J. Pediatr. Endocrinol. Metab. 16(Suppl. 3):651–659.
69. Witchel, S. F. (2010) The medical home concept and congenital adrenal hyperplasia: a comfortable habitat! Int. J. Pediatr. Endocrinol. 2010:561526. Epub 2010 Jun 8.
70. Auchus, R. J. (2010) Management of the adult with congenital adrenal hyperplasia. Int. J. Pediatr. Endocrinol. 614107. Epub 2010 May 30.
71. Loechner, K. J., Patel, S., Fordham, L. Decreased bone mineral density and vertebral compression fractures in a young adult male with 21-hydroxylase deficiency congenital adrenal hyperplasia (CAH): is CAH an unrecognized population at risk for glucocorticoid-induced osteoporosis? J. Pediatr. Endocrinol. Metabol. 23(1–2):179–187.
72. Auchus, R. J. (2010) Congenital adrenal hyperplasia in adults. Curr. Opin. Endocrinol. Diabetes Obes. 17:210–216.
73. Ambroziak, U., Bednarczuk, T., Ginalska-Malinowska, M., Małunowicz, E. M., Grzechocińska, B., Kamiński, P., Bablok, L., Przedlacki, J., Bar-Andziak, E. (2010) Congenital adrenal hyperplasia due to 21-hydroxylase deficiency – management in adults. Endokrynol. Pol. 61(1):142–55.
74. Nebesio, T. D., Eugster, E. A. (2010) Growth and reproductive outcomes in congenital adrenal hyperplasia. Int. J. Pediatr. Endocrinol. 298937. Epub 2010 Feb 1.
75. Frisén, L., Nordenström, A, , Falhammar, H., et al. (2009) Gender role behavior, sexuality, and psychosocial adaptation in women with congenital adrenal hyperplasia due to CYP21A2 deficiency. J. Clin. Endocrinol. Metabol. 94:3432–3439.
76. Kim, M. S., Merke, D. P. (2009) Cardiovascular disease risk in adult women with congenital adrenal hyperplasia due to 21-hydroxylase deficiency. Semin. Reprod. Med. 27:316–321.
77. Weissberg-Benchell, J., Wolpert, H., Anderson, B. J. (2007) Transitioning from pediatric to adult care: a new approach to the post-adolescent young person with type 1 diabetes. Diabetes Care 30:2441–2446.

9 Adolescents and adults with inborn errors of metabolism

Carolyn Bay, Carol Reidand Ashley Daub

Inborn errors of metabolism (IEM), also known as "metabolic diseases" are a broad group of disorders that share the feature of an abnormality (commonly an enzymatic abnormality) affecting the intermediary metabolism of proteins, carbohydrates and fats. This review providesa summary of metabolic diseases and discusses current and recent advances in diagnostic and treatment options. We provide an overview of the fundamental types of IEM and divide them into functional categories. Using phenylketonuria (PKU) as an example, we will outline the history of treatment in this prototype metabolic disease, and describe some of the challenges clinicians and scientists successfully embraced (as well as the ongoing challenges we continue to face). Improved identification and definitive diagnosis, combined with ongoing efforts to maximize treatment options, has resulted in increased survival and reduced morbidity in IEM patients. As a result, patients with IEM are surviving into the teen years and adulthood. With the provision of care, we expect this trend to continue hopefully well into the geriatric age groups.

9.1 Introduction

IEM, also known as "metabolic diseases" are a broad group of disorders that share the feature of an abnormality (commonly an enzymatic abnormality) affecting the intermediary metabolism of proteins, carbohydrates and fats (▶ Tab. 9.1). Classic examples are PKU, galactosemia, methylmalonic aciduria (MMA), Fabry's disease, and Lesch–Nyhan disease. Newer classes of metabolic diseases include fatty acid oxidation defects such asmedium-chain AcylCoA dehydrogenase deficiency (MCAD) and mitochondrial DNA (mtDNA) diseases, resulting in insufficient energy (e.g., mitochondrial encephalopathy with lactic acid and strokes (MELAS)).

Clinical experience and continued research into the etiology of genetic and metabolic disorders has provided more specific diagnoses, and increasingly, more treatment options. As more disease treatments became available, expansion of the number of disorders screened for in the newborn period was warranted. In fact, "Expanded Newborn Screening" is now carried out in all 50 states in the USA, and increasingly worldwide. This has dramatically increased the number of children with IEM identified in the first few days of life, resulting in earlier treatment and fewer life-threatening crises. The combination of earlier diagnosis and more effective treatments has resulted in improved survival and outcomes. Many more patients will survive to teenage years and adulthood with chronic management of their metabolic disease.

We will provide an overview of metabolic diseases; discuss current and recent advances in diagnostic and treatment options; summarize the fundamental types of IEM and divide them into functional categories.

Tab. 9.1: Types of inborn errors of metabolism and classic examples.

1. Organic acidurias
   Propionic acidemia
   Methylmalonicacidemia
2. Disorders of amino acid metabolism
   Phenylketonuria (PKU)
   Maple syrup urine disease (MSUD)
3. Hyperammonemia/urea cycle disorders
   Ornithine transcarbamylase deficiency (OTC deficiency)
   Citrullinemia
4. Disorders of fatty acid oxidation
   Medium-chain Acyl CoA dehydrogenase deficiency (MCAD)
   Very-long chain Acyl CoA dehydrogenase deficiency (VLCAD)
5. Disorders of energy metabolism and lactic acidosis
   Mitochondrial encephalopathy with lactic acidosis and strokes (MELAS)
   Kearns–Sayre syndrome
6. Disorders of carbohydrate metabolism
   Galactosemia
   Glycogen storage diseases, von Gierke, (type I); Pompe's (type II)
7. Peroxisomal disorders
   Adrenoleukodystrophy
   Zellweger's syndrome
8. Disorders of purine metabolism
   Lesch–Nyhandisease
   Adenosine deaminase deficiency (aka severe combined immunodeficiency (SCID))
9. Disorders of transport and mineral metabolism
   Cystinosis
   Wilson's disease
10. Mucopolysaccharidoses
    Hurler's disease
    Hunter's disease
11. Mucolipidoses
    I-cell disease (mucolipidosis, II)
12. Disorders of cholesterol and neutral lipid metabolism
    Familial hypercholesterolemia
    Mevalonicaciduria
13. Lipid storage disorders
    Fabry disease
    Gaucher disease
14. Miscellaneous disorders
    Congenital disorder of glycosylation, type 1a
    Disorders of creatinemetabolism

Taken from Nyhan et al. (9)

Tab. 9.2: Classification of inborn errors of metabolism and examples.

1. Disorders that give rise to INTOXICATION

a) Examples of disorders:
   1) Some amino acid disorders (PKU, MSUD, homocystinuria, tyrosinemia)
   2) Almost all organic acidurias
   3) Congenital hyperammonemia/urea cycle abnormalities
   4) Sugar intolerances (galactosemia)
   5) Metal intoxications (Wilson's disease, Menkesdisease)
   6) Porphyrias

b) Acute and/or progressive

c) Accumulation of toxic compounds proximal to metabolic block

d) Symptom-free intervals alternated with acute, often life-threatening episodes of intoxication

e) Episodes of intoxication provoked by: intercurrent illness, intake of offending precursers in diet; fever; catabolism prompted by insufficient nutritional/caloric intake

2. Disorders involving ENERGY METABOLISM

a) Examples of disorders: etiology is a mitochondrial defect
   1) mtDNA abnormalities: (MELAS, MERRF, NARP, Kearns–Sayre)
   2) Abnormalities of pyruvate catabolism
   3) Disorders of electron transport chain

b) Examples of disorders: etiology is a cytoplasmic defect
   1) Disorders of glycolysis
   2) Disorders of gluconeogenesis
   3) Hyperinsulinism
   4) Disorders of glycogen

c) Symptoms due to deficiency of energy affects most frequently the brain, myocardium, muscle, liver

d) With a few exceptions, treatment options are limited and geared towards supportive care

3. Disorders involving COMPLEX MOLECULES

a) Disorders:
   1) Lysosomal storage disorders, mucopolysaccharidoses
   2) Peroxisomal disorders
   3) Disorders of intracellular protein trafficking and/or processing (alpha-1-antitrypsin deficiency, carbohydrate deficient glycoprotein (CDG) syndrome); disorders of cholesterol biosynthesis)

b) Usually involves organelles within the cytoplasm of the cell

c) Abnormalities in the synthesis or catabolism of complex molecules in the intermediary metabolism

d) Unrelated to dietary intake or intercurrent illness

e) Progressive and permanent without treatment

Taken from Saudubray (10)

Using PKU as an example, we will outline the history of treatment in this prototype metabolic disease, and describe some of the challenges clinicians and scientists successfully embraced (and the ongoing challenges we continue to face). We will summarize current treatment options, and outline the challenges in implementation of treatments, most importantly dietary treatment. We will outline successful strategies to improve compliance in dietary management (especially in the most challenging disorders). Lastly, we have referenced singularly useful textbooks, articles, and internet resources for review.

In 2006, Saudubray and colleagues published a series of articles emphasizing the new era of treatments possible for IEM (10). They broke down this large classification of disorders into three basic groups based upon with similar pathophysiologic characteristics as seen from the therapeutic perspective. This grouping (summarized in ▶ Tab. 9.2), can be useful in the diagnostic evaluation of suspected IEM and guide evaluation of therapeutic options. The article also provides tables of disorders presenting at different ages (including adulthood); signs and symptoms based upon involvement of organ systems; and a listing of medications used in the treatment of inherited metabolic disease.

9.2 Historical perspective of IEM

The initial identification of IEM as a class of disease occurred at the turn of the twentieth century with the identification of alkaptonuria and other disorders by a group of Physician–Scientists, most notably Garrod. As early as 1917, a report was published on the success of restricting milk intake in the treatment of an infant with galactosemia.

As more metabolic diseases were discovered (and the causes of each disease identified), clinicians proposed treatments. Prior to 1950, most of the proposed treatments were not feasible with the technology available. That all changed in the 1950s with PKU.

9.3 Prototype IEM: classic PKU

The diagnosis and development of treatments for classic PKU was the first of many successes in the field of IEM. However, PKU remains a very challenging disease to treat. Some of the ongoing issues are a good example of the challenges for teenage and adult patients with metabolic diseases in general.

Classic PKU is a good example of a disease which has undergone profound changes in diagnosis and management since it was originally identified. Classic PKU is due to a deficiency of the enzyme phenylalanine hydroxylase, which results in the inability of the liver to convert phenylalanine to tyrosine. Patients with untreated classic PKU are blonde or lightly pigmented. Without treatment started in the first few weeks of life, patients have significant cognitive impairment, and can have additional findings of an eczematous rash, hyperactivity and seizures.

9.3.1 PKU: the beginning

Classic PKU was first described in 1934 by the Norwegian Physician and Biochemist Ivar Asbjørn Følling (1888–1973). He described testing the urine of two affected siblings with ferric chloride, and noted that the urine developed a deep green color which indicated the presence of phenylpyruvic acid. In 1937, Penrose named the disease PKU based on urinary findings, and noted the association of mental retardation with a chemically-based problem. Clinicians studying patients with PKU noted elevations of phenylalanine in urine and plasma. In 1953, Jervis reported that *in-vitro* preparations obtained from the liver of PKU patients could not convert phenylalanine to tyrosine, providing insight into the site of the metabolic blockage in PKU.

9.3.2 PKU: Dietary treatment begins: 1950s

Clinicians proposed nutritional therapy that would reduce dietary phenylalanine in an effort to reduce plasma phenylalanine levels, which they hoped might improve cognitive and neurological outcomes. However, implementation of the proposed diet was not possible until the early 1950s. Methods to accomplish a reduced phenylalanine diet were proposed by Wolff. Once a phenylalanine-restricted diet was available, Bickel and colleagues (1953) demonstrated in patients with PKU that reducing dietary intake of phenylalanine resulted in reduced blood phenylalanine levels and was associated with improvement in outcomes.

Clinical experience with the special diet overcame the significant initial difficulties of determining how much phenylalanine was necessary in daily intake to allow normal growth and development without producing inadequate or excessive plasma phenylalanine levels. Clinicians worked out what would be now considered "acceptable blood phenylalanine levels" during ongoing monitoring. They determined necessary total daily nutritional content (which had to be individualized to allow for adequate growth) and it became clear that not all patients with hyperphenylalaninemia had classic PKU. Cooperation from several drug manufacturers was significant because they produced limited quantities of a very expensive formula, often at no cost to families. Further studies demonstrated that prevention of significant cognitive impairment required starting the phenylalanine dietary restrictions in the first few weeks of life of infants with PKU.

The need to identify newborns with hyperphenylalaninemia as neonates so that treatment could be initiated within 7–14 days of life resulted in one of the greatest achievements in modern pediatric medicine: screening for treatable diseases in newborns.

9.3.3 PKU: 1960s: Start of newborn screening and improvements in dietary therapy

In the early 1960s, the American Microbiologist Robert Guthrie (1916–1995) developed an inexpensive (yet sensitive) test for blood phenylalanine in newborn infants using heel stick drops of blood on filter paper. Trial screening programs quickly documented the feasibility of Dr. Guthrie's methodology in large numbers, with sufficient accuracy to identify newborns with elevated plasma phenylalanine. The rapid initiation of dietary therapy was proven to result in markedly improved outcomes in infants. As a result, newborn screening programs were rapidly mandated, and implemented within 5 years throughout the USA. Specialized metabolic disease programs (usually in a University Hospital setting) quickly emerged to care for these patients. From that point on, PKU was considered a treatable condition, with excellent outcomes in children receiving early and appropriate dietary management. Mental retardation in children born with classic PKU became a thing of the past. There are now many teens and adults, fully functional in society, who have classic PKU. The success of newborn screening and treatment programs for PKU prompted the addition of additional disorders screened for in newborns, most notably galactosemia and hypothyroidism, and then later the hemoglobinopathies.

9.3.4 PKU: Maternal PKU syndrome

An unexpected challenge was identified in the early 1960s for women with PKU: elevated phenylalanine levels were found to be teratogenic to the developing fetus (6). Mabry championed the "maternal PKU syndrome" to educate others about the findings of microcephaly, severe cognitive impairment, and congenital heart disease in children born to mothers with PKU untreated prior to and during the pregnancy. Unfortunately, the symptoms of maternal PKU have been observed even when the phenylalanine-restricted diet is reinitiated by the mother during the first and second trimesters of pregnancy. Current recommendations are for women with PKU to continue or reinitiate a strict phenylalanine restricted diet prior to conception and during the entire pregnancy to reduce the chance of having a child with maternal PKU syndrome.

9.3.5 PKU from 1965 to 2000: challenges in dietary treatment

Once diagnosis and dietary treatment for classic PKU were initiated, the next challenges rapidly became apparent. This diet was extremely difficult for parents and patients to comply with once the child was past 12 months of age, when they would normally advance to "real" foods. The "medical food" did not taste good. This led to the inevitable question: how long does a patient with classic PKU have to stay on the diet? Initially, it was felt that the diet needed to continue only as long as the brain was continuing to grow (until the age of ~5 or 6 years). Many patients were taken off of dietary restrictions completely or were prescribed a diet with a milder dietary restriction of phenylalanine. Continued monitoring of classic PKU patients demonstrated that patients taken off dietary restrictions after age 5–6 years demonstrated lower intelligence quotient (IQ) results than those who remained on dietary restrictions. Nyhan observed behavioral problems which could impact school and life issues, even in individuals with normal IQs who were treated appropriately since infancy (9). Dietary restrictions for classic PKU have been the mainstay of treatment (especially in infants and young children). However, Metabolic Centers have found that many patients cannot comply with severe dietary restrictions, and want to eat more "natural" foods. Efforts to find ways to allow for more protein intake, and a more normal lifestyle have been ongoing, but the "best" outcomes from cognitive and behavioral perspectives have occurred in patients with blood phenylalanine levels maintained within a recommended range.

9.3.6 PKU in 2007: cofactor therapy with BH4 in classic PKU and hyperphenylalaninemia

Recently, cofactor therapy with BH4 has been shown to significantly improve the activity of PAH in ≥30% of hyperphenylalaninemia patients. They are currently challenged with BH4 to see if they respond to the cofactor. If they respond with an improved tolerance of phenylalanine intake, oral BH4 supplementation can allow significant liberalization of the dietary phenylalanine intake, with acceptable blood phenylalanine levels. Current challenges with BH4 supplementation include the high cost of the medication.

9.4 Advances in the diagnosis and therapies of IEM

As a diverse group of disorders, IEM are not rare, especially to physicians specializing in metabolic diseases and intensive care. However, individual diseases may be rare. Each disorder has evolved individually with respect to identification as a distinct disease entity, recognition of phenotypic variability, enzymatic and/or molecular documentation of the abnormalities leading to the disease state, and treatment options. References are provided which can provide clinical details about individual diseases and current treatment options. Identification of treatable IEM has been dramatically increased in the past decade as implementation of Expanded Metabolic Screening has unfolded throughout the USA and the world.

9.4.1 2000 to 2006: Expanded Metabolic Screening of newborns

Using newer technologies, including tandem mass spectroscopy, Expanded Metabolic Screening has been mandated in all states of the USA, and is currently being implemented throughout the world. Expanded Metabolic Screening technology greatly increases the capabilities to identify many treatable IEM, including many organic acid disorders and fatty acid oxidation defects. Early identification and treatment often prior to an episode of acute illness can dramatically improve outcomes. Many disorders are under investigation to be added to the list of disorders identifiable by Expanded Newborn Screening.

9.4.2 Metabolic diseases are invariably hereditary

Most frequent: autosomal recessive

Most metabolic diseases (particularly those in which the pathologic abnormality is an enzyme deficiency) are autosomal recessive. This means that siblings, male and female, are also at risk to have the disease. The risk to each pregnancy to the same parentsis 25%. This is particularly important in disorders in which children have not been exposed to a catabolic fasting state such as the fatty acid oxidation disorders. Timely evaluation of siblings in autosomal recessive disorders may identify a pre-symptomatic individual, thereby allowing appropriate treatment. Provision of clinical and molecular genetic diagnoses and appropriate professional genetic counseling allows additional options which parents and family members can utilize.

Also possible: X-linked and other forms of inheritance

There are clear examples of metabolic diseases that are X-linked recessive, such as the E1 subunit of pyruvate dehydrogenase complex. In some cases, depending upon lionization, females can demonstrate expression. Pedigree analysis can be invaluable in assessing these cases, and further investigations to determine whether the case is *de novo* or potentially familial are important aspectsin evaluation of the child and family.

Rare, but highly hereditary: disorders of energy metabolism and mtDNA

Mitochondrial diseases, particularly disorders such as MELAS where the underlying abnormality is a point mutation in mtDNA, can be highly hereditary. In a family with a point mutation in mtDNA, the "carrier" mother will pass on the mutation to all offspring because it is cytoplasmically inherited. However, the percentage of abnormal mtDNA compared with "wild-type" DNA in each patient will be best correlated with the development of symptoms. Providing accurate clinical and molecular genetic diagnosis as well as prognostic and genetic counseling for such cases is challenging. The forefront of our understanding of disorders of energy metabolism is that many cases involve abnormalities of nuclear DNA genes. An example would be mtDNA depletion. Thus, careful investigations into the underlying etiology are necessary to determine an accurate diagnosis, prognosis, and the provision of accurate genetic counseling to family members.

9.5 Treatment teams

Management of IEM has traditionally been the domain of physicians with pediatric, genetic, biochemical genetic and/or endocrine training. Board certification is now possible for physicians in laboratory expertise and medical management of IEM. In the USA, doctoral-level board certification is provided through the American Board of Medical Genetics. Currently, in addition to physicians with specialized training in genetics and metabolism, Metabolic Centers now include a complete team containing Metabolic/Genetic Physicians, Metabolic Dieticians, Metabolic Laboratory Scientists, Newborn Screening Coordinators, Metabolic Nurses, Metabolic Genetic Counselors and Metabolic/Genetic Assistants working together to provide care, education and support to patients with IEM, their families, and colleagues in the medical community.

9.6 Pediatric patients are surviving and thriving

More patients with IEM are surviving childhood, often with markedly improved outcomes. As a result, Metabolic Centers increasingly have patients with various IEM who are now in their teens and adult age groups. The normal developmental stages for teenagers (especially those who seek more independence) can dramatically impact dietary management, and can be quite challenging. Metabolic Team Specialists now have additional challenges as patients seek normal teen and adult experiences and responsibilities. Patients with IEM are now a part of the growing group of subjects with complex diseases who have survived the pediatric age group to adulthood. In these ages they now need clinicians familiar with the specific metabolic disease, and also the usual problems facing teen and adult age groups. The diagnosis and treatment of adolescents and adults by clinicians familiar with metabolic disease and adolescent and adult medicine (as well as other specialties) is one of the new frontiers of genetic and metabolic disease. With new diagnostic capabilities and education, more individuals are being diagnosed with IEM for the first time in adolescence and adulthood. Many may have more residual enzyme activity, and thus become symptomatic at an older age. Thus, an adult may be diagnosed with a disease that is thought to primarily present in childhood, particularly if they were born prior to the advent of Expanded Newborn Screening.

Additional challenges are occurring when patients with metabolic diseases, particularly women, have their own children. Incorporating pre-conceptual and pregnancy treatment to the regimen for pregnant (or soon to be pregnant) patients with IEM can dramatically decrease the potential for harm due to the teratogenic aspects of abnormal maternal metabolism on an unborn baby. The provision of genetic evaluation and counseling can provide individuals with IEM with appropriate knowledge and options for having healthy families.

9.7 Advances in diagnosis and treatment are ongoing

- Expanded Newborn Screening with advanced technologies designed to identify many treatable IEM is now available in all 50 states of the USA. Screening is coupled with coordinated programs to provide definitive diagnoses and early treatment.
- Educational programs within Medical School and Residency programs are providing additional training in the underlying biochemical pathways, diagnosis and management of IEM.
- A coordinated educational effort by Medical and Biochemical Geneticists has resulted in readily accessible online emergency care guidelines for the acute stabilization and emergency management of patient with IEM.
- Laboratory scientists and clinicians specially trained in the diagnosis and management of IEM provide investigation of patient samples, providing access to definitive diagnosis.
- Several excellent textbooks are now available with easily understood information about IEM.
- Research into the etiology, diagnosis, and treatment of IEM is ongoing.

Thus, survival of patients with IEM into adolescence and adulthood, and the recognition of IEM in the older patient groups is going to be increasingly common.

9.7.1 Treatment strategies in IEM

A greater understanding of the mechanisms which result in the specific diseases has led to improved treatments of the acute and chronic aspects of IEM. Current treatment options for IEMare shown below.

- Metabolite-altering nutritional therapy
  - reduction in "offending" amino acids or substrates
  - supplementation of a necessary product not produced due to thedisease
  - supplementation with cofactors (often vitamins) to alleviate effects of abnormal cofactor binding or lack of production
  - examples of diseases amenable to nutritional therapy include: PKU, maple syrup urine disease, homocystinuria, tyrosinemia, lysinuric protein intolerance, urea cycle disorders, proprionic acidemia, methylmalonic academia and many organic acidurias, galactosemia and hereditary fructose intolerance

- Medications to stimulate alternative pathways, for example, betaine in homocystinuria
- Detoxifying medications
  - these agents convert toxic metabolites to non-toxic, readily excretable compounds. For example, carnitine is useful in many IEM, including several organic acidurias, glutaric aciduria and MCAD. Benzoate and phenylacetate are extremely useful in the acute management ofpatients with urea cycle disorders with hyperammonemia
- "Chaperone" therapy
  - this is one of the newest categories of treatment in IEM. Medications increase the residual activity of an enzyme, and may have wide utilization in IEM.
    - BH4 therapy in hyperphenylalaninemic patients
    - Chaperone therapy for neuronopathic lysosomal diseases is currently being investigated. In neuronopathic diseases, some chaperone medications have been shown to enter the brain through the blood–brain barrier. Disorders that may be amenable to this type of treatment include the neuronopathic disorders GM1 gangliosidosis, and Gaucher's disease, as well as other lysosomal storage diseases with central nervous system (CNS) involvement (11).
- Enzyme replacement therapy (ERT)
  - Provision of an active form of the enzyme missing in the patient currently via regular infusions. Enzyme replacement has successfully alleviated symptoms in part or all of the body. ERT is now available for: Hurler syndrome (mucopolysaccharidosis, type I), Hunter syndrome (Mucopolysaccharidosis, type II), Gaucher's disease, Fabry disease and Pompe disease
- Organ transplantation is possible in several disorders, including selected urea cycle disorders such as citrullinemia. Some genetic disorders are amenable to bone-marrow transplantation.
- Gene therapy designed to provide a functional gene and resulting gene product. This is a promising (but very challenging) area of treatment.

9.8 Rigors of maintaining treatment: compliance issues

Compliance with dietary therapy is an ongoing challenge. Some diseases are more difficult to treat than others. Using PKU as our prototype disorder, we wanted to outline an example of the issues in this area, and provide examples of strategies that may be more universally successful.

9.8.1 Dietary challenges in the management of PKU

New challenges in the management of PKU include achieving optimal growth, optimal nutritional status, optimal compliance and QoL of the patients (4). As clinicians, our goal should be to make sure each patient grows and develops normally with good health into adulthood.

Issues

- The PKU diet is very high in carbohydrate and fat. Careful monitoring by a Metabolic Dietitian can increase compliance with the diet prescription, which is

intended to maximize growth and development. It is important to ensure adequate intake of formula as well as essential fatty acids. New amino-acid formulas and low-phenylalanine peptides taste better and promote compliance. Large neutral amino acid (LNAA) therapy and BH4 therapy should also be optimized to provide the least restrictive diet possible (4).
- Nutritional complications such as osteoporosis and vitamin B12 deficiency.
- Pregnancy – adolescent girls with PKU and their guardians should be informed of the issue of maternal PKU syndrome to prevent the condition in offspring.
- Socioeconomic issues: most adult patients have felt that medical expense to continue dietary therapy is a significant economical burden, which often leads to withdrawal from the therapy.

Barriers to following diets for the adult with PKU

- Leaving home and having to be responsible for food preparation, obtaining medically modified low-protein foods and formula, and mailing in blood samples on filter paper for phenylalanine measurement (3).
- Maintaining a career and a social life while also complying with diet restrictions (3).
- Inadequate resources available specifically tailored to their needs (3).
- Poor organoleptic properties of the formula can affect compliance, especially if the patient has been off the diet for a period of time. Formula companies are continuously working on solutions for this. For example, there are various new products available that may improve compliance. There are convenient ready-to-use preparations that might be easier and less "noticeable" than powdered formulas. Palatability of formulas has also improved (4, 12).

Tips for improving outcomes in this population

Lifelong adherence to a low-phenylalanine diet is essential for improved cognitive, behavioral and health outcomes, so establishing phenylalanine tolerance as an adult is especially important. We need to assess phenylalanine tolerance in adults because it is likely to be changed from what they tolerated as children. We need to ensure adequate intake of phenylalanine to support protein synthesis and to prevent catabolism. The results of a recent study looking at the changing requirements for phenylalanine in the adult population suggest that phenylalanine tolerance may be affected by the body mass index (BMI) and change when individuals become overweight. Being male and having a lower BMI, consistent with a lower fat mass, were more predictive of a higher phenylalanine tolerance than genotype alone. Therefore, one strategy that can be used to improve outcomes in the adult population is to promote the increase and maintenance of fat-free mass and avoid accumulation of excess fat. Healthcare providers should prescribe and carefully monitor energy intake, physical activity and weight in PKU patients (7).

Some subjects in the study could increase their phenylalanine tolerance from the initial to final time point. Increased frequency of consumption of modified amino-acid formulas was the best single predictor of the extent to which subjects could increase their phenylalanine tolerance. Emphasis should be placed on spreading the formula intake throughout the day to prevent catabolism (7).

Ongoing communication with a metabolic dietitian can help improve compliance. The dietitian can act as a resource to educate and re-educate patients on various aspects of the diet, providing support and guidance that is crucial to long-term success. A dietitian can also help in the area of weight management (7).

Offering all possible treatment options that might make following the diet a little easier is recommended. For example, offering new formulas and phenylalanine-free peptides, BH4 trial, and LNAA therapy.

Glycomacropeptide is an intact, low-phenylalanine protein formed during cheese production. Used in place of synthetic amino acids, it can improve the palatability, variety, and convenience of the diet (12).

LNAA therapy blocks phenylalanine transport into the brain. Important for adults and adolescents who are off-diet or do not adhere to phenylalaninerestriction (4, 12).

BH4 therapy: some patients respond to a synthetic form of the PAH co-factor BH4. If patients respond, they may be able to increase their phenylalanine tolerance by 50–100% (4).

Offering guidance in a non-judgmental manner involvesrelating to the patient on their level. Starting with small changes and offering praise and encouragement for efforts to improve is the key.

9.9 Unique features of IEM that are helpful in the diagnosis and management of adolescents and adults

- A subclass of IEM, classified by Saudubray (10) as disorders of "intoxication" (e.g., fatty acid oxidation defects and disorders of organic acid metabolism), can be associated with acute, life-threatening episodes requiring intensive care. Recurring episodes strongly suggest this class of disorder. Some IEM, often the organic acidurias, fatty acid oxidation defects, lactic acidosis, and disorders associated with hyperammonemia, are associated with intermittent, severe episodes of acute illness, often requiring intensive care for supportive management. Prior knowledge of the specific diagnosis and effective early treatment usually results in significantly reduced morbidity and mortality. Once diagnosed, patients with these disorders can have additional episodes. Definitive treatment early in an episode can, in some cases, prevent the need for hospitalization. Care, coordinated between Metabolic Physicians, Primary Care Physiciansand Emergency Physicians combined with education of the family in the early recognition of symptoms and prompt initial management of acute episodes, can dramatically improve outcomes.
- IEM can present at any age. Classic IEM are often associated with deficient activity of a key enzyme. Most of the very severe cases involve younger patients who have absent or severely deficient enzyme activity. Milder cases of the same disease usually have some residual enzyme activity. Age at presentation can be later (occasionally much later), including into the adult age groups. Adults with the same disease and enzyme abnormality, but higher residual enzyme activity, might present with a very different phenotype than that seen in infancy, including neurological and/or psychiatric disease.
- "Mild" cases of certain metabolic diseases can be life-threatening in certain circumstances, especially with a serious intercurrent illness, in all age groups.

Children with IEM, most notably those that give rise to intoxication, can be followed for years, with a history of seemingly mild metabolic disease. However, under certain circumstances, they can present as a life-threatening acute illness, and this illness can occur at any age. In children with IEM with residual enzymatic activity, acute metabolic crisis usually occurs in conjunction with an intercurrent illness, such as varicella. For children born prior to the implementation of Expanded Metabolic Screening, they may be completely unrecognized as having an IEM. However, with a significant intercurrent illness, the disease process can be life-threatening. If, a catabolic state ensuesduring hospitalization or prior to evaluation, severe metabolic decomposition can rapidly occur. Delay in recognition of the underlying metabolic disease as a separate diagnosis from the intercurrent illness results in delayed definitive treatment and poorer outcomes. One clue to the underlying diagnosis of an IEM is recurrent acute episodes of illness, or unexpected setbacks in the face of prolonged intravenous therapy. Crises associated with catabolism are extremely suggestive of an underlying metabolic diagnosis. Treatments are becoming increasingly available, so it is important to keep IEM in the differential diagnosis of acutely ill children.

- The age at presentation can influence the phenotype of the disease. Some metabolic diseases present more commonly in adolescence or adulthood, or have a different presentation depending upon the age of onset of the symptoms.

  The classic age of presentation of the mtDNA disorder known as MELAS is mid-childhood, and usually includes seizures and strokes. However, family members with the same mutation but who have a smaller percentage of the mutation ("heteroplasmy"), can present at any age and with very different phenotypes including, among other problems, renal failure, migraines, and symptoms suggestive of fibromyalgia. In our experience, analyses of the extended family pedigree has been extremely helpful in identifying individuals with this disease.

  Wilson's disease (an autosomal recessive disorder of abnormal copper deposition in tissues with deficient ceruloplasmin) can present between childhood years through to adulthood. The classic phenotype usually includes neurologic disease, liver disease or both. There are two typical neurologic presentations. The dystonic form is more frequent in children, and the pseudosclerotic form (characterized largely by tremors) is more common in adults. However, the frequency of neurologic disease is higher in adults (40%), than in children (28%) (9). The phenotype of Wilson's disease is highly variable, and is quite challenging for diagnosticians. Children can present with anemia and liver disease, whereas adults often present with hepatitis, cirrhosis, neurologic disease, and occasionally psychiatric disease. Helpful diagnostic clues are the finding of a Kayser–Fleischer ring in the limbus area of the cornea, and also a sibling with similar or related symptoms. The common feature in all patients with Wilson's disease is abnormal copper deposition and low ceruloplasmin in blood. Effective treatment is available.

9.10 Conclusion

We have provided a brief overview of the broad group of disorders known as IEM. Improved identification and definitive diagnosis, combined with ongoing efforts to maximize treatment options, has resulted in increased survival and reduced morbidity of IEM patients. As a result, patients with IEM are surviving into the teen years and adulthood. We expect this trend to continue, with the provision of care, hopefully well into the geriatric age groups.

Acknowledgements

We thank our colleague C. Charlton Mabry, M. D. for his lifelong commitment to patients with IEM and his seminal work on maternal PKU.

References

1. American College of Medical Genetics. ACT sheets and confirmatory algorithms. Accessed 2010 Jun 05. URL: http://www. acmg. net//AM/Template. cfm?Section=Terms_and_Conditions&termsreturnurl=Section%3DACT%5FSheets%5Fand%5FConfirmatory%5FAlgorithms%26Template%3D%2FCM%2FHTMLDisplay%2Ecfm%26ContentID%3D5661
2. Desnick, R. J., editor. (1991) Treatment of genetic diseases. New York, USA: Churchill Livingstone, p. 331.
3. Durham-Shearer, S. J., Judd, P. A., Whelan, K., Thomas, J. E. (2008) Knowledge, compliance and serum phenylalanine concentrations in adolescents and adults with phenylketonuria and the effect of a patient-focused educational resource. J. Hum. Nutr. Diet 21:474–485.
4. Giovannini, M., Verduci, E., Salvatici, E., Fiori, L., Riva, E. (2007) Phenylketonuria: dietary and therapeutic challenges. J. Inherit. Metab. Dis. 30:145–152.
5. Hoffmann, G. F., Nyhan, W. L., Zschocke, J., Kahler, S. G., Myatepek, E. (2002) Inherited metabolic diseases. Philadelphia, USA: Lippincott Williams Wilkins.
6. Mabry, C. C., Denniston, J. C., Nelson, T. L., Son, C. D. (1963) Maternal phenylketonuria: a cause of mental retardation in children without the metabolic defect. New Engl. J. Med. 269:1404–1408.
7. MacLeod, E. L., Gleason, S. T., van Calcar, S. C., Ney, D. M. (2009) Reassessment of phenylalanine tolerance in adults with phenylketonuria is needed as body mass changes. Mol. Genet. Metabol. 98:331–337.
8. Martins, A. M. (1999) Inborn errors of metabolism: a clinical overview. Sao Paulo Med. 117:251–265.
9. Nyhan, W. L., Barshop, B. A., Ozand, P. T. (2005) Atlas of metabolic diseases, 2nd ed. London, UK: Hodder Arnold.
10. Saudubray, J. M., Sedel, F., Walter, J. H. (2006) Clinical approach to treatable inborn metabolic diseases. J. Inherit. Metab. Dis. 29:261–274.
11. Suzuki, Y., Ogawa, S., Sakakibara, Y. (2009) Chaperone therapy for neuronopathic lysosomal diseases: competitive inhibitors as chemical chaperones for enhancement of mutant enzyme activities. Perspect. Medicinal Med. 3:7–19.
12. Van Calcar, S. C., MacLeod, E. L., Gleason, S. T., Etzel, M. R., Clayton, M. K., Wolff, J. A. et al. (2009) Improved nutritional management of phenylketonuria by using a diet containing glycomacropeptide compared with amino acids. Am. J. Clin. Nutr. 89:1068–1077.

10 Grownups who had kidney disease in childhood

Aftab S. Chishti and Stefan G. Kiessling

A young adult male who recently turned 21 years of age has been followed by a group of Pediatric Kidney Specialists since birth because he was born with a single dysplastic kidney. He progressed towards end-stage renal disease (ESRD) and started hemodialysis in a Pediatric Inpatient Center at the age of 19 years. Due to being significantly overweight, he is not a suitable candidate for renal transplant. He lives at home with his mother (who is his primary caregiver) and his brother. He dropped out of school before the age of 18 years and has currently no intention to finish High School. He has short stature because he refused daily GH injections in the past. During healthcare visits he has always been passive and his mother is making decisions for him. During the last several visits, he and the mother have requested initiation of transition into adult care because he feels it is now time. Patient and mother also start to ask questions about the adult implications of his chronic kidney disease (CKD). Chronic kidney disease in children is quite complex and the implications for adults living with advanced kidney disease since childhood are significant. Optimal care of the adult patient who has been affected by advanced kidney disease since childhood requires a solid understanding of three main domains with significant overlap: (i) the underlying type of kidney disease and the multiple effects that chronic kidney disease has on the body and mind of a child, (ii) the process of care transitioning from the pediatric to the adult environment and (iii) the physical and psychosocial effects of the disease on the adult patient.

10.1 Introduction

Advances in our understanding of renal disease and urinary tract disease, early recognition and improved technology (especially in all forms of renal replacement therapies have led to improved outcome of affected children. Since the 1970s, when the first pediatric kidney transplant was done, kidney transplantation has become routine. It is now the preferred treatment method for children with ESRD. As the medical and technical aspects of dialysis and transplantation have improved and survival of children with CKD and ESRD has increased over the last 25 years, concerns have risen regarding the impact of pediatric kidney disease on adult life in all aspects, including physical health, cognitive function and psychosocial consequences. As reported by Kramer et al. (1), these days we see an increasing number of young adults who started renal replacement therapy as a child. A growing number of studies and publications have tried to shed light on the effects of advanced childhood kidney disease on adults, and some have mentioned the possible detrimental effects of advanced kidney disease in childhood on cognition, educational attainment and employment in this patient population.

The exact incidence of CKD in children is unknown, but the prevalence is estimated to be 1.5–3 per million children < 16 years of age (2). The incidence of ESRD was recently reported to be 14.6 per million of total population for children between 0 years and 19 years of age with 1,245 children who started ESRD therapy in 2007 (3). The most common causes of CKD in adults are DM and hypertension, even though their origin may have been in childhood years because they do not seem to have effects on renal function until later in life. The current epidemic of obesity and DM in young children will result in escalation of the incidence of adult CKD.

Pediatric CKD management involves extensive attention to not only the medical aspects of renal disease but also toward physical and psychological growth and family dynamics. Even though renal transplantation (Rtx) is the ideal treatment option for children with ESRD, quite a few children are dialysed chronically for prolonged periods of time.

This review will discuss important aspects of CKD in children, the process of optimal transitioning into adult care, as well as the major implications of childhood kidney disease for the grownup individual.

10.2 Spectrum of kidney diseases in children

As briefly mentioned above, the etiologic factors leading to kidney disease in children are quite different from those seen in the adult population. Whereas acquired and sometimes preventable diseases such asDM and hypertension are leading causes of renal insufficiency in adults, congenital abnormalities of the urologic and nephrologic system (or acquired diseases for which there is no possible prevention) dominate in children. Understandably, the complexity of the disease can be quite high, and the approach of the healthcare team very different. As children undergo various vulnerable phases of their lives such as early infancy and puberty, their relationship with the team of healthcare providers becomes very close.

The North American Pediatric Renal Trials and Collaborative Study (NAPRTCS) was established in 1987 and is the largest registry of children in North America. It now includes > 15,000 children divided into three categories: chronic renal failure, dialysis, and RTx. The most recent report (published in 2006) shows that renal disease is divided into five major categories:

- Obstructive uropathy
- Renal aplasia, dysplasia or hypoplasia
- Reflux nephropathy
- Focal segmental glomerulosclerosis
- Polycystic kidney disease

CKD in childhood differs from adults in its etiology, management and possibly outcome. The typical etiologies include mainly congenital diseases of the kidney in younger children while they are acquired in young adults. The most common pediatric diseases leading to ESRD are aplasia/dysplasia/hypoplasia in 16% (M=F), obstructive uropathy in another 16% (M > F), focal segmental glomerulosclerosis (FSGS) in 12% and reflux accounts for 5% according to NAPRTCS data (4).

These categories comprise ~60% of all children with CKD. Other diagnoses include chronic or familial glomerulonephritis, hemolytic-uremic syndrome, or cystinosis, and each of those represent < 3% of the total number of enrolled children. The degree of complexity of renal disease varies depending on the time of diagnosis and the underlying etiology. Children with primary renal disease are mostly managed by a team led by the Pediatric Nephrologist, whereas patients with associated urologic abnormalities (e.g., posterior urethral valves) always require the expertise of a Pediatric Urologist to optimize care and outcomes, starting at the time of diagnosis until after successful renal transplantation. The NAPRTCS report from 2006 also showed a sex distribution of 64% male versus 36% female. This is mainly due to the increased incidence of obstructive uropathy in male children. Most children enrolled are Caucasian (61%) with 18.8% African–Americans and 13.7% of Hispanic background.

10.3 Physical health aspects of chronic kidney disease in the child

Just as the etiologies of CKD are very different between children and adults, so are the main clinical concerns that require focus of the Healthcare Team. These include the need for healthy, linear physical growth as well as optimization of neurocognitive development (5).

Several physical health aspects are associated with CKD in childhood. A recent publication by Fadrowski et al. (6) reported a parent-observed decline in physical health-related QoL in adolescents with progressive decrease in glomerular filtration rate. These physical health aspects include (but are not limited to) poor growth, abnormal bone health, hypertension and cardiovascular disease, and changes to physical appearance, including surgical scars and arteriovenous fistulas, for dialysis access.

Growth failure remains the hallmark and a challenging problem in the management of children with CKD. Despite significant advances in the therapeutic methods of CKD, > 50% of the children grow up to be short adults. Growth failure not only hampers social integration but is also associated with increased mortality. Growth failure is multifactorial, arising from renal dysfunction and specific disease-related comorbidities secondary to therapeutic methods and their untoward effects.

Thirty-six percent of patients interviewed in one study were found to be dissatisfied with their height in comparison with only 4% in age-matched healthy controls.

The effects of chronic anemia on physical health have been studied by several investigators. Anemia can affect different areas of physical health, including decreased participation in school activities and general activities (7). Children on dialysis seem to be more affected than Rtx recipients. Another important physical health aspect is the prevalence of cardiovascular disease in children with CKD. A recent comprehensive review by Mitsnefes (8) focused on the high prevalence of cardiovascular abnormalities in children with CKD; recommendations for identification of risk factors and treatment guidelines are provided.

10.4 Mental health aspects of chronic kidney disease in the child

There are multiple variables which factor in development and exacerbation of mental health problems. These include type and severity of the underlying disease, age of onset, methods of therapy and timing of their initiation, and disease-associated problems such as anemia, hypertension and cerebrovascular accidents. These might influence the final outcome in a child suffering from CKD from early life. Hence, a multidisciplinary approach is required to address these issues. In addition to Pediatric Nephrologists, it involves special attention from Psychiatrists, Psychologists, teachers, social workers, parents and family members.

Any insult to the developing brain may have far-reaching detrimental effects. About 20–25% of very young children with ESRD show general developmental delays, and neurodevelopmental impairments appear to be greater in more severe renal dysfunction. These developmental concerns appear to persist even after the transplant. School-age children with ESRD developing after pre-school years show a lower total, verbal and performance IQ in comparison with healthy controls or siblings. Among various therapeutics, RTx patients tend to have a more preserved IQ, especially for non-verbal activities, as compared with dialysis-dependent children. On the social and behavioural domain, young survivors of childhood ESRD have fewer friends, are less likely to participate in extracurricular activities, and are less likely to establish intimate relationships as compared with age-matched healthy peers. These young adults are more likely to be with their parents and tend not to have stable partners in their life.

In the later half of the 1990s, a Dutch study of the late physical, psychological and social effects of renal insufficiency in children (LERIC) showed that prolonged dialysis during childhood may negatively influence the ability to achieve highly skilled jobs. The unemployment level was double in such patients as compared with healthy people but fortunately these adults do better than if they develop ESRD as adults because having grown up with a chronic disease gives them a better chance of adaptability. The overall employment rate of young adults with childhood ESRD is ~67–73%, better that in patients with adult-onset ESRD (49–77%). Psychiatric diseases commonly reported in children with CKD include anxiety and depression. There has been no difference among various methods of therapy. Interestingly, adults with ESRD as children have been reported to have better mental health perceptions than if ESRD is acquired as an adult.

10.5 CKD: special implications related to the transitioning from pediatric to adult care

As in other subspecialties dealing with chronic disease, a particular area of interest in nephrology in the more recent past has been the complexity of the process of healthcare transitioning form the pediatric to the adult patient. To successfully accomplish transition, providers and families need to not only be familiar with different transitioning strategies but also with the impact of chronic disease, including the impact of renal disease on the course of life of young adult patients. Stam et al. (9) reported that young adults with chronic disease seem to achieve significantly fewer milestones or achieve them at an older age compared with controls. There is also less autonomy when compared with healthy peers. These are key issues that providers need to be familiar with as they make the transition into adult care, which is a complex task.

Unfortunately, very little outcome data are available to support a specific approach to transitioning. One approach, suggested by Watson and named PREP, focuses on four key areas and strongly recommends an individualized approach (10):

- Sufficient **p**reparation time before transfer
- **R**eassurance of young patients that they will be listened to
- Expressed **e**mpathy by new medical and nursing staff
- Support by **p**eers who have already made the transition

Successful transition requires a team approach, including the Pediatric and Adult Specialist, family and a patient who is ready to move to self-directed care (11). The process of transitioning is quite similar for different types of chronic disease, so specifics can be found in a separate chapter elsewhere in this book.

10.6 The adult patient with CKD as a child

With increased survival of children with CKD, focus has over the recent years been more and more on adult sequelae and outcome of pediatric renal disease rather than demographics. Most information that is currently available looks at adults who received dialysis, RTx or a combination of both during childhood. Very little information is available on the effects of CKD at stages when the primary treatment is by supplementation of medications. It appears intuitive that the outcome for adults who are treated primarily medically during childhood should be different from healthy controls but data are scarce. As for all children who live with chronic disease, children with CKD also need to learn that compliance with medications is key to successful outcome; they are often restricted in their diet and physical activity, and require frequent visits to healthcare providers. Once kidney function deteriorates enough to require renal replacement therapy or RTx, the issues become far more complex.

Even though pre-emptive RTx is frequently preferred given the better outcome compared with children who undergo dialysis treatment for prolonged periods of time, a significant fraction of children are on dialysis at the time they become adults. This can be due to various factors: RTx might not be an immediate option for children with no suitable live donor; prolonged waiting time for a deceased donor transplant; a recent history of graft loss; patients are medically or psychologically not ready for a transplant. This in turn can be related to several factors, including an insufficiently prepared urinary tract to accept a graft readiness or the inability to comply with the strict post-transplant immunosuppressive regimen.

As outlined by Kramer et al. (1), different structures of Pediatric and Adult Dialysis Units, new Healthcare Provider Teams with different approaches to patient care and expectations, and the expected increase in responsibility for the now adult patient can cause significant stress for the patient and their support system as they transition into adulthood. Even though the adult patient needs to be looked at as a whole, it makes sense, as before, to discuss the physical health aspects and psychosocial outcome separately.

10.7 Physical aspects of grownups with renal disease since childhood

There is overall very little but increasing information available on the overall physical health of adults with CKD. Rosenkranz et al. reported a sample of 39 patients with ESRD who were significantly less satisfied with their health compared with the general population (12). Bartosh et al. (13) reported concerns of hypertension, bone and joint symptoms, fractures, hypercholesterolemia and cataracts as results of a questionnaire given to adult patients who received a renal transplant in childhood. Also, nearly half of the patients had short stature and 27% were obese.

Short stature is a very important concern. A significant fraction of adults with childhood kidney disease would prefer to be taller as an adult and would even trade in years of expected life for an increase in stature (14). A report by Broyer et al. (15) found that the educational level, paid employment, marital life and independent living correlates with personal adult height in individuals who have received RTx in childhood.

Cardiovascular disease is a major cause of mortality of adult RTx recipients, with almost 50% of deaths in patients with functioning grafts being attributed to heart disease. The concerns about cardiovascular disease are significant, and heart disease continues to be a major concern in children with advanced renal disease who transition into adulthood. Data from the Australian and New Zealand Dialysis and Transplant Registry show a 10-year and 20-year survival prevalence of 78% and 66%, respectively, in individuals who developed ESRD before the age of 20 years. Forty-five percent of deaths could be attributed to cardiovascular disease, including cardiac arrest, cerebrovascular accident, myocardial ischemia and pulmonary edema (16).

Hypercholesterolemia, a well-known risk factor for ischemic heart disease, was found in > 50% of pediatric RTx recipients at a mean of 7.4 years post-transplantation (17). Though there are no concensus guidelines available on how often to monitor and when to treat hypercholesterolemia in this patient population, it is important for the provider team assuming care of the adult patient with a pediatric RTx to be aware of this issue. Bone and joint disease is common in children with advanced kidney disease and can significantly affect the adult health status as well.

Little is known about the adult effects of chronic anemia in children with advanced kidney disease. Guidelines on anemia management should be followed in children with CKD or undergoing dialysis therapy once transition into adulthood has occurred (18). Of interest is a recently observed increased incidence of anemia in children after RTx that adult providers need to be aware of (19).

Another very important physical health aspect is the occurrence of malignancies in adulthood because cancer is a well-known complication after solid-organ transplantation. The pattern of cancer in children with RTx is different from the general pediatric population and from adult RTx recipients. Post-transplant lymphoproliferative disorder (PTLD), a malignancy closely linked to the Epstein–Barr virus, is the most common neoplasm in pediatric transplant recipients, occurring in 1–10% of pediatric RTx recipients (20). Other cancers, some of them rare and known to occur later in adulthood, include Burkitt's and Hodgkin's lymphoma, renal papillary carcinoma, and skin cancer. A recent study by Kourkourgianni et al. has shown a cumulative incidence of cancer of 6.9% and 10.2% at 10 and 15 years after RTx (20). For the provider caring for adults who received RTx in childhood, it is very important to keep a high index of suspicion to allow early cancer detection.

Lastly, even though the overall incidence is low, providers need to be aware of post-transplant DM in pediatric RTx recipients because it has been shown to affect long-term patient survival and graft survival.

10.8 Psychosocial issues in adults with childhood-onset kidney disease

There are several areas of psychosocial adjustment that are important to discuss in adults who have kidney disease that started in childhood. These include cognition and intelligence, education, employment, social life and friendships as well as close partnerships. As discussed by Reynolds et al. (21), despite improvements in dialysis treatments and RTx with the associated increase in life expectancy, a normal state of health is never restored; providers taking care of this patient population need to always keep that in mind. Overall, RTx recipients seem to have a better psychosocial outcome when compared with dialysis patients (22). Impaired cognition is one of the major concerns of physicians treating children with CKD, so the long-term outcome in this area has been of interest for several researchers. In a study that involved 126 patients with the onset of ESRD between ages 0 years and 14 years in 1972 to 1992, Groothoff et al. found a lower educational level compared with the general population and the control group (23).

Kaerrfelt (24) interviewed 42 adults who received a RTx during childhood. School performance was nearly identical when compared with the general population but the unemployment prevalence was almost three-times higher in the transplant group (14% vs. 5.3%). Seventy-eight percent of patients who had functioning grafts considered themselves "well", 19% "neither ill nor well", and only 3% as "ill". The score for QoL (between 1 and 10) was encouragingly high: 8. Also, adult follow-up data from the Dutch LERIC study showed a statistically significant difference in the involuntary unemployment rate in adults independent of dialysis or transplant status in former children with ESRD (22). In the same study, adults with childhood ESRD were found to be living alone or with parents more often and were less often in marital relationships. It was concluded that this might be due to delays in autonomy development because parents sometimes develop a dominant pattern of interacting when they take care of a child with a significant chronic disease, as well as due to slower psycho-sexual development. Related to social life and friendship, Reynolds et al. (21) reported that renal patients were not concerned about lack of friends or social isolation but reported some limitation in this area when compared with healthy controls. In this study, twice as many healthy controls were married or cohabitating (48% vs. 24%) and significantly fewer adults with childhood renal disease had experience with close relationships when compared with a healthy control population.

10.9 Conclusions

CKD in children is quite complex and the implications for adults living with advanced kidney disease with childhood onset are significant. Optimal care of the adult patient who has been affected by advanced kidney disease since childhood requires a solid understanding of three main domains with significant overlap:

- The underlying type of kidney disease and the multiple effects that CKD has on the body and mind of a child
- The process of care transitioning from the pediatric to the adult environment
- The physical and psychosocial effects of the disease on the adult patient

Heightened awareness of the complexity of the transition of the pediatric to the adult patient and an increased focus on the needs of the adult patient are very important steps in improving physical, mental and socioeconomic outcome in grownups with childhood kidney disease. To do so, Pediatric and Adult Generalists and Specialists need to work as a team that is familiar with, and focuses on, the special needs of this patient population. As more children with advanced kidney disease survive into adulthood, it will be important to assess current practices and strategies related to the care process. It will also be important to continue to collect information on QoL, psychosocial status and physical health parameters to identify areas that require additional attention.

References

1. Kramer, A., Stel, V. S., Tizard, J., Verrina, E., Ronnholm, K., Palsson, R., et al. (2009) Characteristics and survival of young adults who started renal replacement therapy during childhood. Nephrol. Dial. Transplant 24:926–933.
2. Whyte, D. A., Fine, R. N. (2008) Chronic kidney disease in children. Pediatr. Rev. 29:335–341.
3. USRDS, Pediatric, ESRD. http://www. usrds. org/2009/pdf/V2_08_09. PDF.
4. North American Pediatric Renal Transplant Cooperative Study Annual Report. (2006) Renal transplantation, dialysis, chronic renal insufficiency. Rockville, USA: NAPRTCS.
5. Greenbaum, L. A., Warady, B. A., Furth, S. L. (2009) Current advances in chronic kidney disease in children: growth, cardiovascular, and neurocognitive risk factors. Semin. Nephrol 29:425–434.
6. Fadrowski, J., Cole, S. R., Hwang, W., Fiorenza, J., Weiss, R. A., Gerson, A., et al. (2006) Changes in physical and psychosocial functioning among adolescents with chronic kidney disease. Pediatr. Nephrol. (Berlin) 21:394–399.
7. Gerson, A., Hwang, W., Fiorenza, J., Barth, K., Kaskel, F., Weiss, L., et al. (2004) Anemia and health-related quality of life in adolescents with chronic kidney disease. Am. J. Kidney Dis. 44:1017–1023.
8. Mitsnefes, M. M. (2008) Cardiovascular complications of pediatric chronic kidney disease. Pediatr. Nephrol. (Berlin) 23:27–39.
9. Stam, H., Hartman, E. E., Deurloo, J. A., Groothoff, J., Grootenhuis, M. A. (2006) Young adult patients with a history of pediatric disease: impact on course of life and transition into adulthood. J. Adolesc. Health 39:4–13.
10. Watson, A. R. (2005) Problems and pitfalls of transition from paediatric to adult renal care. Pediatr. Nephrol. (Berlin) 20:113–117.
11. Ferris, M. E., Mahan, J. D. (2009) Pediatric chronic kidney disease and the process of health care transition. Semin. Nephrol. 29:435–444.
12. Rosenkranz, J., Reichwald-Klugger, E., Oh, J., Turzer, M., Mehls, O., Schaefer, F. (2005) Psychosocial rehabilitation and satisfaction with life in adults with childhood-onset of end-stage renal disease. Pediatr. Nephrol. (Berlin) 20:1288–1294.
13. Bartosh, S. M., Leverson, G., Robillard, D., Sollinger, H. W. (2003) Long-term outcomes in pediatric renal transplant recipients who survive into adulthood. Transplantation 76:1195–1200.
14. Busschbach, J. J., Rikken, B., Grobbee, D. E., De Charro, F. T., Wit, J. M. (1998)Quality of life in short adults. Horm. Res. 49:32–38.
15. Broyer, M., Le Bihan, C., Charbit, M., Guest, G., Tete, M. J., Gagnadoux, M. F., et al. (2004) Long-term social outcome of children after kidney transplantation. Transplantation 77:1033–1037.

16. McDonald, S. P., Craig, J. C. (2004) Long-term survival of children with end-stage renal disease. New Engl. J. Med. 350:2654–2662.
17. Sharma, A. K., Myers, T. A., Hunninghake, D. B., Matas, A. J., Kashtan, C. E. (1994) Hyperlipidemia in long-term survivors of pediatric renal transplantation. Clin. Transplant. 8(3 Pt. 1):252–257.
18. KDOQI Clinical Practice Guideline and Clinical Practice Recommendations for anemia in chronic kidney disease: 2007 update of hemoglobin target. Am. J. Kidney Dis. 50:471–530.
19. Mitsnefes, M. M., Subat-Dezulovic, M., Khoury, P. R., Goebel, J., Strife, C. F. (2005) Increasing incidence of post-kidney transplant anemia in children. Am. J. Transplant. 5:1713–1718.
20. Koukourgianni, F., Harambat, J., Ranchin, B., Euvrard, S., Bouvier, R., Liutkus, A., et al. (2009) Malignancy incidence after renal transplantation in children: a 20-year single centre experience. Nephrol. Dial. Transplant. 2010 Feb; 25(2):611–616. Epub 2009 Oct 10.
21. Reynolds, J. M., Morton, M. J., Garralda, M. E., Postlethwaite, R. J., Goh, D. (1993) Psychosocial adjustment of adult survivors of a paediatric dialysis and transplant programme. Arch. Dis. Child. 68:104–110.
22. Groothoff, J. W., Grootenhuis, M. A., Offringa, M., Stronks, K., Hutten, G. J., Heymans, H. S. (2005)Social consequences in adult life of end-stage renal disease in childhood. J. Pediatrics 146:512–517.
23. Groothoff, J. W., Grootenhuis, M., Dommerholt, A., Gruppen, M. P., Offringa, M., Heymans, H. S. (2002) Impaired cognition and schooling in adults with end stage renal disease since childhood. Arch. Dis. Child. 87:380–385.
24. Karrfelt, H. M., Berg, U. B. (2008) Long-term psychosocial outcome after renal transplantation during childhood. Pediatr. Transplant. 12:557–562.

11 Adult survivors of childhood cancer

Sherry Bayliffand Jeffrey A. Moscow

Approximately 80% of childhood cancer patients become survivors in need of long-term follow-up for the monitoring and management of residual and late-onset sequelae of their cancer diagnosis and its treatment. Late effects include any physical and/or psychological outcome that develops and/or persists beyond 5 years from the diagnosis of cancer. Childhood cancer survivors often have difficulty accepting their post-therapy health risks and their therapy-related physical and neurocognitive limitations. Parents have reported a consistently poorer health-related QoL for their childhood cancer survivor than population controls of the same age and sex. Though late effects are frequent and may be serious for the childhood cancer survivor, the implementation of risk-based care and the education of care providers in the early recognition of long-term sequelae offers opportunity for intervention and improved outcomes. Though the Pediatric Oncologist remains an integral part of the survivor's care plan, the Primary Care Physician is essential in the ongoing care of the survivor. Efforts to provide resources and educate all care providers remain an important part of the process.

11.1 Introduction

For childhood cancer survivors, "care" does not end with "cure". As summarized best by Aziz and Rowland (1): "cancer today is a curable disease for many and a chronic illness for most". Taken one step further, the definition of "survivor" includes all patients who have been diagnosed with cancer – from the "time of diagnosis through the balance of his or her life" (2). Approximately 80% of childhood cancer patients become survivors in need of long-term follow-up for the monitoring and management of residual and late-onset sequelae of their cancer diagnosis and its treatment (3). Late effects include any physical and/or psychological outcome that develops and/or persists beyond 5 years from the diagnosis of cancer (4).

Pediatric cancers differ when compared with adult cancers in their histopathologic subtypes, origin, incidence and treatment. In addition, treatment toxicities known from the adult cancer experience can be amplified by the developmental stage of the childhood cancer patient. Such distinctive characteristics, as well as young survivor age and expected longevity, lend to the many long-term sequelae that healthcare providers can recognize to ensure optimal healthcare delivery to the childhood cancer survivor.

Cancer is the second leading cause of death in adolescents and children in the USA, and is the number-one cause of death due to disease (5). It was estimated in 1997 that there were ~270,000 survivors of childhood cancer in the USA, and that 1 in 1,000 individuals was a childhood cancer survivor. The Surveillance, Epidemiology, and End Results (SEER) Registry of the National Institutes of Health predicted that, by the year 2010, 1 in every 250 adults would be a childhood cancer survivor. Considering that > 20.000 new childhood cancer diagnoses are made each year, ~80% of which are expected to survive 5 years from diagnosis and about 75% at 10 years, childhood cancer survivors are clearly becoming a growing adult population that will require specialize continued care (6).

The long-term sequelae that arise after childhood cancer therapy may appear 5, 10, and even 20 years after the completion of treatment. Of > 10,000 adult (mean age, 26.6 years) childhood cancer survivors who participated in the Childhood Cancer Survivor Study (CCSS), the largest most comprehensive cohort study of childhood cancer survivors, 73% were noted to have developed at least one chronic health problem by 40 years of age, > 40% of which would be categorized as severe, life-threatening, or fatal (8, 9). When compared with their sibling participants, survivors were 3.3-times as likely to have a chronic health condition of any grade and 4.9-times as likely to have two or more chronic health conditions. Increased riskcorrelated with treatment intensity and cancer diagnosis.

In addition, childhood cancer survivors were 8-times as likely as their sibling counterparts to have severe or life-threatening chronic conditions, especially in three apparently high-risk groups: bone tumors, CNS tumors, and Hodgkin's disease. Of greatest concern is that the incidence of chronic conditions increases over time and does not *plateau*, and that the intensity of childhood cancer treatment has gradually increased to provide improved treatment outcomes at the expense of a higher risk of long-term complications.

11.2 Hereditary considerations in cancer survivorship

With continued advances in cancer genetics research, it is now recognized that genetics, both constitutional (host-related hereditary) and acquired somatic (disease specific), play an important part in survivorship outcomes for childhood cancer survivors. Their impact may be noted at multiple points during the course of the cancer diagnosis. Such impact dictates outcomes related to cancer progression, death during induction, resistance to chemotherapy, relapse of disease, and even the risk for comorbidities and long-term adverse effects (10). The discussion of specific genetic influences on survivorship is not included here, though the potential effect of genetics on survivorship must be considered as a part of the "big" picturewhich includes not only the therapy utilized, but the unique characteristics of the host and his/her disease.

11.3 Comprehensive long-term follow-up care initiatives

Childhood cancer patients require the cooperative efforts of a large team of experts for the diagnosis and treatment of their disease, including Pediatric Oncologists, Surgeons, and Radiation Oncologists. Many others, however, provide insight and management recommendations that have significantly contributed to the advancement in childhood cancer survival rates by controlling therapy-related toxicity and comorbidities, including Cardiologists, Nephrologists, Endocrinologists, Nutritionists, Psychologists/Psychiatrists, and Geneticists. When therapy ends, it is through only the coordinated efforts of all of the above that the success of a "cure" can be sustained. After the completion of their cancer therapy and initial off-therapy observation period, most childhood cancer survivors continue their care not at their Cancer Center but with a primary care provider (11, 12). Most primary care providers lack the knowledge base needed to ensure optimal follow-up care for the childhood cancer survivor (12). In addition, most childhood cancer survivors lack the understanding of their previous therapy, and are unaware of their risks for late effects that may occur (13). For these reasons, a movement toward the provision of comprehensive long-term follow-up care has led to the development of multidisciplinary comprehensive long-term follow-up care programs and the utilization of "risk-based" care plans. Risk-based care of the childhood cancer survivor is intended to provide a systematic life-long plan for screening, surveillance, and prevention of late effects from cancer treatment. Categorization of risks is based on the cancer diagnosis itself, therapy received, genetic predispositions, lifestyle behaviors, and comorbidity (13–15).

There are many long-term follow-up care plan models that may be utilized when developing a risk-based care plan for childhood cancer survivors, the details of which are important here only in recognizing the role of the primary care provider within that care model (16). Most Each patient must have a comprehensive treatment summary that details the diagnosis (date, location, history of relapse), age at diagnosis, number of years from diagnosis and from the end of therapy, and treatment specifics (including surgical procedure utilized for the diagnosis and local control and associated morbidity, dosing and chemotherapy agents used, dosing of radiation and fields treated, and hematopoietic stem cell transplant specifics). A summary of other health complications that may have been present at the time of presentation or occurring during or after therapy – i.e., hypothyroidism, infections, graft-versus-host disease – is also extremely important. Ideally, this summary would be provided to survivors upon completion of their therapy or at the end of their initial off-therapy surveillance period. Utilizing this patient-specific treatment summary, a long-term follow-up plan may be created that defines expected long-term sequelae, the expected interval to their onset, and how best to monitor for their occurrence such that early detection and intervention may be optimized. Once a care plan has been established, most care providers, regardless of their training background, can provide continued care for the childhood cancer survivor.

11.4 Overview of adverse late effects as a function of therapy type

An important part of the evaluation of the childhood cancer survivor is the recognition of individual treatment exposures (i.e., surgery, chemotherapy, radiation) and their potential roles in the development of late effects. Appreciation of the multifactorial risk escalation of different cancer therapies as they relate to each other is extremely important. For instance, the neurocognitive sequelae associated with intrathecal chemotherapy for the treatment of acute lymphoid leukemias (ALLs) are significantly less than those in patients who also receive cranial irradiation because of the high-risk of CNS disease. Furthermore, it is important to recognize that each treatment method not only contributes to organ-specific adverse health effects, but that all the long-term sequelae combined have a significant impact on the childhood cancer survivor's QoL.

Late effects of surgery are related to local injury to tissue (17). Resection of bone tumors may result in functional abnormalities, physical deformities that may contribute to poor body image or other adverse psychological outcomes, and even chronic pain.

Surgical removal of abdominal and pelvic tumors may result in organ-specific damage such as an increased risk of infection after splenectomy, nutritional deficits after bowel surgery, and altered sexual maturation and/or function. A wide range of neurological deficits may arise after the resection of (or even biopsy of) brain tumors depending on their location (18). With careful preoperative imaging and planning, and the increasing utilization of laparoscopic procedures for cancer surgeries, reduction in potential late effects as they relate to surgery may be avoided.

Radiation is also utilized for local control in many childhood cancer treatment plans. Though similar to surgery in its ability to cause tissue-specific damage, radiation has the added adverse effect of potentially causing damage to DNA. Because of this latter effect, significant efforts to minimize radiation exposure and to "tailor" the delivery of radiation to a limited target area have evolved (17, 18). In each of the long-term sequelae sections that follow, the specific effects of radiation will be discussed.

Like radiation, several chemotherapy agents damage the DNA of normal cells as well as tumor cells. These agents are considered to be carcinogens and produce the risk of secondary malignancies. In addition, the late effects of tissue-specific toxicities can be exaggerated by exposure to these agents during early childhood development.

Hematopoietic stem cell transplant (SCT) survivors have what may loosely be considered a two-fold risk for long-term sequelae. However, in many cases, the long-term sequelae of SCT is only the intensification of some component of the initial diagnosis and the treatment methods used to induce remission and prepare for transplantation. Late effects associated with SCT will be discussed as they relate to each of the long-term sequelae, with additional information included if necessary. Please note, however, that a complete discussion of the late effects that may result after SCT is not appropriate for discussion in this forum.

11.5 Secondary malignancies

The overall prevalence of secondary malignancies in childhood cancer survivors is 12.6% within the first 25 years from diagnosis, and as high as 12–20% at 20 years after the end of therapy (17, 19, 20). Childhood cancer survivors have a 10–20-fold lifetime risk of developing a second cancer when compared with age-matched controls (4). Secondary malignancies are surpassed only by recurrence of the primary cancer as the leading cause of death in long-term survivors of childhood cancer. The development of secondary neoplasms is probably multifactorial and a result of interactions between host factors (genetics, immune function, hormonal status), primary cancer therapy, environmental exposures and lifestyle factors.

Acute myeloid leukemia (AML) is the most common therapy-associated leukemia, though ALLmay also occur. The association with a specific chemotherapy agent has been greatest with the alkylating agents (i.e., carboplatin, cisplatin, cyclophosphamide, busulfan, ifosfamide), though the extended usage of the topoisomerase II inhibitors (especially the epipodophyllo-toxin etoposide) is also associated with an increased risk of leukemia as a secondary malignancy (21). There is a delay to onset that may be as short as 2–3 years with the epipodophyllotoxins or even 5–10 years after alkylating agents, though the risk *plateaus* after 10 years (21–23). The cumulative risk of leukemia as a secondary cancer is ~1% at 20 years.

Whereas the risk of secondary leukemias after alkylating agents is dose-related, the risk associated with epipodophyllotoxins correlates with the intensity and schedule of dosing (and is further increased with unique chromosomal aberrations of chromosomes 11q23 and 21q22). Multimodal chemotherapy regimens, such as the mechlorethamine, oncovin, procarbazine, and prednisone (MOPP) regimen (historically used for the treatment of Hodgkin's lymphoma) have an increased risk of a secondary cancer as a late effect, and the risk increases with each additional course utilized. Furthermore, other treatment and host factors may also contribute, such as a history of splenectomy and/or radiation history in patients with Hodgkin's lymphoma treated with MOPP (22).

Almost always the onset of an acute leukemia is preceded by the development of myelodysplasia, therefore, follow-up of abnormal findings (i.e., macrocytosis, evolving cytopenias) on routine blood count with microscopic review is extremely important. Cytogenetic abnormalities (such as abnormalities associated with the long arm of chromosome 5 and/or 7) recognized in the peripheral blood or upon evaluation of bone marrow at the end of therapy may also increase the risk for development of a secondary leukemia. If present, serial bone marrow aspiration/biopsy may be useful in facilitating the early transition from myelodysplasia to acute leukemia.

Radiation therapy is associated with an increased risk of secondary leukemias, but the risk is significantly less than that associated with chemotherapy. This is in part related to the reverse association with dosein that increased risk is associated with low-dose radiation because higher doses of radiation result in cell death. The risk of secondary leukemias peaks 4–9 years after radiation (21). Though advances in the treatment of secondary leukemias continue, the prognosis remains extremely poor, and the treatment of choice is hematopoietic SCT.

Solid tumors as secondary malignancies in childhood cancer survivors are most often associated with a history of radiation therapy as a part of their primary treatment plan. The Childhood Cancer Survivors Study documented 108 sarcomas out of 751 secondary cancers reported by > 14,000 patients who self-reported their secondary cancers. This demonstrated a 9-fold higher incidence than that in the general population matched for age (24). Seventy-nine percent of patients who reported sarcomas as second neoplasms had received radiation, though only 56% received radiation to the primary site of the secondary sarcoma(24). The delay to onset peaks > 10 years after administration of radiation therapy, with a median of 7 years, and does not *plateau*.

Several factors are associated with an increase in the risk of secondary sarcomas: radiotherapy > 30 Gy; higher doses of anthracyclines or alkylating agents; having a primary diagnosis of soft-tissue sarcoma, bone tumor or Hodgkin's lymphoma; family history of cancer or genetic cancer predisposition syndrome (increases risk by 50%); or history of other secondary malignancies (24, 25). Benign and low-grade malignancies such as non-melanomatous skin cancer and meningiomas may also present as late sequelae of radiation therapy for the treatment of childhood cancers (19, 21).

Though risk data regarding chemotherapy and the development of second neoplasms are limited, it is recognized that the risk of bone sarcoma as a second neoplasm increases with the use of alkylating agents. This risk increases linearly as the cumulative dose increases. Furthermore, it is also apparent that the risk of second malignancies is greater if chemotherapy and radiation are used concomitantly instead of sequentially (19, 26).

Breast cancer is the most common secondary solid tumor in female survivors of Hodgkin's lymphoma. The use of radiation therapy in the treatment plan increases the prevalence by 10–20% at 20 years post-irradiation such that the cumulative incidence at 20–25 years post-radiation therapy is 35% (19, 27). An extended volume of radiation delivery, as in "T-mantle" radiation, greatly increases the risk and becomes excessive if the treatment delivery was prior to the age of 30 years. The risk of breast cancer as a secondary cancer is decreased, however, if prior treatment results in premature menopause (i.e., alkylating agents at higher cumulative doses and/or ovarian radiation > 5 Gy). The risk of secondary breast neoplasms begins to increase 8 years after radiation, which is often at a much younger age than the 40 years of age in the general population.

History-taking and physical examination remain the greatest tools for the detection of secondary neoplasms, with appropriate imaging only if new concerns arise. In women who have received mediastinal radiation, breast cancer screening is recommended 8 years after the completion of radiation therapy. Mammography is often difficult to interpret in young women because of the increased density of the breast tissue, so breast MRI may be considered for women < 30 years of age. Nearly 50% of malignant breast tumors were detected with palpation while patients were undergoing mammography screening (27–29), suggesting that mammography alone may not be sufficient for this childhood cancer survivor population.

11.6 Cardiopulmonary complications

The risk of cardiopulmonary complications is increased selectively in childhood cancer survivors (30). It is well recognized that certain chemotherapy agents are associated with adverse long-term cardiac effects, a result of subclinical injury that leads to significant morbidity as time progresses after the completion of cancer therapy (21, 30, 31). In addition to the alterations of cardiovascular structure and function that result from prior radiation and chemotherapy, factors that increase the risk for the development of cardiovascular late effects may also include GH deficiency, obesity, poor exercise habits (32). Pulmonary morbidity that is clinically significant often presents itself sooner, though it is limited to high-risk groups such as hematopoietic SCT survivors (21, 33).

Survivors of Hodgkin's lymphoma have an increased risk of heart disease that presents 5–10 years after primary cancer therapy and which increases over time. The association of anthracycline use and late-onset heart disease is well recognized. Though many chemotherapy agents may contribute to the development of early heart disease, the anthracyclines (doxorubicin, daunorubicin, epirubicin, and idarubicin) and high-dose cyclophosphamide have the greatest risk. This risk is cumulative dose-related (i.e., above certain cumulative dosing levels the risk of cardiotoxicity increases significantly). For example, a doxorubicin dose > 450 mg/m^2 result in a risk of cardiac disease of 5–11%. At doses > 400 and < 600 mg/m^2, the risk is nearly 23%. At doses > 800 mg/m^2 the risk is 100%. The appropriate conversion factor for different anthracyclines into "doxorubicin equivalent" cardiotoxic cumulative doses is controversial, but the concept is similar in that the risk of heart disease increases significantly as cumulative dose increases. Anthracycline-associated heart disease most often presents as a ventricular dysfunction (27), though this may be asymptomatic (i.e., evident on echocardiography only) in many patients (27, 34).

Chemotherapy-associated chronic pulmonary toxicity is rare. Bleomycin, nitrosurea, cyclophosphamide, cisplatinum, and methotrexate have been recognized as potential contributors to long-term pulmonary toxicity. Pulmonary adverse effects may present as pneumonitis or fibrosis (the most common adverse late pulmonary finding), acute hypersensitivity, or non-cardiogenic pulmonary edema. Again, the cumulative dose of chemotherapy is important. For example, there is a 10% increased risk of pulmonary fibrosis at cumulative doses of bleomycin > 400 U(4, 30). The risk of significant pneumonitis is increased with exposure to supplemental oxygen (i.e., after surgery or during scuba diving), especially if the exposure is within 12 months of bleomycin therapy (though may be as late as 2 years after therapy). Other factors that increase the risk of pulmonary fibrosis as a long-term sequela of bleomycin therapy include older age, smoking, renal dysfunction, infections, and mediastinal radiation.

Cardiopulmonary late effects after primary radiation therapy occur most often after mediastinal radiation. The primary form of cardiac toxicity after radiation presents as coronary artery disease (though pericarditis, ventricular dysfunction, and valvular disease may also occur). The risk of clinically significant cardiac disease in patients who have received radiation for the treatment of Hodgkin's disease was demonstrated to decrease as the patient agessuch that patients who are < 20 years of age have the greatest risk and patients > 50 years of age have no increased risk over that of the general population (30, 35). The development of pericarditis as a late effect of radiation therapy is between a few months and (uncommonly) several years, and most often resolves in little over 1 year. Only rarely will radiation-induced pericarditis progress to symptomatic constriction requiring surgical release. Cardiomyopathy as a late effect of mediastinal radiotherapy is most often mild and subclinical. At doses of < 25 Gy, subclinical cardiomyopathy may present; symptomatic myocardial dysfunction often will not present without doses of radiation > 60 Gy. Again, the combination of mediastinal radiation and anthracycline doses of < 300 mg/m^2 is additive, but does not seem to be clinically relevant with doses of radiation between 20 Gy and 40 Gy (30, 36). Valvular disease as a result of radiation therapy for the treatment of childhood cancers, while present on imaging, is rarely clinically significant. Abnormalities may present as early as 7 years after radiation therapy, though the incidence increases with time (especially for the aortic valve).

Radiation-induced pneumonitis occurs most frequently after radiotherapy for the treatment of lung cancer (risk, 5–15%). This risk increases with concomitant chemotherapy, prior history of lung irradiation, and corticosteroid therapy. The cumulative dose of radiation and higher daily fractions is associated with this risk increase. The risk is lower for Hodgkin's lymphoma (< 3%) and breast cancer (< 1%) survivors who receive radiation. Young age (< 3 years) at the time of radiation delivery is also associated with increased toxicity. This is probably secondary to the altered growth and maturation of alveoli, as well as impaired growth of the chest wall and lungs. Impaired production of surfactant due to damage of type-II pneumocytes also plays a part (4). Progressive alveolar septal fibrosis with collapsed alveoli and destruction of connective tissue is a late pulmonary sequela related to radiation therapy.

History-taking and physical examination are very important in the monitoring of cardiotoxicity as long-term sequelae for childhood cancer survivors. A review of systems should always include questions regarding shortness of breath, fatigue, exercise intolerance, and/or pedal edema. An intercurrent diagnostic history and clinical signs of congestive heart failure (sinus tachycardia, pleural effusions, an S3 gallop, hepatomegaly, and/or elevated jugular venous distension) are also indicative of a cardiac abnormality (37). Echocardiographyis recommended in patients who receive mediastinal radiation or anthracyclines approximately every 2–5 years, the frequency being dependent upon the age of exposure and the doses of both therapies. Fractional shortening of > 29% is considered normal. In patients with an increased BMI, radionuclide cardiac cineangiocardiography (MUGA) may be used to evaluate cardiac function. Left ventricular end-diastolic function (LVEF) is assessed by MUGA and > 55% are normal. Evidence that cardiac function is deteriorating includes a decrease in fractional shortening or LVEF of 10% of the previous measured value and/or fractional shortening < 29% or LVEF < 55% (4, 30). ECG findings are often late and non-specific, and may include sinus tachycardia, low voltage, poor R wave progression, non-specific T-wave changes, and prolonged QTc (≥0.45 s and is associated with doses of anthracyclines > 300 mg/m^2). Incidentally, female survivors of childhood cancer who received combined modality therapy, thoracic radiation doses > 30 Gy, or anthracycline doses > 300 mg/mg^2 should have echocardiography in the third trimester of pregnancy (when the associated increase in fluid load may induce cardiac dysfunction). Management of cardiac disease in the childhood cancer survivor is the same as that for cardiac disease due to any other etiology. Treatment-related cardiomyopathy is often progressive, and may be managed medically with ACE inhibitors, beta-blockers, and/or diuretics.

Symptoms of late pulmonary toxicity in the childhood cancer survivor include a history of shortness of breath, dyspnea with exertion, persistent cough, and/or recurrent pneumonia, and increase the suspicion of underlying pulmonary disease. Pulmonary function testing (PFT) is important in the assessment of suspected pulmonary disease, though PFT generally improves (but rarely normalizes) over time after mediastinal radiation and/or bleomycin therapy. Baseline PFT isdone 6–12 months after the completion of therapy, and is repeated usually at 2–5-year intervals if unremarkable at that time. If pulmonary abnormalities are found, PFT demonstrates a restrictive ventilatory defect with hypoxia, hypercapnia and evidence of chronic hyperventilation as measured by the diffusing capacity of the lung for carbon monoxide (D_LCO) test. The chest radiograph in patients with bleomycin toxicity may show interstitial pneumonitis with a reticular or nodular pattern, and CT can assess further alterations. Nuclear medicine scans (i.e., ventilation/perfusion (V/Q) scans and gallium scans) may also be used to assess alveolar blood flow and lung volume/ventilation data. If the differentiation of metastatic recurrence versus chronic fibrosis as a late effect is difficult, lung biopsy may be helpful. Increasing the awareness of survivors such that they decrease additional risk factors such as smoking is important. Corticosteroids, bronchodilators, expectorants, antibiotics, and supplemental oxygen may be used to manage symptoms but have no curative potential.

11.7 Endocrine complications

The most common endocrine abnormalities that occur in childhood cancer survivors are related to GH deficiency and thyroid dysfunction. These long-term effects may present as decreased linear growth (delayed or accelerated growth, growth failure, or short stature), abnormal musculoskeletal development and skeletal maturation, or signs and symptoms of thyroid disease. A history of radiation to the hypothalamic–pituitary–GH hormone axis or the musculoskeletal axis at a younger age imposes the greatest risk (4, 13) for abnormalities of growth and development. A history of radiation to the neck (or mantle irradiation for the treatment of Hodgkin's disease) imposes the greatest risk for thyroid abnormalities.

Growth failure may occur in the childhood cancer survivor without GH deficiency (i.e., after radiation at a young age to the linear skeleton or musculoskeletal structures). However, ifGH deficiency is detected, GH may be given. It is important to wait until the cancer survivor has been cancer-free for 1–2 years after the end of therapy, and that the risks related to its use are understood. GH supplementation may worsen the degree of scoliosis if present, induce reversible benign intracranial hypertension, and increase the risk of inducing a secondary cancer (though this hypothesis is controversial) (38, 39).

Hypothyroidism is the most common long-term sequela of radiation therapy delivered to the neck (40). Even with low-dose radiation the prevalence is 10–28%. Hypothyroidism as a late effect of radiation therapy may present as early as 5 years, and increases until 20 years, post-therapy. The prevalence is nearly 66% in survivors of Hodgkin's lymphoma who receive mantle irradiation. Doses > 20–30 Gy impose the greatest risk (4, 30). Screening for thyroid abnormalities begins with physical examination. A palpable thyroid is abnormal and warrants an ultrasonography and nuclear scanning for functional status. Ultrasonography serves to detect the location, number, and density of nodules. If a nodule is present, a biopsy is necessary. Screening for thyroid deficiency includes evaluation of thyroid-stimulating hormone (TSH) beginning 1 year after the end of therapy for the detection of subclinical hypothyroidism. If the TSH level is increased, free triiodothyronine (T3)/thyroxine (T4) should be sent. Hypothyroidism is managed with supplementation treatment. Papillary thyroid cancer is managed with total thyroidectomy, radioactive iodine, and/or TSH suppression with thyroxine.

Other endocrinopathies may occur, though infrequently, in the childhood cancer survivor. Adrenocortical deficiencies, gonadotropin deficiencies, and other hypothalamic–pituitary axis disturbances result due to direct damage to tissue from the tumor or surgery, doses of radiation > 30 Gy, but rarely as a result of prior chemotherapy exposure. It is important that suspicions for these late effects are further evaluated by Endocrinologists so they may be managed effectively (4, 30, 40).

11.8 Adverse outcomes in the CNS

Neurologic long-term sequelae are most significant for childhood brain tumor survivors, though survivors of ALL may also experience difficulties after their cancer therapy (30, 41). Neurocognitive dysfunction is associated with the greatest morbidity related to CNS late effects in childhood cancer survivors because of the impact it has on QoL. Brain tumor survivors are particularly susceptible to the adverse effects of therapy on intellectual function and emotional–social maturation (21). Female sex, age < 3 years, and increased time from treatment of childhood cancer with CNS-directed therapies have the greatest predisposition to cognitive deficits (8, 21, 42). Neuropathies, new-onset seizures that present during therapy, and even chronic fatigue may also be described as late effects (30, 41).

Radiation to the CNS results in several pathologic changes (damage to the vasculature, demyelination, damage to supporting tissue, and focal destruction of white matter) that ultimately lead to increased susceptibility to more damage by chemotherapy and abnormal functioning. There are four primary pathologic subtypes of CNS damage related to cancer therapy: leukoencephalopathy, mineralizing microangiopathy, subacute necrotizing leukoencephalopathy, and secondary brain tumors (4, 43).

Leukoencephalopathy may present as early as 4 months after cranial irradiation as new-onset seizures, ataxia, lethargy, slurred speech, spasticity, dysphagia, and confusion. A decrease in IQ scores and memory confusion may also be noted. Patients who received ALL therapy with intrathecal methotrexate, > 40 mg/m^2 weekly methotrexate, and 20 Gy of cranial radiation for treatment of CNS disease are at greatest risk. Imaging may demonstrate cerebral atrophy and hyperdensity of white matter on MRI. Subclinical leukoencephalopathy may be seen in up to 55–60% of patients who get CNS prophylaxis only (seen incidentally on CT/MRI but without clinical signs or symptoms). Mineralizing microangiopathy may present with seizures with associated electroencephalography(EEG) abnormalities, incoordination/gait disturbances, memory deficits, learning disorders, decreased IQ scores and behavioral problems. Presentation may be 10 months-to-several years post-CNS prophylaxis, though earlier presentation is associated with CNS radiation in combination with intrathecal and systemic methotrexate. Gray-matter changes in the area of the basal ganglia are most frequently seen on imaging as a result of calcium deposits in small blood vessels with occlusion of the lumen by debris.

Subacute necrotizing leukoencephalopathy presents as focal myelin necrosis on the posterior and/or lateral columns of the spinal cord after cranial or craniospinal irradiation in combination with intrathecal methotrexate. Brain tumors as a second malignancy are a greater risk for patients treated at a young age and with CNS radiation. ALL survivors with a history of CNS radiation for the treatment of CNS disease have a 1% risk of a secondary malignant brain tumor within 10 years after therapy if they were treated before the age of 5 years. Children < 6 years of age treated with CNS radiation have an increased risk of high-grade gliomas. Meningiomas may occur 10, even 20, years after CNS radiation in this age group.

Chemotherapy-associated CNS late effects are not well understood but appear to be related not only to damage of glial tissue and capillaries, but also to impaired functioning of neurotransmitters. The pathogenesis is the same as that seen in radiation-induced CNS damage. Intrathecal methotrexate and/or cytarabine and high-dose systemic methotrexate and/or cytarabine have the greatest incidence of adverse sequelae in the form of abnormal intellectual functioning. Despite this understanding, studies have recognized that survivors of childhood ALL who received chemotherapy only do not demonstrate adverse neurocognitive sequelae by 5 years after therapy (though a later onset may occur) (44). When found, deficits are mild and not significantly different from those of their healthy siblings. Other chemotherapy agents (e.g., 5 fluorouracil, ifosfamide, carmustine, cisplatin, vincristine, L-asparaginase, procarbazine) may also be associated with neurologic late effects such as encephalopathy, seizures, and neuropathies.

All patients who received cranial irradiation, intrathecal chemotherapy, and/or high-dose methotrexate therapy at < 10 years of age should have neurocognitive testing to evaluate for learning disabilities (4, 45). Ideally, all such patients should have been tested at baseline (i.e., within in the first several weeks after their diagnosis and start of therapy) and twice yearly during therapy. In reality, most patients that begin their long-term follow-up care have only been tested at the end of therapy. Hence, patients at high risk should have repeat testing at the time of transition to long-term follow up and every 2–3 years until early adulthood. Imaging for the detection of neurotoxic late effects was described previously because it relates to specific pathologic CNS damage.

Neurocognitive impairment in one or more areas occurs in ≤40% of childhood cancer survivors (8, 45). The areas most commonly affected include attention and concentration, processing speed, visual perceptual skills, executive function and memory (8, 45, 46). Recognition of dysfunction in these areas is important so that interventions may be put in place before global deficits lead to poor academic and job performance, and the psychological and emotional disorders that are associated with both. If abnormal neuropsychological findings are present on testing facilitated by the care provider they should be used to guide appropriate interventions (8, 47).

11.9 Reproduction and fertility

Multiple therapy methods for the treatment of childhood cancers may contribute to adverse reproductive late effects. The impact on fertility and preservation of sexual development is age-specific and sex-specific. Surgery may impact fertility by reducing the numbers of germ cells available (after surgical removal of one or both ovaries/testicles) or may result in sexual dysfunction (after pelvic surgery for both sexes). Chemotherapy and radiation have similar end results, though the risk differs based on sex and the time at which therapy is delivered. Though it would be ideal for most childhood cancer patients receiving therapy that may affect fertility, so that appropriate preventative efforts such as cryopreservation may be pursued, the reality is that many childhood cancer survivors are unaware of, or do not completely understand, their risks.

Ovarian function is preserved at much higher doses of alkylating agents in the pre-pubertal female versus the post-pubertal female because of an increased number of follicles (21, 48, 49). At standard combination chemotherapy doses, however, most females recover or retain ovarian function. For instance, females treated with 2.8–9.0 gm/m^2 of cyclophosphamide for Burkitt's lymphoma between the ages of 3 years and 17 years have a 1-year delay in menarche, but 94% have unimpaired fertility. In contrast, females who receive an increased cumulative dose of cyclophosphamide in preparative regimens for hematopoietic SCT have a substantial risk of acute ovarian failure and premature menopause (8). In patients who receive MOPP therapy for Hodgkin's lymphoma, age is a predictor of ovarian failure – teenagers maintain regular menses and women treated at ages > 30 years have a higher incidence of amenorrhea (risk increases as the number of cycles increases to 5–6 cycles). Though patients who have received chemotherapy alone for the treatment of germ cell tumors retain fertility, the combination of chemotherapy and abdominal or pelvic irradiation has a 30% cumulative incidence of non-surgical menopause (50).

Radiation to the pelvis in pre-pubertal females has a reduced risk of inducing ovarian failure and infertility, though it is dose-dependent. Pelvic radiation doses of > 20 Gy result in permanent ovarian failure for most females regardless of age, whereas doses of 20–30 Gy may only stall or delay pubertal development in the pre-pubertal female (8, 51).

Evaluation of the childhood cancer survivor who presents with primary or secondary amenorrhea includes bone age and ultrasonography of the ovaries. Laboratory testing includes assessment of thyroid function (TSH, FT3/FT4) as well as levels of dehydroepiandrosterone sulfate (DHEAS), testosterone, prolactin, FSH, luteinizing hormone(LH), and estradiol. An elevated FSH/LH will be seen in 95% of patients after craniospinal irradiation and involved field abdominal/pelvic irradiation. If evident, premature menopause may not always be treated in the post-pubertal female survivor because of the increased risk of breast cancer with progestin supplementation.

Boys are much more sensitive to the effects of alkylating agents on gonadal function. This effect is dose-related for chemotherapy and testicular radiation, but age and pubertal status have little impact because damage to germ cells is very common. Cyclophosphamide doses of 300–350 mg/kg result in sterility in boys and oligospermia/azoospermia in pre-pubertal/pubertal boys. MOPP therapy for Hodgkin's lymphoma results in 80–100% azoospermia after 5–6 cycles for pre-pubertal and adult males. Though 20% may recover 7 years after therapy, nearly 50% remain sterile (even after as few as 3 cycles). Radiation of the testes at 1–3 Gy is often associated with reversible decreases in spermatogenesis, but not at doses that exceed 3 Gy (regardless of age/pubertal status) (21, 52, 53). Because Leydig cell function is preserved after most therapies that affect fertility, testosterone production continues and the progression of puberty is unaffected. Increased cycles of MOPP therapy may be associated with Leydig cell damage for boys between 11 years and 16 years of age (4, 54). Signs of Leydig cell dysfunction may include gynecomastia, reduced testosterone levels, and increased levels of FSH/LH. Physical examination with Tanner staging is important in the assessment of boys with a history of childhood cancer therapy. Further assessment should include bone age and sperm count, morphology, and motility testing by fertility experts.

Importantly, for those patients who do not have impaired fertility, there are no adverse sequelae of childhood cancer therapy for their offspring (21, 55). No increase in the incidence of birth defects or adverse pregnancy outcomes is evident, unless there is a history of radiation to the uterus. However, radiation-induced vascular uterine insufficiency is associated with an increased risk of spontaneous abortions, neonatal death, low birth-weight infants, fetal malposition and premature labor (21, 56).

11.10 Other late effects

Genitourinary late effects as a result of treatment for childhood cancer are markedly reduced by implementation of limited cumulative dosing of cisplatinum and ifosfamide. These agents are known to cause hemorrhagic cystitis if given in high doses without protective mesna administration and hydration or concurrently with bladder irradiation. Acute tubular dysfunction may also occur after giving alkylating agents at high cumulative doses or radiation doses of 20–30 Gy to the kidneys. Nephrotic syndrome (Fanconi syndrome) is considered significant if the associated increase in excretion of potassium, phosphorus and magnesium leads to the following findings: glucose

< 150, urinary protein: creatinine < 0.2, phosphorus < 3.5 mg/dL, potassium < 3 mEq/L, bicarbonate < 17 mEq/L, and 1+ glycosuria. Hypophosphatemic rickets may result from a prolonged decrease of phosphorus after ifofamide therapy. Radiation of the pelvis in the treatment of rhabdomyosarcoma may also result in dribbling and nocturnal enuresis in 27–100% of patients (4).

Total body irradiation in preparation for hematopoietic SCT may be associated with a myriad of dose-related adverse ocular late effects (4). At doses > 50 Gy, neovascularity, glaucoma, atrophy of the iris, retinal infarction, exudates, hemorrhage, optic neuropathy, and decreased tearing and fibrosis of the lacrimal glands may occur. At doses of 40–50 Gy, ulceration, neovascularization, keratinization, and edema of the cornea may occur. Cataracts may develop after doses of radiation of only 10–15 Gy, or with corticosteroid therapy. The childhood cancer survivor should maintain regular health maintenance visits to the ophthalmologist at least every 1–2 years (and more frequently as clinically indicated).

Radiation-induced chronic otitis and sensorineural hearing loss may occur at doses to the middle ear of 40–50 Gy (4). Sensorineural hearing loss may also follow cisplatin chemotherapy and be further exacerbated by concomitant use of aminoglycosides (used for management of infection for many childhood cancer patients). Hearing evaluations are a part of any treatment regimen thought to be associated with an increased risk of hearing loss, and continued follow-up as directed by the Audiologistis important. If severe hearing loss occurs, cochlear implants have been useful in returning some element of hearing to the childhood cancer survivor.

Radiation-induced enteritis, fibrosis of the esophagus through the colon, and hepatitis fibrosis/cirrhosis may occur at doses > 40 Gy. This effect is intensified by the concurrent use of dactinomycin and/or doxorubicin. Hepatic effects are also increased by the use of methotrexate, 6-mercaptopurine, and 6-thioguanine. Early colorectal screening for patients who receive pelvic or abdominal radiation doses > 25 Gy is recommended starting 15 years after treatment or at age 35 years (whichever is later). Screening by fecal occult blood with/without sigmoidoscopy or colonoscopy is adequate (4, 21).

11.11 Psychosocial support

Childhood cancer survivors often have difficulty accepting their post-therapy health risks and their therapy-related physical and neurocognitive limitations. Parents report a consistently poorer health-related QoL for their childhood cancer survivor than population controls of the same age and sex (8, 21, 57). Seventeen percent of 9, 535 young adult survivors of childhood cancer in the Childhood Cancer Survivors Study had depressive, somatic, or anxiety symptoms (58). Ten percent reported moderate-to-extreme pain. With the development of long-term follow-up programs, education of the childhood survivor is increasingly more advanced. Utilization of health links specific to the survivor's diagnosis and treatment further provide educational materials. Finding appropriate psychosocial support for the childhood cancer survivor poses one of the greatest challenges for the healthcare provider.

Promoting self-care is essential in the care of childhood cancer survivors. Primary prevention of secondary cancers with the tools mentioned above in this chapter is important, but so is the importance of encouraging smoking cessation, alcohol abstinence, dietary modification, exercise and sunscreen use. By increasing awareness and providing access to screening, secondary prevention of cancer as a late effect is also provided. Though the focus has been on the late effects of cancer therapy, it is important to maintain routine health screening as well.

11.12 Future considerations

Though late effects are frequent and may be serious for the childhood cancer survivor, the implementation of risk-based care and the education of care providers in the early recognition of long-term sequelae offers opportunity for intervention and improved outcomes. Though the Pediatric Oncologist remains an integral part of the survivor's care plan, the Primary Care Physician is essential in the ongoing care of the survivor. Efforts to provide resources and educate all care providers remain an important part of the process.

11.13 Resources available to the healthcare provider

11.13.1 Clinical guidelines

- Children's Oncology Group long-term follow-up guidelines for survivors of childhood, adolescent, and young adult cancers. Children's Oncology Group Version 2.0, 2006.
- Available: www. survivorshipguidelines. org

11.13.2 Patient education materials

- Keene, N., Hobbie, W., Ruccione, K. (2007) Childhood cancer survivors: a practical guide to your future, 2nd ed. Sebastopol, USA: O'Reilly Media.
- Currently available free of charge to "needy" patients at the following Internet address: www. candlelighters. org/Book_Order_Form. pdf
- Children's Oncology Group Health Links, 2006
- Available: www. survivorshipguidelines. org

11.13.3 Textbooks and other publications

- Schwartz, C. L., Hobbie, W. L., Constine, L. S., Ruccione, K. S., eds. (2005) Survivorsof childhood and adolescent cancer: a multidisciplinary approach. Heidelberg, Germany: Springer.
- Wallace, W. H. B., Green, D. M., eds. (2004) Late effects of childhood cancer. London, UK: Arnold.
- Hewitt, M. E., Weiner, S. L., Simone, J. V., eds. (2003) Childhood cancer survivorship: improving care and quality of life. Washington, USA: National Academies Press.

References

1. Aziz, N. M., Rowland, J. H. (2003) Trends and advances in cancer survivorship research: challenge and opportunity. Semin. Rad. Onc. 13:248–266.
2. National Coalition for Cancer Survivorship. http://www. canceradvocacy. org.
3. Horner, M. J., Ries, L. A. G., Krapcho, M., Neyman, N., Aminou, R., Howlader, N., et al., eds. (2009) SEER Cancer Statistics Review, 1975–2006, National Cancer Institute. Bethesda, USA. Based on November 2008 SEER data submission, posted to the SEER website, http://seer. cancer. gov/csr/1975_2006/. Accessed 28 October 2009.
4. Lanzkowsky, P. (2005) Manual of pediatric hematology and oncology, 4th ed. New York, USA: Elsevier.
5. Jemal, A., Siegel, R., Ward, E. et al. (2006) Cancer statistics, 2006. CA Cancer J. Clin. 56:106–130.
6. Ries, L. A. G., Smith, M. A., Gurney, J. G., et al, eds. (1999) Cancer incidence and survival among children and adolescents: United States SEER Program 1975–1995. Bethesda, USA: National Cancer Institute.
7. Oeffinger, K. C., Mertens, A. C., Sklar, C. A., et al. (2006) Chronic health conditions in adult survivors of childhood cancer. N. Engl. J. Med. 355:1572–1582.
8. Oeffinger, K. C., Nathan, P. C., Kremer, C. M. (2008) Challenges after curative treatment for childhood cancer and long-term follow up of survivors. Pediatr. Clin. N. Am. 55:251–273.
9. Oeffinger, K. C., Mertens, A. C., Hudson, M. M., et al. (2004) Health care of young adult survivors of childhood cancer: a report from the Childhood Cancer Survivor Study. Ann. Fam. Med. 2:61–70.
10. Allan, J. M. (2008) The genetics of cancer survivorship. Hematol. Oncol. Clin. North Am. 22:257–269.
11. Oeffinger, K. C., Wallace, W. H. (2006) Barriers to follow-up care of survivors in the United States and the United Kingdom. Pediatr. Blood Cancer 46:135–142.
12. Kadan-Lottick, N. S, Robison, L. L., Gurney, J. G., et al. (2002) Childhood cancer survivors' knowledge about their past diagnosis and treatment: Childhood Cancer Survivor Study. JAMA 287:1832–1839.
13. Oeffinger, K. C., Hudson, M. M. (2004) Long-term complications following childhood and adolescent cancer: foundations for providing risk-based health care for survivors. CA Cancer J. Clin. 54:208–236.
14. Landier, W., Bhatia, S., Eshelman, D. A., et al. (2004) Development of risk-based guidelines for pediatric cancer survivors: The Children's Oncology Group long-term follow-up guidelines from the Children's Oncology Group Late Effects Committee and Nursing Discipline. J. Clin. Oncol. 22:4979–4990.
15. Hewitt, M., Weiner, S. L., Simone, J. V., eds. (2003) Childhood cancer survivorship: improving care and quality of life. Washington, USA: National Academies Press.
16. Landier, W., ed. (2007) Establishing and enhancing services for childhood cancer survivors: LTFU Program Resource Guide, 2007. http://www. survivorshipguidelines. org/pdf/LTFUResourceGuide. Accessed 28 Oct 2009.
17. Goldsby, R. E., Taggart, D. R., Ablin, A. R. (2006) Surviving childhood cancer: the impact on life. Pediatr. Drugs 8:71–84.
18. Pizzo, P. A., Poplack, D. G. (2002) Principles and practice of pediatric oncology, 4th ed. Philadelphia, USA: Lippincott Williams Wilkins.
19. Neglia, J. P., Friedman, D. L., Yasui, Y., et al. (2001) Second malignant neoplasms in five-year survivors of childhood cancer: childhood cancer survivor study. J. Natl. Cancer Inst. 93:618–629.

20. Robison, L. L., Mertens, A. (1993) Second tumors after treatment of childhood malignancies. Hematol. Oncol. Clin. North Am. 7:401–415.
21. Hudson, M. M. (2008) Survivors of childhood cancer: coming of age. Hematol. Oncol. Clin. North Am. 22:211–231.
22. Meadows, A. T., Obringer, A. C., Marrero, O., et al. (1989) Secondary malignant neoplasms following childhood Hodgkin's disease: treatment and splenectomy as risk factors. Med. Pediatr. Oncol. 17:477–484.
23. Smith, M. A., Rubinstein, L., Anderson, J. R., et al. (1999)Secondary leukemia or myelodysplastic syndrome after treatment with epipodophyllotoxins. J. Clin. Oncol. 17:569–577.
24. Henderson, T. O., Whitton, J., Stovall, M., et al. (2008) Secondary sarcomas in childhood cancer survivors: a report from the Childhood Cancer Survivor Study. J. Natl. Cancer Inst. 99:300–308.
25. Atwal GS, Rabadan R, Lozano G, Strong LC, Ruijs MWG, Schmidt MK, et al. (2008) An information-theoretic analysis of genetics, gender and age in cancer patients. PLoS ONE 3(4):e1951.
26. Guerin S, Guibout C, Shamsaldin A, et al. (2007) Concomitant chemo-radiotherapy and local dose of radiation as risk factors for second malignant neoplasms after solid cancer in childhood: A case-control study. Int. J. Cancer 120:96–102.
27. Hodgson, D. C. (2008) Hodgkin lymphoma: the follow-up of long-term survivors. Hematol. Oncol. Clin. North. Am. 22:233–244.
28. Lee, L., Pintilie, M., Hodgson, D. C., et al. (2008) Screening mammography for young women treated with supradiaphragmatic radiation for Hodgkin's lymphoma. Ann. Oncol. 19:62–67.
29. Diller, L., Medeiros Nancarrow, C., Shaffer, K, et al. (2002) Breast cancer screening in women previously treated for Hodgkin's disease: a prospective cohort study. J. Clin. Oncol. 20:2085–2091.
30. Yahalom, J., Portlock, C. S. (2008) Long-term cardiac and pulmonary complications of cancer therapy. Hematol. Oncol. Clin. North Am. 22:305–318.
31. Lipshultz, S. E., Lipsitz, S. R., Sallan, S. E., et al. (2005)Chronic progressive cardiac dysfunction years after doxorubicin therapy for childhood acute lymphoblastic leukemia. J. Clin. Oncol. 23:1629–1636.
32. Greving, D. M., Santacroce, S. J. (2005) Cardiovascular late effects. J. Pediatr. Oncol. Nurs. 22:38–47.
33. Gower, W. A., Collaco, J. M., Mogayzel, P. J., Jr. (2007) Pulmonary dysfunction in pediatric hematopoietic stem cell transplant patients: non-infectious and long-term complications. Pediatr Blood Cancer 49:140–147.
34. Krischer, J. P., Epstein, S., Cuthbertson, D. D., et al. (1997) Clinical cardiotoxicity following anthracycline treatment for childhood cancer: the pediatric oncology group experience. J. Clin. Oncol. 15:1544–1552.
35. Hancock, S. L., Tucker, M. A., Hoppe, R. T. (1993) Factors affecting late mortality from heart disease after treatment of Hodgkin's disease. JAMA 270(16):1949–1955.
36. Glanzmann, C., Huguenin, P., Lutolf, U. M., et al. (1994) Cardiac lesions after mediastinal irradiation for Hodgkin's disease. Radiother. Oncol. 30:43–54.
37. Adams, M. J., Lipsitz, S. R., Colan, S. D., et al. (2004) Cardiovascular status in long-term survivors of Hodgkin's disease treated with chest radiotherapy. J. Clin. Oncol. 22:3139–3148.
38. Fletcher, D. B. (1997) Effects of pediatric cancer therapy on the musculoskeletal system. Pediatr. Radiol. 27:623–636.
39. Rutter, M. M., Rose, S. R. (2007) Long-term endocrine sequelae of childhood cancer. Curr. Opin. Pediatr. 19:480–487.
40. Schmiegelow, M., Feldt-Rasmussen, U., Rasmussen, A. K., et al. (2003) Assessment of the hypothalamo-pituitary-adrenal axis I patients treated with radiotherapy and chemotherapy for childhood brain tumor. J. Clin. Endocrinol. Metab. 88:3149–3154.

41. Langeveld, N., Ubbink, M., Smets, E. (2000) 'I don't have any energy': the experience of fatigue in young adult survivors of childhood cancer. Eur. J. Oncol. Nurs. 4:20–28.
42. Waber, D. P., Tarbell, N. J., Kahn, C. M., et al. (1992) The relationship of sex and treatment modality to neuropsychologic outcome in childhood acute lymphoblastic leukemia. J. Clin. Oncol. 10:810–817.
43. Moore, I. M., Packer, R. J., Karl, D., et al. (1994) Adverse effects of cancer treatment on the central nervous system. In: Schwartz, C. I., Hobbie, W. L., Constine, L. S., Ruccione, K. S., editors. Survivors of Childhood Cancer: Assessment and Management. St. Louis, USA: Mosby, pp. 81–95.
44. Jansen, N. C. A. J., Kingma, A., Schuitema, A., et al. (2008) Neuropsychological outcome in chemotherapy-only-treated children with acute lymphoblastic leukemia. J. Clin. Oncol. 26:3025–3030.
45. Krull, K. R., Okcu, M. F., Potter, B., et al. (2008) Screening for neurocognitive impairment in pediatric long-term survivors. J. Clin. Oncol. 26:4138–4143.
46. Mulhern, R. K., Palmer, S. L. (2003) Neurocognitive late effects in pediatric cancer. Curr. Probl. Cancer 27:177–197.
47. Butler, R. W., Mulhern, R. K. (2005) Neurocognitive interventions for children and adolescents surviving cancer. J. Pediatr. Psychol. 30:65–78.
48. Muller, J. (2003) Impact of cancer therapy on the reproductive axis. Horm. Res. 1(Suppl. 59):12–20.
49. Thomson, A. B., Critchley, H. O., Kelnar, C. J., et al. (2002) Late reproductive sequelae following treatment of childhood cancer and options for fertility preservation. Best Pract. Res. Clin. Endocrinol. Metab. 16:311–314.
50. Sklar, C. A., Mertens, A. C., Mitby, P., et al. (2006) Premature menopause in survivors of childhood cancer: a report from the childhood cancer survivor study. J. Natl. Cancer Inst. 98:890–896.
51. Bath, L. E., Wallace, W. H., Critchley, H. O. (2002) Late effects of the treatment of childhood cancer on the female reproductive system and the potential for fertility preservation. BJOG 109:107–114.
52. Muller, J. (2003) Impact of cancer therapy on the reproductive axis. Horm. Res. 1(Suppl. 59):12–20.
53. Thomson, A. B., Critchley, H. O., Kelnar, C. J., et al. (2002) Late reproductive sequelae following treatment of childhood cancer and options for fertility preservation. Best Pract. Res. Clin. Endocrinol. Metab. 16:311–334.
54. Leventhal, B. G., Halperin, E. C., Torano, A. E. (1994) The testes. In: Schwartz, C. I., Hobbie, W. L., Constine, L. S., Ruccione, K. S., eds. Survivors of Childhood Cancer: Assessment and Management. St Louis, USA: Mosby, pp. 225–244.
55. Nagarajan, R., Robison, L. L. (2005) Pregnancy outcomes in survivors of childhood cancer. J. Natl. Cancer Inst. Monogr. 34:72–76.
56. Sinorello, L. B., Cohen, S. S., Bosetti, C., et al. (2006) Female survivors of childhood cancer: preterm birth and low birth weight among their children. J. Natl. Cancer Inst. 98:1453–1461.
57. Speechley, K. N., Barrera, M., Shaw, A. K., et al. (2006) Health-related quality of life among child and adolescent survivors of childhood cancer. J. Clin. Oncol. 24:2536–2543.
58. Hudson, M. M., Mertens, A. C., Yasui, Y., et al. (2003) Health status of adult long-term survivors of childhood and adolescent cancer: The Childhood Cancer Survivor Study. JAMA 290:1583–1592.

12 Adults with genetic syndromes

Jacqueline A. Noonan and Michelle A. Grenier

New problems may arise as patients with genetic syndromes age. This review will consider six of the more common genetic syndromes likely to survive to adulthood, and suggests appropriate management strategies. In this review we will consider multiple malformation syndromes that are relatively common, likely to survive to adulthood and able to live independently or with some supervision. We will limit our discussion to four chromosomal malformations and two dominantly inherited disorders due to gene mutations.

12.1 Introduction

In this review we will consider multiple malformation syndromes that are relatively common, likely to survive to adulthood and able to live or with modest supervision independently. We will limit our discussion to four chromosomal malformations and two dominantly inherited disorders due to gene mutations.

12.2 Velo-cardio facial syndrome: deletion of chromosome 22q11.2

Velo-cardio facial syndrome (VCFC) is due to a heterozygous deletion of chromosome 22q11.2. This syndrome was considered to be at least three district syndromes because of the very wide clinical findings that encompass this condition and which include Di George syndrome, cono-truncal anomaly face syndrome and VCFS (1, 2). In 1992, a deletion of chromosome 22q11.2 was found to be present in all three syndromes. The DNA procedure fluorescent *in situ* hybridization (FISH) a allows a definitive diagnosis to be made.

The incidence of this syndrome is estimated between 1:2,000 and 1:7,000. About 70% have congenital heart disease involving cono-truncal and aortic arch defects. Among infants with an interrupted aortic arch, more than half will have the deletion; nearly half of cases will have truncus anteriosus. More than 15% of newborns with tetralogy of Fallot and about one-third of posterior malalignment VSDs are also affected. Newborns with these correlations are frequently screened at birth using FISH analyses. VCFC is also common among individuals with palatal anomalies (especially submucous cleft palate) and the often unrecognized occult submucous cleft palate. These conditions lead to hypernasal speech in affected individuals. A pharyngoplasty is recommended if there is moderate or severe hypernasal resonance and/or nasal escape. Major vascular anomalies (including abnormal placement of carotid, vertebral, chest and brain arteries) may become a potential risk if palatal surgery is required (3).

Some affected individuals have a characteristic facial appearance which may include narrow palpebral fissures, small mouth, hypoplastic mandible and a square-appearing nose due to hypoplastic ala nasi. The facial appearance is most pronounced during childhood but is more subtle in the newborn and in adults.

Deletion of chromosome 22q is frequently associated with hypoparathyroidism due to congenital agenesis on hypoplasia of the parathyroid glands. Hypocalcemia frequently occurs in infancy but often resolves. About 70% of patients with VCFC have some degree of hypocalcemia. Hypocalcemia which resolves in infancy may recur later in life. There are several reports of hypocalcemia presenting with seizure in adults with VCFC as the first manifestation of the syndrome (4, 5). Hypoparathyroidism may become manifest later in life, so regular and continuous monitoring of serum calcium and parathyroid status is warranted.

Mal-development of the thymus may rarely result in severe T-cell immunodeficiency in infancy. In many others, T-cell counts in the peripheral blood diminish over time, leading to recurrent infections. Most patients, however, generate an adequate antibody response to allow the usual immunizations.

Most individuals with VCFS have some cognitive impairment, with resulting learning disabilities. The mean IQ is ~75. Speech is a particular problem if palatal abnormalities are present. Unfortunately psychiatric disorders may develop in adolescence or adulthood. It is estimated the rate of psychoses in VCFS in 25-times greater than in the general population. The prevalence of schizophrenia is 20–30% in VCFS compared with 1% in the normal population (6). Other brain disorders such as bipolar disorders, early-onset Parkinson's disease and early-onset dementia have all been reported (6). Adults need careful evaluation for mental and neurologic status on follow-up visits.

The Physician assuming care of an adult with VCFS needs knowledge of the medical history and the medical procedures that have been carried out. It is becoming more apparent that a number of individuals remain undiagnosed until adulthood (7, 8). This may occur if an infant is born with a severe cardiac defect and found to have VCFS. Close evaluation of both parents may reveal that one parent has a previously undiagnosed VCFS. VCFS is an autosomal dominant disorder, so an affected individual has a 50% chance of having an affected offspring. Although 90% of cases are *de-novo* mutations, as more individuals survive after successful medical treatment it is likely that the number of newborns inheriting the disorder will increase. About 30% of individuals do not have a cardiac defect and may have subtle findings, so many patients may go undiagnosed. Physicians caring for adults need to consider this diagnosis (9).

Ongoing care for adults with VCFS requires close attention to mental status for early recognition of any of the psychiatric illnesses of significant risk in adults. Hearing tests need to be done regularly. Genetic counseling is necessary if newly diagnosed or if a pregnancy is planned. A baseline ionized calcium parathyroid hormone level should be assessed and followed. In addition, a CBC and TSH level should be obtained. An initial bone density test should be ordered and followed as needed. Ongoing cardiology follow-up is essential.

12.3 TS

TS is a sex chromosomal abnormality due to the absence or partial absence of one X chromosome. It occurs in ~1 in 2,500 live born infants. TS is often suspected prenatally because of a prominent cystic hygroma. The newborn may have prominent webbing of the neck, peripheral edema and evidence of a left-sided obstructive cardiac lesion such as coarctation of the aorta, aortic stenosis, bicuspid aortic valve or hypoplastic left heart syndrome. A chromosome karyotype is undertaken for the diagnosis.

TS is characterized by short stature, webbing of the neck, low-set ears, low hairline, small mandible, and cubitus valgus. All patients require complete cardiovascular evaluation to look for a bicuspid aortic valve, coarctation of the aorta as well as the less common (but very serious) hypoplastic left heart syndrome. Lifelong cardiac follow-up is required.

Once a diagnosis is made the child requires a multidisciplinary approach for care. Pediatric specialists in endocrinology, audiology ophthalmology, genetics, cardiology and nephrology are required for all cases, but other specialists such as otolaryngology or speech therapy may be added as needed. Growth failure is a constant in TS, and GH therapy is a routine recommendation. Although the ideal age GH should be started is undecided, treatment starting between 4 years and 9 years of age is common. Absent pubertal development is very common although 30% will show some pubertal development. Estrogen therapy is generally started at about 12 years of age and is continued until the usual time of menopause. Gonadal failure is the rule, but a few undergo spontaneous pubertal development and 2–5% may achieve normal pregnancy.

Most girls with TS have normal intelligence but learning difficulties in mathematics, as well as visual, spatial and executive functions are common. Although most girls with TS are diagnosed shortly after birth or in childhood, some are not recognized until adolescence or even as adults.

Adult women with TS require lifelong careful medical follow-up (10). All the medical problems identified in childhood (e.g., cardiac, thyroid, celiac, hearing loss) require continued periodic assessment. Screening for osteoporosis, DM, hypertension and dyslipidemia are indicated because all are increased in TS. Evaluation of hearing on a regular basis is needed because~60% of adults with TS have senoneural hearing losses (11). Unfortunately, obesity and sedentary lifestyles increase the risk for DM, hypertension and osteoporosis. The recommended need for mammography, breast examination and papanicolaou (PAP) smears is similar to that for the general population.

Some women with TS have elevated liver enzymes, but this usually does not progress to hepatic disease. If the enzymes remain elevated or progress, further studies by a Hepatologist is recommended.

Osteoporosis is an increased risk for TS women, so a baseline bone density study is indicated. If the woman is taking adequate estrogen replacement, the BMD should be normal. If BMD is low, one must be sure estrogen replacement is adequate and that tobacco use, excessive intake of alcohol, or possible celiac diseases is not a contributing factor. Vitamin D level should be obtained and adequate amounts of calcium and vitamin D prescribed to maintain a normal BMD. Exercise should be encouraged.

These women often have risk factors for coronary artery disease. Hypertension is common, as well as T2DM and dyslipidemia. This is in addition to the frequent associated cardiovascular abnormalities which will require lifelong follow-up.

Patients who had repair for coarctation of the aorta in the past or have an abnormal aortic valve need follow-up by a Cardiologist knowledgeable in congenital heart defects. If the adult has never had a cardiac evaluation in the past, cardiac ultrasonography is needed to evaluate the aortic valve, ascending aorta and the presence of any other structural cardiac abnormality. If transthoracic cardiac ultrasound is not satisfactory, MRI should be recommended.

A study from Great Britain of 3, 439 women with TS showed that overall mortality was threefold higher than for the general population (14). Although the greatest mortality was in cardiovascular disease, other major contributors to the increased mortality included DM, epilepsy, liver disease, non-infective enteritis and colitis, renal and ureteric disease, and pneumonia.

Patients with TS have a significant risk for aortic root dilation and the resulting risk for ascending aorta dissection and rupture (12). The thoracic aorta must be evaluated in relation to the body surface area because dissection with an aorta diameter as low as 3.7 cmhas been reported. If the ascending aorta is normalized to body surface area, about one-third of TS women have an area greater than the 95th percentile of 2.0 cm/m^2. TS women with an aortic size index ≥2.5 cm/m^2 are at the highest risk for dissection (13). Unfortunately, unlike MFS (where progressive dilation of the aorta is helpful in following patients at risk for dissection), in TS, rupture may occur without any progressive increase in the ascending aorta diameter. Hence, all women with TS should be informed that, if severe pain in the chest or back occurs, they should go to an Emergency Room and request a computed axial tomography (CAT) scan of the aorta to look for dissection of the aorta. Early identification can be life-saving.

12.4 Noonan syndrome

Noonan syndrome (NS) (15–17) is a relatively common genetic syndrome due to several germline mutations in the Ras-MAPK pathway. A mutation in the PTPNII gene is present in 50% whereas SOS1, RAF1, and SHOC2 mutations are the next most common (with a rare KRAF and BRAF mutation as well). Additional genes in the pathway will probably be found to explain the ~20% unidentified genes causing this syndrome. The estimated incidence is 1:1000 to 1:2500. It is transmitted as an autosomal dominant by affected individuals but is more frequently sporadic. The clinical phenotype is variable, with many mild cases undiagnosed. Distinctive facial features include hypertelorism, downslanting palpebral fissures, low-set posteriorly rotated ears, ptosis and malar hypoplasia. About 70% are short in stature, and some form of congenital heart disease is found in ~80% (with pulmonary valve stenosis most frequent (70%)) and hypertrophic cardiomyopathy in ~20%. Chest deformity and undescended testes are also commonly found. Children with NS usually do quite well (although feeding problems may be present in infancy). Some have learning difficulties but most graduate from High School, many graduate from College, and a few have received higher degrees. Most become employed and live productive lives.

Easy bruising is common in NS and may result in epitasis, menorrhagia or excessive bleeding with surgical procedures. Several coagulation factor deficiencies have been described. Partial factor X1 occurs in ~25% and other factors such as XII, VIII and occasionally XI have been deficient. Thrombocytopenia and platelet dysfunction have also been reported. A screening CBC with differentials should be done at the time of diagnosis, as well as prothrombin time (PT)/activated partial thromboplastin time (aPTT). If abnormal consultation with a Hematologist is recommended, aspirin and aspirin-containing medications should be avoided.

The phenotype of NS changes with age (18). The short neck and flat nasal bridge seen in infancy is replaced in adolescents with a more triangular face and lengthening of the neck so that webbing becomes more obvious. As adults, the facial features become sharper and the nose has a pinched root and a high thin bridge. The older adult has prominent nasal labial folds and the skin appears transparent and wrinkled. Adults with NS are often difficult to recognize. It is now quite common for an adult with NS to be diagnosed after an affected child is born. Careful evaluation of each parent will quite often reveal one parent to have some features of NS not previously recognized. Often the affected parent has relatively mild findings, but genetic studies can now confirm the diagnosis in baby and parent. The condition can be transmitted as an autosomal dominant genetic disorder, so genetic counseling should be carried out. A newly diagnosed adult with NS should have a thorough evaluation, including a cardiac ultrasound and ECG even if a murmur is not heard.

There is surprisingly little literature available on the long-term follow-up of individuals with NS (19, 20). In one study (20), cardiac status was available for 45 adult NS patients; 93% had some form of cardiac disease; 57% had pulmonary valve stenosis and had balloon valvuloplasty or surgery in childhood. Four patients had died at 30–49 years of age. One had been treated for severe pulmonary valve stenosis with good relief of the obstruction. He developed cardiac failure and an arrhythmia, and died at age 48 years (some 30 years after surgery). Two others who had a repair of an ostium primum defect required mitral valve replacement and died in their thirties some years later. Another patient underwent a myectomy to relieve a left and right ventricular obstruction due to cardiomyopathy at age 12 years. She developed atrial fibrillation in her early thirties which was successfully treated, but she recently had a sudden collapse from ventricular-fibrillation and, after successful cardioversion, is stable with an implanted defibrillator. There is another patient with a defibrillator and 2 cases with pacemakers. In all, 31% of the 45 patients have ongoing cardiac problems, indicating a significant need for long-term follow-up of the cardiac status of adults with NS.

Lymphedema which may be present at birth is usually not a problem in childhood but may become a problem in adolescence or adulthood. Leg edema is not uncommon and 1 adult developed intestinal lymphangiectasia. Arthritis, fibromyalgia and back pain are frequent complaints among adults. Psychological problems such as depression requiring medication were frequent in one study of 51 patients (20). Twenty-three percent of patients were on antidepressant medications, a bipolar disorder was present in 1 subject, and 3 cases were recovering alcoholics.

The presence of a symptomatic Arnold–Chiari malformation appears to be increased in NS. After surgery and good relief of symptoms, several patients have had recurrence of symptoms requiring additional surgery. Excessive formation of scar tissue is the probable cause of the recurrence. Seizures are uncommon but may develop in adolescence. Fortunately, so far an increased risk of malignancy has not been noted in adults (19, 20). We have little knowledge of if or how the germline mutation in the important RAS-MAPK pathway will affect aging in a patient with NS.

Ongoing care should include genetic counseling because the condition is transmitted as an autosomal dominant. Regular cardiac follow-up is needed. Neurologic symptoms such as headache, spastic weakness of the legs, or cerebellar ataxia should prompt consideration of Arnold–Chiari malformation. The Physician should be alert to the relatively frequent occurrence of depression.

12.5 Down syndrome (trisomy 21)

Down syndrome occurs in 1.36 of every 1,000 infants born, or ~5,500 births per year (21, 22). Down syndrome is due to complete trisomy of chromosome 21 in 95% of patients, with the remainder affected by chromosomal translocation or mosaicism. Many of the phenotypic features of Down syndrome vary by ethnicity, and change as the patient ages, sometimes making it difficult to identify patients as having an abnormality. There are varying degrees of developmental disability in these patients, which may be related to the specific area of mutagenesis. Distinct regions of mutagenesis have been mapped for eight common Down syndrome features (23).

Common facial features of Down syndrome include microbrachycephaly, sparse hair, mid-facial hypoplasia, upward-slanting eyes with epicanthal folds, and Brushfield spots. The extremities are remarkable for transverse palmar creases, clinodactyly/brachydactyly, and gaps between the first and second toes. The following musculoskeletal abnormalities may occur: atlantoaxial instability, hypoplastic pelvis and joint laxity. Neurodevelopmental abnormalities include hypotonia, visual impairment, hearing impairment (sensorineural and conductive), moderate intellectual impairment, and delay in development. There may be a predisposition to gastrointestinal abnormalities (e.g., duodenal atresia and annular pancreas), structural and functional abnormalities of the genitourinary system, a predisposition to leukemia (Philadelphia chromosome and leukemoid reactions), a predisposition for thyroid abnormalities, sleep apnea and dental abnormalities.

Survival has improved over the years. The median age of death for a person with Down syndrome has varied from 25 years to 49 years (24), with a mean life-expectancy now approaching the late fifties to early sixties. Factors that affect survival in patients with Down syndrome include the presence of cardiovascular disease, blood and immune disorders, gastrointestinal and thyroid abnormalities, and the development of neurofibrillar disease and amyloid plaques.

Structural heart disease is common in patients with Down syndrome, affecting ~40–60% (25). One-half of these are endocardial cushion defects, a distinctive arrest of normal cardiac development resulting in a spectrum of abnormalities. These include the common atrioventricular canal, primum ASD with cleft mitral valve, inlet VSD, and the transitional canal. The risk of endocardial cushion defects is increased ~1000-fold with respect to the non-Down syndrome population, and accounts for 70% of all atrioventricular canal-type defects (23). The distribution of structural cardiac defects which may be seen at a high frequency in patients with Down syndrome are: common atrioventricular canal (45%), primum ASD (8%), PDA (7%), tetralogy ofFallot (4%), double outlet right ventricles, tet/canals and unbalanced/hypoplastic left and right ventricles (<1%). Some forms of heart disease, such as MVP, are not observed until adulthood, and are progressive overtime. Candidate genes involved in the promulgation of congenital heart defects in Down syndrome have been proposed (23). These include a 1.7-Mb DSCHD critical region which contains 10 genes (including the promoter), and a portion of the Down syndrome cell adhesion molecule (DSCAM) gene.

Infants and children with Down syndrome appear to be more severely affected by pulmonary hypertension due to hemodynamically significant shunts (large ASDs, large VSDs, leaking atrioventricular valves), which may have long-term effects on adolescents and adults. This pulmonary vascular hyper-reactivity has prompted aggressive medical and surgical treatment at a young age (27, 28) and as such, may provide better long-term outcome. However, earlier surgical repair of smaller individuals may carry other long-term risks. This may include further damage to the atrioventricular node (which may have been congenitally abnormal to begin with) resulting in dysrhythmia; and/or pacemaker implantation as these patients age; residual atrial or ventricular level shunts which would require subacute bacterial endocarditis prophylaxis (29, 30); residual tricuspid or mitral regurgitation; or surgically induced tricuspid or mitral valve stenosis.

Although these residual lesions may not prevent the patient from participating in physical activities (with the possible exceptions of those with dysrhythmias and/or significant pulmonary hypertension), they do require long-term follow-up and, in some instances of atrioventricular valvar regurgitation and continued pulmonary hypertension, may require chronic medical therapy, such as ACE inhibitors and/or endothelial receptor protagonists (31, 32). Some adults with Down syndrome have unrepaired defects, whereas those that have been repaired may have undergone repair after they developed significant pulmonary hypertension, or have residual valvar regurgitation.

Young adult patients with Down syndrome should be screened periodically for the development of valvar dysfunction. This may be due to surgical treatment or develop over time (e.g., MVP and aortic insufficiency). They may be managed medically with ACE inhibitors or ARBs: enalapril, captopril, cilazapril, or lisinopril (31). The effects on the rennin–angiotensin–aldosterone axis are thought to be similar to those of non-Down syndrome adults, i.e., lowering aortic pressure and systemic vascular resistance. Tachyphylaxis does not appear to be a problem. These medications are frequently used in concert with diuretic therapy, occasionally low-dose digoxin and beta-blockers. In the event of optimal medical management and patient compliance without significant clinical improvement, surgical intervention should be entertained. Endothelial cell receptor blockers are indicated for pulmonary hypertension (32).

Pregnancy in females with Down syndrome has produced healthy infants. If chronic cardiac medications are used, the adult Down syndrome patient with or without the patient's guardian must understand that the ACE/ARB categories carry a real risk of teratology. Those women with pulmonary hypertension/Eisenmenger syndrome should be discouraged from reproducing due to the very high risk of morbidity and mortality to the mother and fetus. Contraception to prevent pregnancy should avoid drugs likely to increase the risk associated with pulmonary hypertension.

Most adolescents and adults with Down syndrome can compete in such activities as the Special Olympics. Encouragement of these sorts of activities may prevent the excess weight gain that may be seen in patients with Down syndrome (35). Pre-pubertal children with Down syndrome have demonstrated an increase in levels of obesity-related hormones such as leptin, a finding that is significant while holding age, sex, ethnicity and further adjustments for percent body fat constant (36). This weight gain may be further potentiated by the hypothyroidism occasionally associated with Down syndrome. The result may be an exaggerated response to the metabolic syndrome with an extreme increase in levels of triglycerides and diminished levels of high-density lipoprotein. These lipid abnormalities have been described (37, 38). They appear to have no correlation with atherosclerosis, which seems to occur less commonly in patients with Down syndrome (although there are case reports of unusually aggressive coronary occlusion in patients with Down syndrome) (39). The lack of evidence for typical coronary atherosclerotic disease in this subgroup of patients may have more to do with their lack of longevity. Alternatively, it may be related to the known elevated activity of cytosolic superoxide dismutase, which is encoded by a gene on chromosome 21, and is known to be elevated in patients with Down syndrome (40).

With increasing lifespans in these patients, atherosclerosis may become more common. Extreme hyperlipidemia should be medically treated in young adults with Down syndrome to avoid other known complications of hyperlipidemia such as pancreatitis, dementia and Alzheimer's disease. Likewise, monitoring and treatment of hypothyroidism is appropriate. Down syndrome patients aged ≥40 years exhibit amyloid plaques and neurofibrillary tangles consistent with Alzheimer's disease. Only a minority of these patients develops clinical Alzheimer's disease, but depression and obsessive–compulsive disorder may present in an atypical fashion. These sorts of neuropsychological decline are a set-up for cardiovascular decompensation, and may be prevented by consistent and expert follow-up in this special population.

Specific approved monitoring guidelines for adults with Down syndrome are lacking. They are reported to have the same healthcare needs as the general population. However, there is a predisposition toward testicular cancer, otolaryngolic diseases (obstructive sleep apnea, conductive and sensorineural hearing loss), and neuropsychiatric, endocrine as well as cardiovascular diseases. Thyroid testing should be carried out every 1–2 years because of the increased incidence of hypothyroidism and hyperthyroidism. The patient with Down syndrome senesces prematurely, and this should be kept in mind with respect to assessment.

12.6 Williams–Beuren syndrome

Williams–Beuren syndrome (WBS) is a rare neurodevelopmental disorder occurring in 1/10–20,000 live births, with most patients surviving into their sixties (42). It occurs sporadically, although it may be transmitted in an autosomal dominant fashion due to a micro-deletion of ~1.5 million DNA base pairs located on chromosome 7q[del(7)(q11.23)] (43, 44). This genetic defect results in the loss of the elastin gene, causing decreased production of elastin protein. Elastin is prevalent throughout the body. Diminished production results in the characteristics of WBS: inguinal hernia, bowel and bladder diverticuli, hoarse voice, and distinctive facial features (e.g., periorbital puffiness, fleshy lips, full nasal tip, fleshy philtrum, wide lips). The cardinal features of the disease are the facial features, as described, as well as the endocrine and growth abnormalities (hypocalcemia, hypothyroidism, abnormal glucose metabolism, short stature, spinal curvature, joint contractures); cardiovascular disease (generalized arteriopathy resulting in supravalvar aortic stenosis, branch pulmonary artery stenosis, renal artery stenosis, mesenteric artery stenosis, coarctation, systemic hypertension, predisposition to ischemic disease secondary to supravalvar narrowing and compromised coronary flow), connective tissue abnormalities (abdominal pain, diverticuli, chronic constipation, gastroesophageal reflux), and neuropsychiatric disease (overfriendliness, impulsivity, ADHD, obsessive–compulsive disease, depression).

Supravalvar aortic stenosis is nearly pathognomonic of WBS, with a reported 75% of infants and children diagnosed with this structural abnormality (45). There is a spectrum of severity of stenosis, with the most severe resulting in left ventricular hypertrophy, heart failure, and myocardial infarction and/or death if the lesion is not addressed soon enough (46). Coronary stenosis occurs and may be due to medial hyperplasia, or may be a sideeffect of the dysplastic aortic valve leaflets' occlusion of diastolic inflow (47). Adults with WBS also appear to be at increased risk for developing MVP, which may be progressive and severe enough to require valve replacement (48).

The vascular stenosis commonly found in WBS (supravalvar aorta, ascending aorta, descending aorta, branches of the aorta) do not typically respond to balloon catheter dilation, but typically require surgical intervention. In fact, the stenosis typically occurs at the proximal portion of the vessels, which originate from the aorta, resulting in renal artery stenosis, mesenteric artery stenosis, and coronary artery stenosis (46–49). Occasionally, the branch and supravalvar pulmonic stenosis which may occur with WBS will cause significant right ventricular hypertrophy necessitating intervention; the response to catheterization is usually modest at best.

Systemic hypertension occurs in nearly half of children and many adults with WBS. Care should be taken to assess the blood pressure in more than the right arm because the Coanda effect (due to supravalvar aortic stenosis) may result in a falsely elevated right-arm blood pressure when compared with the left arm (50). In evaluating newly recognized systemic hypertension, a renovascular etiology should be sought and appropriately addressed. If not related to renal artery stenosis, the systemic hypertension seems to respond to standard modes of anti-hypertensive therapy. Given the predisposition for systemic hypertension and coronary anomalies, adult WBS patients should be followed up regularly to evaluate for ischemic heart disease. The risk of coronary stenosis has been described to be 25–100-fold greater for WBS patients than it is for the general population (46). Non-invasive assessment for ischemic disease is substandard in exercise testing and 24-h ambulatory blood pressure assessment in the WBS population (51). It seems this population fatigues early, making data difficult to interpret. Nonetheless, close follow-up for ischemic heart disease is warranted.

Sudden death related to implementation of anesthesia has been described in WBS patients (52). The cause and relationshipwith cardiovascular disease is unknown. Therefore, cardiovascular status should be thoroughly assessed in this population prior to administration of anesthesia.

There are few case reports of pregnancy in females with WBS. However, in the cases reported, there is increased morbidity and mortality in mother and fetus (53, 54). Pregnancy can be complicated by previously diagnosed and treated supravalvar stenosis (particularly aortic), vascular stenosis, systemic hypertension and heart failure. Premature delivery growth retardation has been reported. It is important to have a clear and concise discussion of these risks with adult WBS patients and the caregivers or guardians.

Most adults with WS will be living with parents, in a group home, or in other sheltered environments. Several studies have shown adults with WS to have a full-scale IQ of 61 (i.e., function at the level of a 6–8-year-old in regard to academic and social skills). Social, emotional and behavioral problems are common. Many are very anxious and isolated. Overfriendliness and the propensity to trust others put them at risk. They are often anxious, obsessive and distractible. The adult provider must be aware of the potential social and behavioral problems these patients face in addition to the known medical risks of obesity, hypertension and cardiac problems.

12.7 MFS and Loeys–Dietz syndrome

MFS and Loeys–Dietz syndrome (LDS) are diseases of connective tissue. They have clinically similar appearances, but are genetically distinct, involving differing mutations and protein abnormalities. LDS is caused by a mutation in transforming growth factor beta-1 (TGFB1) or transforming growth factor beta-2 (TGFB2). MFS involves an abnormality in the formation and production of the protein fibrillin (a major building block of microfibrils), which is the structural component of ocular, pulmonary, cardiovascular and gastrointestinal systems. Fibrillin serves to keep TGFB bound to its extracellular matrix. Mutant fibrillin, caused by one of 600 mutations of the FBN-1 gene, has an impaired ability to keep the latent TGFB in its inactive form. The presence of free TGFB causes the features seen in MFS (55). LDS is caused by a mutation in TGFB1 or TGFB2. There is much phenotypic overlap (56) if any of these genes do not function correctly.

The incidence of MFS is reported as 1/5000 live births(56), regardless of ethnicity or sex. The gene is transmitted in an autosomal dominant fashion, with a 50% chance of affected offspring; there is much intrafamilial variability. The penetrance of the gene is high. The Ghent criteria (57) were developed to facilitate the diagnosis of MFS, allowing appropriate supervision and treatment of the disorder.

Besides the tall stature and lax joints, other common problems include dislocated lenses (which may not be recognized early in life). There is an increased risk of retinal detachment, and continued follow-up by an Ophthalmologist is required. Skeletal deformities such as kyphoscoliosis, pectus excavation and pectus carinatium are common. In addition, the lax joints lead to several joint problems that require orthopedic follow-up. The risk of spontaneous pneumothorax is significantly increased in MFS.

Ninety percent of those diagnosed with MFS has cardiovascular involvement (56). Hence, appropriate and early diagnosis of MFS patients allows appropriate restriction from overly strenuous activity and appropriate medical and surgical treatment. This has increased the mean lifespan of those affected by MFS to ≥70 years as last reported in 1995 (58). Prior to the implementation of these measures, > 90% of all deaths in MFS patients were due to abnormalities of the cardiovascular system.

The MFS phenotype evolves, necessitating long-term follow-up of patients from infancy through adulthood. The occasional presentation during infancy is due to severe cardiovascular manifestations of MVP and resultant regurgitation, as well as possible aortic root dilation and resultant aortic insufficiency. While aortic root dissection occurs rarely in childhood, aortic root dilation and MVP are common. The degree of left ventricular dysfunction, which may be associated with MVP and resultant mitral regurgitation, seems disproportionate, leading to the hypothesis that some patients with MFS suffer from primary cardiomyopathy (59).

Mitral valve repair (and sometimes aortic root replacement) may be necessary during childhood, requiring long-term follow-up of adults who have undergone surgical repair. Absolute measurements of the dimensions of the aorta are taken into consideration regarding the need for surgical intervention. However, it is important to relate the aortic dimensions to age, sex, and body surface area over time (60) because escalating aortic root dilation in a child or smaller person may not meet the published absolute criteria for surgical intervention. The use of Z scores (a statistical portrayal of standard deviation from the mean) allows appropriate tracking of root dilation in comparison with other patients of same age, sex, and size. This affords the practitioner a means of plotting the Z score over time. For example, if the patient's Z score of 3 suddenly changes to 7, this is a significant variance in comparison with previous measurements. The rate of change is the impetus for further investigation by an alternative imaging method, or immediate surgical intervention. Z scores may even be used in adults because there is extreme variability in height and weight by ethnic groups.

Patients with MFS significantly dilated aortic roots are treated by prophylactic means with beta blockade (61), or an ARB such as losartan (62). The beta-blocker is usually given at a dose that produces a negative chronotropic/inotropic effect. Based on murine data, trials are ongoing to evaluate the effects of losartan versus nebivolol (a selectivebeta-blocker) or both on dilation of the aortic root in MFS with the FBN-1 gene mutation (63). As mentioned above, TGFB is bound to the extracellular matrix; there is more bound TGFB than free-form TGFB. Losartan directly blocks the receptor and nebivolol exerts an "anti-stiffness effect" in addition to its chronotropic effect. The results of this trial are pending.

Patients with MFS who are interested in sports participation should be referred to the guidelines from the 36th Bethesda Conference. These guidelines are specific for those individuals with aortic root dilation (Z score > 2 mm diameter or > 4 mm diameter in a "normal-sized" fully grown individual), and moderate MVP restricting them from highly competitive, strenuous sports (64). Those with mild dilation or evidence of phenotypic evidence of MFS without significant cardiovascular involvement are discouraged from participating in contact sports. This is often a source of difficulty in the tall, thin, asthenic patient who is coveted by local basketball teams. However, these forms of activity restriction have been shown to reduce the incidence of sudden cardiac death (65). The most common cause of death in these patients is vascular rupture or dissection. Therefore, it is imperative that patients with MFS be followed up closely with echocardiography and other, newer forms of non-invasive imaging (e.g., MRI CT). The latter imaging of the entire aorta and its branches.

The most common form of aortic dissection in patients with MFS is typeA (the root and ascending aorta) and is correlated to the dimension of the root. Type-B dissection (beyond the subclavian artery) has been described. There have also have been reports of dissection of brachiocephalics and aortic dissection, although this is more likely to occur in patients with the vascular form of Ehlers–Danlos syndrome or LDS.

There also may be progressive dilation of the main pulmonary artery, which does not seem to show a high preponderance for dissection.

In addition to the predisposition to aortic dissection, progressive aortic root dilation also predisposes the patient to aortic insufficiency, due to "stretching" of the sinuses of valsalva and lack of coaptation. Aortic insufficiency results in left ventricular dysfunction and heart failure, particularly if it is associated with mitral valve disease. The current recommendations state that surgery should be consideredif the aortic diameter reaches 45–55 mm. Valve-sparing surgery is always entertained, but may not be possible if the entire root is involved. Attempts are being made to carry out this type of surgery before the sinotubular junction dilates severely. Long-term results are being tracked in the National Marfan Foundation Registry. It is not known if adults with MFS are more predisposed to inflammatory heart disease resulting in abdominal aortic dissection. However, it is highly recommended that this group be followed up aggressively, and that they make the appropriate lifestyle changes.

Pregnancy is discouraged in females with MFS if the aortic root dimension is > 40 mm. Valve-sparing surgery is recommended if pregnancy occurs. In general, if the root measures < 40 mm, the patients and infants are closely monitored. Delivery should be by the route that causes the least amount of rapid fluid swings. Aortic dissection, type A or type B (which can occur without dilation of the aortic root), can occur any time during the third trimester of pregnancy, parturition, or up to 6 months post-partum.

Through the study of MFS, a differential diagnosis for vascular abnormalities has developed. There is a subset of patients with the cardiovascular appearance of MFS, with aortic and pulmonic root dilation, without other/differing clinical features. The importance in distinguishing these disorders, which are not fibrillin disorders but rather disorders TGFB1 and TGFB2, is that the underlying mutant substrate is different (66). These patients manifest mutations in the receptors for TGFB, and are much more predisposed to dissection/rupture of the aorta and dilation of the pulmonary arteries than patients with MFS. They also dissect/rupture in parts of the aorta where MFS patients are usually unaffected, such as branches of the aorta.

The most common syndrome associated with the TGFB abnormalities is LDS (66). MFS and LDS share a wide variety of phenotypes beginning at any age. MFS and the vascular forms of Ehlers–Danlos syndrome must be included in the differential diagnosis, but the other clinical phenotypic features of each disease differ. Just as in MFS, patients with LDS may differ phenotypically within families. The vascular fragility described in patients with Ehlers–Danlos syndrome is not found in patients with LDS.

The prevalence of this disease is not known because it was first described in 2005 and has clinical overlap with MFS patients. Therefore, the likelihood is high that some of these patients previously diagnosed as "atypical MFS" have LDS *in lieu*. LDS has no sex or ethnic predilection; it may be a spontaneous mutation, or it may be inherited.

Aortic dilation has been noted as early as in fetal life (67), but can present and progress at any age. The arterial pathology differs from MFS, including dissection of aortic branches and arterial tortuosity, so it is important that any patient being evaluated for LDS undergo thorough MRI or CT imaging (68). Echocardiography is still necessary in the assessment of related MVP, ASDs, PDA and bicuspid aortic valves. A patient with known TGFB receptor abnormality without the phenotypic presentation should be followed up expectantly with thorough evaluations because LDS patients exhibit a high predisposition to dissection/rupture. These patients are treated similarly (although possibly more aggressively) than MFS patients. As mentioned above, there are ongoing and novel trials evaluating the benefits of beta blockade and/or ARB (losartan) (62, 63). The animal and preliminary data appear favorable, although whether these agents are sufficient to attenuate dilation and dissection in humans remains to be seen.

Any patient carrying the diagnosis of LDA should refrain from contact sports. There are no specific physical activity restrictions (not addressed in the 36th Bethesda conference), but criteria similar to those used to restrict patients with MFS should be considered.

Certainly, any patient with tortuous arteriopathy and multiple areas of aortic aneurysms should be evaluated for LDS, particularly in the absence of some of the cardinal features of MFS, such as ectopia lentis (69). Bifid uvula is thought to be pathognomonic of LDS. These patients should undergo testing for TGFB receptor mutations for a definitive diagnosis because there are serious health implications. Surgery is advocated at a lower threshold in patients with LDS than in patients with MFS (40 mm *in lieu* of 50 mm in adults) (71), and prophylactic root repair should be strongly considered.

This disease has been described only recently and interventions such as surgery are undertaken aggressively, so the natural history/normal lifespan of a patient with LDS is not known. The scrupulous use of efficacious medical therapy, aggressive surgical intervention and restriction from contact and over-vigorous sports is likely to prolong the lifespan of these individuals.

Women with LDS are prone not only to the same and maybe higher prevalence of complication as those with MFS, but also risk uterine rupture or hemorrhage in pregnancy or peripartum at a prevalence of ~50% (66). Women known to carry TGFB receptor abnormalities should be advised appropriately along the guidelines used for pregnancy in women with MFS. Aggressive use of MRI or CT should be use before conception, during pregnancy (MRI) and in the peripartum period for appropriate anticipatory care.

12.8 Summary

Adults with MFS and LDS require the same ongoing care as any adult. We have discussed the special needs to be considered in each of these unique syndromes. There are hundreds of other very rare syndromes which a provider of adult care may encounter. The National Organization for Rare Disorders can be contacted to obtain information on all the known rare disorders. This would be very useful to a provider of adult care who assumes care of such a patient.

References

1. Yamagishi, H. (2002) The 22q11.2 deletion syndrome. Keio J. Med. 51:77–88.
2. Shprintzen, R. J. (2008) Velo-cardio-facial syndrome: 30 years of study. Dev. Disabil. Res. Rev. 14:3–10.
3. Lai, J. P., Lo, L. J., Wong, H. F., Wang, S. R., Yun. C. (2004) Vascular abnormalities in the head and neck area in velocardiofacial syndrome. Chang. Gung. Med. J. 8:586–593.
4. Johnston, P. C., Donnelly, D. K., Morrison, P. J., et al. (2008) DiGeorge syndrome presenting as late onset hypocalcaemia in adulthood. Ulster Med. J. 77:201–202.
5. van den Berge, K., Diderich, K., Poddighe, P., Berghout, A. (2009) Symptomatic hypoparathyroidism based on a 22q11 deletion first diagnosed in a 43 year old woman. J. Med. 67:102–104.
6. Vorstman, J. A. S., Chow, E. W., Ophoff, R. A., van Engeland, H., Beemer, F. A., Kahn, R. S., et al. (2008) Association of the PIK4CA schizophrenia-susceptibility gene in adults with the 22q11.2 deletion syndrome. Am. J. Med. Genet. 150B:430–433.
7. Zaleski, C., Bassett, A. S., Tam, K., Shugar, A. L., Chow, E. W. C., McPherson, E. (2009) The co-occurrence of early onset Parkinson disease and 22q11.2 deletion syndrome. Am. J. Med. Genet. 149A:525–528.

8. Evers, L. J., Vermaak, M. P., Engelen, J. J., Curfs, L. M. (2006) The velocardiofacial syndrome in older age: dementia and autistic features. Genet. Couns. 17:333–340.
9. McDonald-McGinn, D. M., Tonnesen, M. K., Laufer-Cahana, A., Finucane, B., Driscoll, D. A., Emanuel, B. S. et al. (2001) Phenotype of the 22q11.2 deletion in individuals identified through an affected relative: cast a wide FIHSing net! Genet. Med. 3:23–29.
10. Bondy, C. A. (2007) Care of girls and women with Turner syndrome: a guideline of the Turner syndrome study group. J. Clin. Endocrinol. Metab. 92:10–24.
11. Hederstierna, C., Hultcrantz, M., Rosenhall, U. (2009) A longitudinal study of hearing decline in women with Turner syndrome. Acta Otolaryngol. :1–8.
12. Carison, M., Silberbach, M. (2007) Dissection of the aorta in Turner syndrome: two cases and review of 85 cases in the literature. J. Med. Genet. 44:745–749.
13. Matura, L. A., Ho, V. B., Rosing, D. R., Bondy, C. A. (2007)Aortic dilatation and dissection in Turner syndrome. Circulation 116:1663–1670.
14. Shoemaker, M. J., Swerdlow, A. J., Higgins, C. D., Wright, A. F., Jacobs, P. A. (2008) Mortality in women with Turner syndrome in Great Britain: a national cohort study. J. Clin. Endocrinol. Metab. 93:4735–4742.
15. Noonan, J. A. (1968) Hypertelorism with Turner phenotype. Am. J. Dis. Child. 116:373–380.
16. Tartaglia, M., Mehler, E. L., Goldberg, R., Zampino, G., Brunner, H. G., Kremer, H., et al. (2001)Mutations in PTPN11, encoding the protein tyrosine phosphatase SHP-2, cause Noonan syndrome. Nat. Genet. 29:465–468.
17. Zenker, M., Buheitel, G., Rauch, R., Koenig, R., Bosse, K., Kress, W., et al. (2004) Genotype-phenotype correlations in Noonan syndrome. J. Pediatr. 144:368–374.
18. Allanson, J. E., Hall, J. G., Hughes, H. E., Preus, M., Witt, R. D. (1985) Noonan syndrome: the changing phenotype. Am. J. Med. Genet. 21:507–514.
19. Shaw, A. C., Kalidas, K., Crosby, A. H., Jeffery, S., Patton, M. A. (2007) The natural history of Noonan syndrome: a long-term follow-up study. Arch. Dis. Child. 92:128–132.
20. Noonan, J. A. (2005) Noonan syndrome. In: Goldstein, S., Reynolds, C. R., eds. Handbook of Neurodevelopmental and Genetic Disorders in Adults. New York, USA: Guilford, pp. 308–319.
21. Bittles, A. H., Glasson, E. J. (2004) Clinical, social and ethical implications of changing life expectancy in Down syndrome. Dev. Med. Child. Neurol. 46:282–286.
22. Centers for Disease Control and Prevention. (2005) Improved national prevalence estimates for 18 selected major birth defects – United States, 1999–2001. MMWR 54:1301–1305.
23. Korbel, J. O., Tirash-Wagner, T., Urban, A. E. et al. (2009) The genetic architecture of Down syndrome phenotypes revealed by high-resolution analysis of human segmental trisomies. Proc. Natl. Acad. Sci. 2009:12031–12036.
24. Yang, Q., Rasmussen, S. A., Friedman, J. M. (2002) Mortality associated with Down's syndrome in the USA from 1983 to 1997: a population-based study. Lancet 352:1019–1024.
25. Freeman, S. B., Taft, L. F., Dooley, K. J. et al. (1998) Population-based study of congenital heart defects in Down syndrome. Am. J. Med. Genet. 80:238–241.
26. Vis, V. J., Duffels, M. G., Winter, M. M. et al. (2009) Down syndrome: a cardiovascular prospective. J. Intell. Disabil. Res. 53:419–425.
27. Brun, H., Holmstrom, H., Thaulow, E. et al. (2009) Patients with pulmonary hypertension related to systemic-to-pulmonary shunts are characterized by inflammation involving endothelial cell activation and platelet-mediated inflammation. Congenit Heart Dis 4:153–159.
28. Simsic, J. M., Coleman, K., Maher, K. O. et al. (2009) Do neonates with genetic abnormalities have an increased morbidity and mortality after surgery? Congenit. Heart Dis. 4:160–165.
29. Reller, M. D., Morris, C. D. (1998) Is Down syndrome a risk factor for poor outcome after repair of congenital heart defects? J. Pediatr. 132:738–741.
30. ACC/AHA Task Force on Practice Guidelines. ACC/AHA guidelines for the patient with valvular heart disease: a report of the American College of Cardiology/American Heart Association Task

Force on practice guidelines (a task force to revise the 1998 guidelines for the management of patients with valvular heart disease); developed in collaboration with the Society of Cardiovascular Anesthesiologists: endorsed by the Society for cardiovascular Angiography and Interventions and the Society of Cardiothoracic Surgeons of Infectious Endocarditis. (2006) Circulation114:e84–e231.

31. Momma, K. (2006) ACE inhibitors in pediatric patients with heart failure. Paediatr. Drugs. 8(1):55–69.
32. Duffels, M. G., Vis, J. C., van Loon R. L. et al. (2009) Effect of bosentan on exercise capacity and quality of life in adults with pulmonary arterial hypertension associated with congenital heart disease with and without Down's syndrome. Am. J. Cardiol. 103:1309–1315.
33. Pueschel, S. M., Werner, J. C. (1994) Mitral valve prolapse in persons with Down syndrome. Res. Dev. Disabil. 15:91–97.
34. Geggel, R. L., O'Brien, J. E., Feingold, M. (1993) Development of valve dysfunction in adolescents and young adults with Down syndrome and no known congenital heart disease. J. Pediatr. 122:821–823.
35. Hawn, J., Rice, C., Nichols, H., McDermott, S. (2009) Overweight and obesity among children with Down syndrome: a descriptive study of children attending a Down syndrome clinic in South Carolina. JS Med. Assoc. 105:64–68.
36. Magge, S. N., O'Neill, K. L., Shults, J. et al. (2008) Leptin levels among prepubertal children with Down syndrome compared with their siblings. J. Pediatr. 152:321–326.
37. Patterson, D. (2009) Molecular genetic analysis of Down syndrome. (2009) Hum. Genet. 126:195–214.
38. Nishida, Y., Araoka, I., Nishizawa, T., Maruki, M., Maruki, K. (1977) Hyperlipedemia in patients with Down's syndrome. Atherosclerosis 26:269–272.
39. Ho, P. C., Nguyen, M. (2003) Acute two-vessel coronary closure in a patient with Down's syndrome. Int. J. Cardiovasc. Intervent. 5:95–97.
40. Akinci, O., Mihci, E., Tacoy, S., Kardelen, F., Keser, I., Aslan, M. (2010) Neutrophil oxidative metabolism in Down syndrome patients with congenital heart defects. Environ. Mol. Mutagen. 51(1):57–63.
41. Vis, J. C., Thoonsen, H., Duffels, M. G. et al. (2009) Six-minute walk test in patients with Down syndrome: validity and reproducibility. Arch. Phys. Med. Rehabil. 90:1423–1427.
42. Stromme, P., Bjornstad, P. G., Ramstad, K. (2002) Prevalence estimation of Williams syndrome. J. Child. Neurol. 17:269–271.
43. Osborne, L. R. (2006) The molecurlar basis of a multisystem disorder. In: Morris, C. A., Lenhoff, L. M., Wang, P., eds. Williams-Beuren Syndrome: Research, Evaluation and Treatment, 1st ed. Baltimore, USA: Johns Hopkins University Press, pp. 18–58.
44. Morris, C. A., Thomas, I. T., Klaiman, C. et al. (1993) Multisystem study of 20 older adults with Williams syndrome. Am. J. Genet. 47:478–481.
45. Eronen, M., Peippo, M., Hiippala, A. et al. (2002)Cardiovascular manifestations in 75 patients with Williams syndrome. J. Med. Genet. 39:554–548.
46. Bird, L. M., Billman, G. F., Lacro, R. V. et al. (1996)Sudden death in Williams syndrome: report of 10 cases. J. Pediatr. 129:926–931.
47. Kececiolgu, D., Kotthoff, S., Vogt, J. (1993) Williams-Beuren syndrome: a 30 year follow-up of natural and postoperative course. Eur. Heart J. 14:1458–1464.
48. Morris, C. A., Lenard, C. O., Dilts, C., Demsey, S. A. (1990) Adults with Williams syndrome. Am. J. Med. Genet. Suppl. 6:102–107.
49. Wessel, A., Gravenhosts, V., Buckhorn, R. et al. (2004) Risk of sudden death in Williams-Beuren syndrome. Am. J. Med. Genet. 127:234–237.
50. French, J. W., Guntheroth, W. G. (1970) An explanation of asymmetric upper extremity blood pressures in supravalvar aortic stenosis: the Coanda effect. Circulation 42:31–36.
51. Giordano, U., Turchett, A., Giannotti, A. et al. (2001) Exercise testing and 24 hour ambulatory blood pressure monitoring in children with Williams syndrome. Ped. Cardiol. 22:509–511.

52. Kaplan, P. (2006) The medical management of children with Williams-Beuren syndrome. In: Morris, C. A., Lenhoff, H. M., Wang, P. P., eds. Williams-Beuren Syndrome: Research, Evaluation and Treatment, 1st ed. Baltimore, USA: Johns Hopkins University Press, 83–106.
53. Van der Tuuk, K., Drenthen, W., Moons, P., Budts, W. (2007) Three live birth pregnancies in a woman with Williams syndrome. Congenit. Heart Dis. 2:139–142.
54. Mulik, V. V., Temple, K. I., Howe, D. T. (2004) Two pregnancies in a woman with Williams syndrome. BJOG 11:511–512.
55. Neptune, E. R., Frishmeyer, P. A., Arking, D. E. et al. (2003) Dysregulation of TGF-beta activation contributes to the pathogensis in Marfan syndrome. Nat. Genet. 33:407–411.
56. Pyeritz, R. E. (2007) Marfan syndrome and related disorders. In: Rimoin, D. L., Conner, J. M., Pyeritz, R. E., Korf, B. R., eds. Principles and Practice of Medical Genetics, 5th ed. Philadelphia, USA: Churchill Livingstone, pp. 3579–3624.
57. DePaepe, A., Dietz, H. C., Devereux, R. B. et al. (1996) Revised diagnostic criteria for the Marfan syndrome. Am. J. Med. Genet. 6:417–426.
58. Silverman, D. I., Burton, K. J., Gray, J., et al. (1995) Life expectancy in the Marfan syndrome. Am. J. Cardiol. 75:157–160.
59. Morse, R. P., Rockenmacher, S., Pyeritz, R. E. et al. (1990) Diagnosis and management of Marfan syndrome in infants. Pediatrics 86:888–895.
60. Roman, M. J., Devereux, R. B., Kramer-Fox, R., O'Laughlin, J. (1989) Two-dimensional echocardiographic aortic root dimensions in children and adults. Am. J. Cardiol. 64:507–512.
61. Shores, J., Berger, K. R., Murphy, E. A., Pyeritz, R. E. (1994) Chronic B-blockade protects the aorta in the Marfan syndrome: a prospective, randomized trial of propranolol. N. Engl. J. Med. 330:1334–1341.
62. Lacro, R. V., Dietz, H., Wruck, L. et al. (2007) Rationale and design of a randomized clinical control trial of B-blocker therapy (atenolol) versus angiotensin II receptor blocker therapy (losartan) in individuals with Marfan syndrome. Am. Heart J. 1544:624–631.
63. Gambarin, F. I., Fava, L. C., Serio, A., et al. (2009) Rationale and design of a trial evaluating the effects of losartan versus nebivolol versus the association of both on the progress of aortic root dilation in Marfan syndrome with FBN-1 gene mutations. J. Cardiovasc. Med. 10:3554–3562.
64. Maron, B. J., Zipes, D. P., Ackerman, M. J., et al. (2005) The 36th Bethesda Conference: Eligibility recommendations for competitive athletes with cardiovascular disease. J. Am. Col. Cardiol. 45:1413–1475.
65. Maron, B. J. (2003) Sudden cardiac death in young adults. N. Engl. J. Med. 349:1064–1065.
66. Loeys, B. I., Chen, J., Neptune, E. R. et al. (2005) A syndrome of altered cardiovascular, craniofacial, neurocognitive and skeletal development caused by mutations in TGFBR1 or TGFBR2. Nat. Genet. 37:275–281.
67. Viassolo, V., Lituania, M., Marasini, M. et al. (2006) Fetal aortic root dilation: a prenatal feature of the Loeys-Dietz syndrome. Prenat. Diagn. 26:1081–1083.
68. Johnson, P. T., Chen, J. K., Loeys, B. L. et al. (2007)Loeys-Dietz syndrome: MDCT angiography findings. Am. J. Roentgenol. 189:W29–W35.
69. LeMaire, S. A., Pannu, H., Tran-Fadula, V. et al. (2007)Severe aortic and arterial aneurysms associated with a TGFBR2 mutation. Nat. Clin. Pract. Cardiovasc. Med. 4:167–171.
70. Williams, J. A., Loeys, B. L., Nwakanma, L. U. et al. (2007) Early surgical experience with Loeys-Dietz: a new syndrome of aggressive thoracic aortic aneurysm disease. Am. J. Thorac. Surg. 83:S757–S763.
71. Loeys, B. L., Schwarze, U., Holm, T. et al. (2006) Aneurysm syndromes caused by mutations in TGF-B receptor. N. Engl. J. Med. 355:788–798.

13 Adult considerations of pediatric urologic care

Stephen E. Strup, Ali M. Ziada and William B. Rogers

Management of pediatric urologic conditions that persist into adulthood or that have long lasting sequelae as a result of their treatment can be a complex task. Fortunately, many urologic disease processes of infancy and childhood do not persist into adulthood. For those scenarios in which significant urologic concerns continue into the later years of life, an urologist will likely be involved in the patient's care, at least for routine checks and for when major issues develop. The intent of this text, as with the rest of the manuscript, is to provide a basic knowledge and understanding of the disease processes themselves, follow-up and "what to watch for" items.

13.1 Introduction

The management of pediatric urologic conditions that persist into adulthood or that have long-lasting sequelae as a result of their treatment can be a complex task, even for the well-trained Urologist. Fortunately, many urologic disease processes of infancy and childhood do not persist into adulthood, are definitively managed within that age group, or have minimal follow-up with passive observation. These conditions may be briefly mentioned only below or, in the case of those that do not present in adulthood, not discussed.

For those scenarios in which significant urologic concerns continue into the later years of life, a Urologist will probably be involved in the patient's care (at least for routine checks and if major issues develop). The intent of this chapter (as with the rest of the book) is to provide a basic knowledge and understanding of the disease processes, follow-up "what to watch for" items, and simple interventions for adult manifestations of these conditions.

13.2 Upper urinary tract

The upper urinary tract consists of the kidneys and ureters. It is separated from the lower urinary tract and external genitalia on an anatomic, embryologic and partially functional basis. There is much overlap in conditions affecting the upper tract and the lower tract. However, for the purposes of dealing with pediatric urologic disease and for reasons of organization, the embryologic origin and development of these systems lends to a separation along these lines. These systems are further subdivided into malignant and non-malignant processes.

13.2.1 Malignant upper tract pediatric urologic disease

Most malignant pediatric upper tract urologic disease of significance is limited to renal neoplasms. This is because ureteric neoplasms of infancy and childhood are virtually unheard of. These include Wilms' tumor (pephroblastoma), neuroblastoma, rhabdomyosarcoma, and other, more rare neoplasms. Adult considerations for these neoplasms are mainly related to post-treatment sequalae and renal insufficiency. These are usually best predicted by the treatment method employed rather than the disease. However, the disease, depending on stage and type, will be a major contributing factor to which treatment and outcomes are most likely.

13.2.2 Current treatment for specified malignancies

Most upper tract pediatric tumors will be neuroblastoma in the younger patient and Wilms' tumor for children aged > 2 years. Neuroblastoma is a malignant tumor of neural crest origin and usually arises in the abdominal cavity or pelvis. More rarely, neruoblastoma can arise in the mediastinum and neck. Wilms' tumor is the most common malignant renal tumor of childhood, and these patients also typically present with abdominal disease. Treatment for both malignancies is generally multimodal. It consists of surgical staging (including resection if possible) followed by chemotherapy and possibly radiation therapy. The chemotherapeutic agents that are typically used for neuroblastoma patients include cyclophosphamide, cisplatin, carboplatin, doxorubicin, and ifosfamide. For patients with Wilms' tumor, the agents include vincristine, actinomicin D, and doxorubicin. Abdominal radiation is used for more advanced stages of both tumors (1, 2).

There are more rare tumors of the upper urinary tract, including clear-cell sarcoma, rhabdoid tumor of the kidney, and renal cell cancer. These are typically treated with a combinationof surgery, chemotherapy and possibly radiation therapy.

13.2.3 Post-treatment sequelae of surgery

The loss of a portion or all of a renal unit is well tolerated, and the development of renal failure is rare unless there is intrinsic renal disease. For patients with bilateral Wilms' tumors, the prevalence of ESRD may be ≤15%. Preservation of normal renal parenchyma is preferred if possible (1). For those with a solitary kidney, it undergoes hypertrophy over time.

13.2.4 Post-treatment sequelae of chemotherapy

Chemotherapy can affect many systems as the child grows. Cardiac toxicity, pulmonary toxicity and endocrine malfunction are some of the problems with childhood chemotherapy. These effects tend to be agent-specific. Urologic issues arising from chemotherapy for upper tract renal tumors include renal insufficiency from the use of cisplatin and, to a lesser degree, carboplatin. Ifosfamide can lead to Fanconi's syndrome (glucoseuria, amino aciduria, hypophosphatemia, and hypochloremic metabolic acidosis). The metabolites from cyclophosphamide can lead to hemorrhagic cystitis. The cystitis can be potentially prevented with the use of mesna. Hydration during the administration of these agents is also helpful. Testicular and ovarian function can also be altered. Germ cells are very sensitive to chemotherapy and gonadal failure can be a consequence. In males, the prevalence of testicular failure from chemotherapy may approach 50%, but generally the hormonal function of the testicular Leydig cells is preserved (3).

13.2.5 Post-treatment sequelae of radiation therapy

Several urologic issues may arise from radiation therapy of the abdominal cavity. Radiation enteritis can occur and be chronic in nature. The kidney also demonstrates dose-related impairment for radiation doses > 12 Gy. Gonadal tissue is also quite sensitive to radiation therapy, with ovarian failure reported in ~68% of patients receiving doses > 25 Gy. The testis is more sensitive, with gonadal failure reported in patients receiving doses as low as 5 Gy (4). Testicular failure is characterized by azospermia and a elevated levels of FSH.

13.2.6 Non-malignant upper tract pediatric urologic disease

Most non-malignant diseases of the upper urinary tract are definitively managed (usually surgically) in the pediatric setting or observed throughout life, and interventions are not pursued unless they become medically necessary. Benign conditions of the upper tracts usually present within the first few years (if not days) of life with the notable exceptions of duplicated collecting systems, variations in anatomic position/form of the kidneys and, in some cases, obstruction of the ureteropelvic junction. These latter entities are much more likely to first become problematic or noticeable in adulthood, if at all.

13.2.7 Vesicoureteral reflux

Vesicoureteral reflux (VUR) is abnormal retrograde pulsion of urine from the bladder proximally back through the ureter and possibly to the kidney. This usually occurs during micturition or with a filled bladder. Primary high-grade reflux is usually unilateral but may be associated with contralateral reflux (usually lower grade). Primary reflux is associated with an abnormality in the way the uretervesical junction develops and/or functions. Secondary reflux is a function of the normal ureterovesical junction anti-relflux mechanism being overwhelmed. Treatment for the latter usually consists of therapy of the underlying mechanism such as neurogenic bladder dysfunction or other forms of urinary retention with associated increased intravesical pressures. Their treatments are discussed elsewhere. Secondary VUR is the term usually employedif reflux develops sometime in life after primary VUR has been effectively ruled out (5).

Primary reflux is graded into five categories for prognostic, treatment, and research purposes. Grading is based upon the degree of reflux and associated abnormalities on voiding cystourethrography. Grade I is reflux into a non-dilated ureter and grade V is reflux into the kidney with gross dilation of the entire urinary collecting system, tortuosity of the ureter, and blunting of the normal intrarenal architecture (6).

The mainstays for management of VUR are observation with prophylactic antibiotic therapy and surgical intervention (unilateral or bilateral). Different centers, different

Urologists, and different articles support slightly different criteria for when each therapeutic option is most appropriate. The general guidelines taken into consideration are age of the patient (resultant renal cortical scarring and parenchymal loss is more likely after reflux-associated pyelonephritis the younger a patient is), frequency of UTI and associated episodes of pyelonephritis, condition of and degree of reflux in the contralateral side, and the grade of reflux within the affected side.

Surgical correction of VUR consists mainly of open re-implantation of the ureters. This can involve direct extravesical re-implantation at a more anatomic and reflux-inhibiting position with tailoring of the dilated ureter or even tunneling the ureters submucosally (with crossing of the ureters to achieve the desired tunnel length) within the bladder to achieve an approximate 5:1 ratio of ureteral diameter to tunnel length buried under the submucosa. The general theme is to provide supporting tissue to buttress the distal ureter and place it into a position where the path of least resistance for urine to flow will be out of the urethra instead of retrograde into the ureter during micturition. Advents in laparoscopic, robotic-assisted and even endoscopic correction of VUR are being utilized and have shown promise (7). Surgical correction is generally indicated in older children (5–10 years) with persistent disease after initial medical prophylaxis and "watchful waiting", or those who have high-grade reflux with persistent infections/ renal cortical scarring (8). Surgical correction is usually delayed as long as medically reasonable in the hope that the reflux will correct with growth as well as to allow for a more definitive and technically less challenging procedure.

Applications to adult life of reflux after surgical correction (barring some form of perioperative morbidity, scarring and obstruction, or persistent reflux after surgery) are usually limited to the knowledge that distal ureteral anatomy may not be where expected (e.g., crossed ureters where the right kidney drains from a ureteral orifice on the left kidney during evaluation by a Urologist by endoscopic or radiographic (e.g., intavenous pyelography) means). Renal cortical scarring on imaging may be a very old process and not related to any current adult presentation.

Medical antibiotic prophylaxis is generally indicated in low grade (I–II) reflux in all age categories and sexes up to about the age of 10 years unless there is resolution of reflux prior to this. Antibiotic prophylaxis is generally the first-line and only line of therapy until about the age of 5 or 6 years except for certain instances such as significant renal scarring with grade-V reflux in children aged < 5 years (8–10).

Follow-up for resolution of VUR in the teenage to early adult years includes cessation of antibiotic therapy without further intervention unless a febrile UTI occurs. Recurrent febrile UTI with cessation of antibiotic therapy at any age may be an indication for surgical correction of VUR (10).

There is much controversy about whether or not surgical correction is indicated for post-pubertal girls with persistent VUR. There is evidence suggesting a significantly higher percentage of women with a history of VUR acquiring pyelonephritis during gestation than those without VUR, but these series show prevalence in the 10–15% range (10). There is insufficient evidence to conclusively support either stance.

13.2.8 Cystic kidney disorders

There are multiple types of cystic diseases of the kidneys. These range from exceedingly rare genetic pleomorphisms resulting in gross glomerular cyst formation to common cystic disorders of the kidney such as autosomal dominant polycystic kidney disease (ADPKD) and simple cysts. A thorough discussion of all the cystic diseases of the kidney (including those that do not develop or present until well into adulthood) is outside the scope of this chapter. Discussed below are the relatively common cystic diseases of infancy and childhood that may affect and sometimes present in later life.

Renal cystic disease of childhood is more readily examined if genetic and non-genetic types are separated. Genetic-linked types of childhood cystic kidney disease include autosomal recessive polycystic kidney disease (ARPKD), ADPKD, mulitple malformation syndromes with renal cysts (including vonHippel–Lindau disease (VHL) and tuberous sclerosis), and very rare entities such as medullary cystic disease. Non-genetic types of childhood cystic renal disease mainly include multicystic dysplastic kidneys and medullary sponge kidney. Non-genetic simple cysts (present in ~50% of the adult population), and acquired renal cystic disease are primarily manifestations in adult patients.

ARPKD is usually discovered at birth or during gestation but may not present until the adolescent years. Polycystic kidney disease (PKD) of the newborn or discovered *in utero* is usually fatal within the first few months of life. The earlier it presents then, usually, the more severe the disease. ARPKD is almost always associated with hepatic fibrosis but this is usually less severe if ARPKD is discovered at a younger age. Older children will have gradual development and worsening of renal failure and hypertension but their clinical picture may be dominated by the signs and symptoms of liver failure (11). ARPKD has no effective cure, and treatment for those patients that survive or present at an older age consists of temporizing measures for hepatic failure and hemodialysis with or without RTx (12).

ADPKD is typically considered a diagnosis with presentation in adults at mid-life. However, ADPKD has been found in newborns and there is evidence to suggest that, with increased genetic screening in families and the more frequent use of imaging methods such as renal ultrasonography, earlier diagnosis of ADPKD is becoming more common. ADPKD is also associated with hepatic involvement in the form of multiple cysts and with cysts in a multitude of body structures, the most significant of which may be berry aneurysms which may lead to subsequent subarachnoid hemorrhage and death. It usually presents with hypertension and may demonstrate hematuria, proteinuria, flank pain, and after significant enlargement of the cystic kidneys and liver, early satiety owing to extrinsic compression of the stomach (9).

ADPKD commonly leads to renal failure and the eventual need for hemodialysis and RTx. Common indications for nephrectomy for PKD include degeneration of cystic structures into potential/probable metastatic lesions, frequent hemorrhage into the cysts necessitating blood transfusion, chronically infected cysts, inability to consume adequate nutrition orally secondary to gastric compression, and pain (relative indication) (13). In our experience, polycystic kidneys may also be removed if they are large enough to inhibit successful renal allograft transplantation in a patient undergoing hemodialysis. One must consider if the patient's native kidneys are contributing significantly to the excretion of excess amounts of fluid volume before considering nephrectomy, even in the patient with severe renal failure or who has undergone RTx.

There are several inherited multiple malformation syndromes such as autosomal dominant tuberous sclerosis and VHL that may lead to renal failure secondary to cystic/mass compression of the kidneys. Tuberous sclerosis is usually associated with mental retardation, seizure disorders, adenoma sebaceum (usually on the mid-face), and cranial calcifications. It usually leads to benign cystic and mass lesions of the kidney, the most common mass being an angiomyolipoma. VHL may lead to a constellation of findings: hemangioblastomas, cysts of multiple structures (including the kidneys, pancreas, and epididymis), epididymal cystadenomas, and renal cell cancer. Pheochromocytomas also appear to be more common in VHL patients. Hemodialysis and RTx may be necessary secondary to renal failure in any of these patients, and resection warranted for renal cell cancer (usually clear-cell type) in VHL patients (13, 14).

Multicystic kidney disease (MCKD), also known as multicystic dysplasia, is a severe form of hydronephrosis and renal cystic dysplasia thought to result from renal obstruction *in utero*. The obstruction may be known in the form of ureteropelvic junction obstruction (UPJO), VUR, congenital megaureter, and atretic ureters. Unlike PKD, MCKD is more frequently unilateral, but may be bilateral in the case of malformations that affect both systems. Bilateral MCKD is usually fatal. A unilateral multicystic kidney usually involutes with time and requires no further monitoring after childhood (15). In rare instances, a multicystic kidney may require surgical removal for development of a Wilms' tumor (usually < 5 years of age), renal cell carcinoma, or uncontrolled hypertension (16). Adult considerations for MCKD are usually limited to those associated with anyone with a solitary functioning kidney. One must also keep in mind that the contralateral renal collecting system may also have varying degrees of abnormalities because entities such as VUR may occur in the contralateral system. The abnormality on the other side tends to be of lesser degree as demonstrated by the lack of multicystic dysplasia forming on that side.

Medullary sponge kidney is a result of numerous dilations of the renal collecting tubules resulting in formation of a cyst-like structure. This results in enlarged kidneys containing what appear to be multiple intrarenal cysts, sometimes with calcifications. Medullary sponge kidney is present at childhood and may present anywhere from a few weeks after birth to the seventh or eighth decade of life. Many patients are asymptomatic and may go undiagnosed. Symptomatic medullary sponge kidney is associated in some patients with hypercalcemia/hypercalciuria and formation of kidney stones, renal colic, recurrent UTI, and hematuria. Asymptomatic medullary sponge kidney requires no intervention. Hypercalciuria may be treated with thiazide diuretics or inorganic phosphates and the associated stones, if of significant size and obstructive, may be managed with appropriate endoscopy and lithotripsy. Chronic or recurrent UTIs are generally managed with frequent urine cultures and appropriate antibiotic treatment and, in some cases, prophylactic antibiotic regimens (17).

13.2.9 Duplicated urinary collecting systems

Duplication of the urinary collecting system including the renal pelvis and ureters is considered common. There is a variance in the reported prevalence of partial or complete duplication, but most autopsy date reveals a value of ~1%. It may be present in one or bothrenal systems, and occurs due to abnormalities in separation, differentiation, or "meeting" of certain urologic structures during embryogenesis. Duplication may refer to separation of an upper and lower pole moiety of the kidney with division of only their renal pelvises and a joined single ureter, complete duplication of the renal pelvicalyceal system with separate ureters with separate terminations in the bladder, and anything in between. Common terms such as a "bifid kidney" or "bifid renal pelvis" are used if two separate calyceal systems are seen draining into one common ureter beginning at the ureteropelvic junction (UPJ), whereas a bifid ureter would indicate continued separation of the upper and lower pole portions of the kidney via separate ureters to any point distal to the UPJ. In the case of separation of the upper and lower poles of the kidney to insertion of the ureter at the bladder, this is termed a "complete duplication" (or "double ureters") as stated above.

Duplication of part or all of the urinary system by itself may not be problematic. Manyduplications are found incidentally on radiographic films or are never diagnosed. There may be loss of functional renal parenchyma within one portion of the kidney (usually the upper pole) secondary to longstanding obstruction but this is not usually clinically significant and no intervention needs to be taken. Situations where duplicated systems usually become problematic in childhood are if they are associated with the other abnormalities discussed below (e.g. ureteroceles, ectopic ureters) (18). With complete duplications, the problematic renal unit is usually the upper pole system. The ureteric insertion is more likely to be abnormal, and obstruction with or without infection may need to be addressed.

In general, symptomatology from duplicated systems in adolescence or adulthood is usually related to infection, stone formation and difficult passage or extraction, or renal colic. Chronically problematic non-functioning renal segments may warrant surgical removal. As indicated above, asymptomatic duplications warrant no further intervention and should cause no significant concern for the patient. However, a familiar predisposition is thought to be present because the prevalence increases to just over 10% in immediate family members of those with duplications (19).

13.2.10 UPJO

UPJO may present or occur at any stage of life. UPJO presenting in adult life may have been undiagnosed in childhood and become symptomatic with growth and development of the patient. Alternatively it or may be secondary to acquired abnormalities of the UPJ such as scarring with stone disease and instrumentation involved in the treatment of stone disease. The discussion below deals with UPJO that is usually present during development and early growth of the kidney and ureters.

UPJO is a decrease in the normal flow of urine from the renal pelvis into the ureter with varying degrees of reduction. In the child it is thought to arise from inborn anatomic and functional anomalies of the UPJ and proximal ureter. These include deficiency in the development of the musculature or supporting tissues, obstructing and narrowing mucosal folds, or extrinsic compression from a crossing lower pole renal vessel lying across the UPJ or proximal ureter. UPJO may also be secondary to gross abnormalities of the kidney and renal pelvis such as found in some duplications and partial duplications, or a manifestation of VUR (20). Congenital, and usually developmental rather than acquired, UPJO is more likely to be associated with some varying degree of contralateral UPJO which may be so severe as to lead to multicystic dysplasia of the kidney (21).

Over time UPJO leads to renal hypertrophy, hydronephrosis, and resultant functional renal parenchymal loss. Symptomatic UPJO presents in older children and adolescents, whereas it is usually found on pre- and post-natal ultrasonography in neonates and infants who cannot effectively report symptoms (22). Ultrasonography is reliable only in ascertaining hydronephrosis of a kidney; radionuclide imaging is usually required to elucidate a finding of obstruction and determine the remaining function of the affected kidney. Symptomatic UPJO in older children, adolescents, and adults may present as most other forms of kidney obstruction in the form of renal colic, infection, and decreased renal function. In the face of any significant decrease in renal function or significant symptoms of the affected kidney, surgical correction is usually warranted. This assumes there is sufficient salvageable functioning parenchyma in the obstructed kidney (22).

Surgical correction of UPJO may be undertaken in an open fashion, endoscopic, or laparoscopic approach. Dilation of the obstruction, dismemberment and re-anastomosis of the affected segment around a source of extrinsic compression, and incision of the obstructed area with restructuring are employed. The method usually depends upon the degree and length of obstruction, age of the patient, and presence or absence of a crossing vessel. Surgical correction of UPJO is generally very successful (23). Appropriate correction is usually defined as stabilization or improvement in the differential function of the afflicted kidney with an improvement of washout time of radionuclide on functional imaging. This will be followed up postoperatively. After successful correction, repeat imaging is generally indicated for ≤3 years, with most follow-up occurring within the first few months to 1 year. There are no specific recommendations for functional assessment of a surgically corrected UPJO without evidence of symptoms or renal failure after this time. However, if symptoms occur or evidence of decline in renal function is found later in life, it may be prudent to evaluate with a diuretic renal scan (24).

13.2.11 Chronic pyelonephritis and renal scarring

Chronic pyelonephritis and renal scarring in late childhood, adolescent, and adult years is associated with late diagnosis and treatment of, or inadequate treatment of, urinary structural abnormalities leading to obstruction and infection. The most common culprit is VUR. As mentioned above when discussing VUR, renal scarring is more likely the younger a patient is and increases with the number of UTIs; treatment should be initiated promptly. The potential for significant renal scarring may persist until puberty (24).

Chronic pyelonephritis induced renal scarring may lead to xanthogranulomatous-pyelonephritis. This is a renal area consisting of necrotic, infected, and non-functioning tissue that may be hard to differentiate from renal cell cancer, and which may necessitate surgical removal. Renal scarring is also associated with a significant increase in the risk of hypertension and renal failure in later years. Early detection and appropriate management of hypertension in these patients has been shown to reduce the likelihood of renal failure (24, 25).

13.2.12 Rotational/ascent/fusion/formation anomalies of the kidney

Formation of the adult kidney from embryologic structures in the lower abdomen and pelvis and its ascent and rotation into its native position within the upper retroperitoneal space create several chances for aberrance in its form, position, and function. Congenital abnormalities of the kidney range from the rare and fatal bilateral renal agenesis to a simple malrotation of the kidney or failure of ascent of the kidney resulting in a pelvic kidney. Abnormalities of the formation and positioning of he kidney are not extremely common but are sufficiently frequent to warrant discussion. The more prevalent renal abnormalities and their impact in later life are discussed below.

Unilateral renal agenesis may be as common as one in a few thousand people. It is usually not associated with adrenal agenesis because this is a separate embryologic structure, and is slightly more common on the left side (26, 27). Assuming appropriate development of the contralateral kidney, adult patients with unilateral renal agenesis should be treated as any other patient with a solitary kidney with judicious use of nephrotoxic agents as well as prompt and immediate intervention for various forms of obstruction. Unilateral renal agenesis may not be discovered until adulthood. There is a strong association of renal agenesis with abnormalities of the internal genital tract as well as some association with malformations of other internal structures such as the heart and GI tract. Absence, duplication, or atresia of various organs such as the vagina, uterus, and vas deferens are relatively common with renal agenesis (26). These may lead problems with infertility and sexual function in adult life.

Just as one can have one less kidney than the norm, a patient may have an additional "supernumerary kidney. " The additional kidney general functions with its own blood supply and collecting system that may be located near or distant from the normally positioned kidney. Generally, the supernumerary kidney is asymptomatic. If it becomes symptomatic secondary to stone formation or other processes, or if it obstructs and inhibits the function of another kidney, then appropriate intervention by a Urologist should be instituted. Otherwise, the additional kidney may be observed without intervention or concern.

Various abnormalities in the position of the kidney may occur and are termed "ectopia" or "rotational abnormalities". The kidney may: fail to ascend and become a pelvic kidney; ascend too high and become a thoracic kidney; not rotate into its normal anatomic relationship with surrounding structures. Occasionally, a kidney may "fuse" with nephrogenic structures from the contralateral system, resulting in "crossed renal ectopia" where the kidney is fused and positioned with the kidney on the contralateral side and its ureter drains into the other side of the bladder. Fusion of the inferior poles (usually) of both kidneys, with the upper pole and remainder of the kidneys staying on the same side as their respective ureters, results in a "horseshoe kidney".

Most renal ectopia remains asymptomatic throughout life. However, like renal agenesis, there is considerable association of renal ectopia and fusion abnormalities with abnormalities of the internal genitalia and reproductive organs. Symptomatic ectopia may be demonstrated with renal stones and obstructive processes. Generally, this changes only surgical planning if these problems manifest. A horseshoe kidney is the most common entity to develop symptoms of renal ectopia and fusion abnormalities. It is the most common form of renal fusion abnormalities, with a prevalence of ~0.25% (28). The fused, midline portion of the horseshoe kidney is likely to catch on the inferior mesenteric artery during ascent in embryogenesis, leading to a more inferior position. Horseshoe kidneys are usually asymptomatic but result in a slightly increased disposition towards stone formation and recurrent UTIs. The latter are usually managed with culture-appropriate antibiotic therapy. The former are managed via endoscopic and percutaneous as other stones are but with a variable degree of increased difficulty due to differences in the position and rotation of the renal collecting system structures (27).

13.2.13 Megatureter, ectopic ureter and ureterocele

By definition, megatureteris dilation of the ureter > 5 mm. The term encompasses several entities and may be primary (due to a defect in the development of the ureter) or secondary (from a distal obstructing source). Secondary megaureter is managed by correction of the distal obstruction. Primary megaureter is treated in a similar fashion to VUR, but megaureter is primarily broken down into obstructing and non-obstructing classifications. Obstructing megaureter subtypes may require surgical intervention (usually in the age range 1–2 years) and/or antibiotic prophylaxis. Non-obstructing megaureter subtypes such as primary non-obstructing and non-refluxing megaureter are usually managed expectantly with spontaneous resolution. Indications for surgical intervention fall along the lines of recurrent infections and evidence of worsening renal function secondary to the megaureter. Primary megaureters found in adults are usually incidental findings on radiography. They do not require intervention because they generally remain stable over time (29).

An ectopic ureter is used to describe an abnormal insertion of the ureter and ureteral orifice. It describes insertion anywhere into the genitourinary system (including abnormal insertions into the urinary bladder) but the definition is usually employed to indicate insertion of the ureter into a structure at the bladder neck (junction of bladder and urethra) or any point distal. In males, the ureteral insertion is more likely to occur within the posterior (proximal) urethra or seminal vesicle. In females, it is more likely to occur within the urethra or the vestibule (2). Most ectopic ureters are associated with duplicated urinary collecting systems, but this phenomenon is much more common in females (as are ectopic ureters). Ectopic ureters may also be associated with a wide range of genitourinary malformations, includingmalformation of the kidneys and uterovaginal agenesis, atresia, and imperforate anus (30, 31).

Ectopic ureters may persist into adulthood without detection, yet if found in early life are associated with findings directly related to obstruction (just as many of the other non-malignant diseases of the upper urinary tract). These include hydronephrosis, infection, renal parenchymal loss, and proximal ureteral dilation. Due to the association with duplicated collecting systems, frequently an ectopic ureter will be associated with heminephric (usually the upper pole system) obstruction and renal cortical loss. It may be treated with heminephrectomy and ureterectomy or reinsertion of the ectopic ureter into the common sheath of the normally positioned ureter. Systems with a solitary ureter with an abnormal termination are generally re-implanted in a more natural position. Most ectopic ureters will be diagnosed by infection (common in males) or vaginal urine leak at an early age and treated appropriately without further intervention in adult life. However, presentation or radiographic findings of these may occur. If no significant association with infections or a patient's QoLis found then intervention is probablynot necessary (30). Any renal loss at that point is probably unrecoverable and, unless there is another indication for intervention (e.g., chronically infected non-functional kidney or kidney segment), there is no need for further intervention.

An ureterocele is a cystic dilation of the end of the ureter (a congenital ureteral diverticulum is a similar entity with similar complications but is very rare). Like ectopic ureters, ureteroceles are commonly associated with duplicated collecting systems and usually arise from the upper pole moiety of the renal collecting system. They are also much more common in females and, like other non-malignant abnormalities of the upper urinary tract, are problematic in childhood and adult life if they result in obstruction and infection (30, 32). Ureteroceles are analogous to ectopic ureters in that they cause distal ureteric obstruction which may necessitate surgical intervention (anywhere from ureteral incision and decompression to heminephrectomy or nephrectomy) and/or antibiotic prophylaxis. However, large ureteroceles near the bladder neck may also result in incontinence or urinary retention (which may be the presenting symptom) and may require intervention for these reasons alone (30, 33). As with megaureter and ectopic ureters, ureteroceles usually manifest in childhood and are treated prior to the patient's transition to adulthood without need for consideration other than the potential long-term loss of functioning renal parenchyma.

13.2.14 Lower urinary tract and genitalia

The lower urinary tract and genitalia are mainly derived from separate embryologic structures than the upper urinary tract, and are readily separated from the upper tract for the purposes of discussion. As stated earlier, there is much overlap and dependency between systems during development and from a lifelong standpoint. One may even argue that the inappropriate development or dysfunction of the lower tracts is mainly problematic due to its impact on the upper urinary tract and the main functioning unit of the entire system: the kidney. This would seem to be applicable to non-malignant processes, at least. As with the upper urinary tract, the abnormalities and their implications on adult life are best subdivided along the lines of malignant and non-malignant disease.

13.2.15 Malignant lower tract and genital associated pediatric urologic disease

As with other malignant disease of the genitourinary tract, most considerations of late childhood, adolescence, and adulthood center around post-treatment and long-term sequelae rather than the disease and its potential follow-up. The two malignant conditions of the lower urinary tract and genitalia that are of greatest concern to the Pediatric Urologist are testicular neoplasms and pelvic sarcomas. We discuss below these disease processes and their treatment with a general emphasis on what these treatments may entail for the patient in later life.

13.2.16 Testicular tumors

Malignant germ cell tumors are fairly rare in children. The most common type of testicular tumor is yolk sac tumor. Adult yolk sac tumors tend to occur as a component of a mixed germ cell tumor, but childhood yolk sac tumors tend to be pure yolk sac. These tumors secrete alpha fetoprotein (AFP), and this marker is helpful for staging and monitoring of this disease. Treatment of yolk sac tumor includes radical orchiectomy as well as chemotherapy utilizing cisplatin, etoposide, and bleomycin. Surgical excision of the retroperitoneal lymph nodes is also utilized in cases such as a persistent retroperitoneal mass after chemotherapy (34).

Other testicular neoplasms include testicular stromal tumors, Leydig cell tumors and Sertoli cell tumors. These tumors tend to behave more benignly (though Leydig cell tumors can cause endocrine dysfunction (precocious puberty) upon presentation). Treatment is typically excision of the primary tumor without additional therapy.

The other important testicular tumor is paratesticular rhabdosarcoma. This tumor arises in the paratesticular region and tends to behave less aggressively than other pelvic sarcomas in childhood. In addition to radical excision of the testis, paratesticular rhabdosarcomas are treated with chemotherapy utilizing agents listed below for pelvic rhabdomyosarcomas. Surgical staging and treatment by undertaking a retroperitoneal lymph node dissection is also done for patients presenting at an older age or if other poor prognostic factors (e.g., high-risk histologic subtypes) are present. Radiation therapy to the retroperitoneum is used only for high-risk cases (35).

13.2.17 Pelvic sarcomas

Rhabdomyosarcoma is the most common sarcoma of childhood. The most common location for the primary lesion is the head and neck, followed by the pelvis in the genitourinary system. Approximately 20% of childhood rhabdomyosarcomas involve the bladder, prostate, vagina, cervix, or paratesticular tissues.

Treatment of rhabdomyosarcoma has changed. Initially, aggressive resection of the pelvic organs with urinary diversion was done. However, after demonstrating the beneficial effects of combination therapy (chemotherapy, radiation, surgery) treatment has shifted to initial chemotherapy and radiation with organ preservation if possible. Chemotherapeutic agents typically utilized are vincristine, actinomycin, cyclophosphamide, and more recently doxorubicin and cisplatinum. Using upfront multimodal therapy, retention of a functional bladder has gone from ~25% (using earlier treatment regimens) to ~60% (36).

13.2.18 Post-treatment sequelae of surgery

Retroperitoneal lymph node dissection for testicular tumors can result in ejaculatory dysfunction. If the sympathetic nerves that run parallel to the aorta and vena cava are injured, ejaculatory dysfunction can persist. Preservation of one or both of these nerve chains can preserve ejaculation function in ≤90% of patients.

Radical excision of the bladder and prostate gland can result in erectile dysfunction due to injury of the cavernosal nerve fibers that coarse along the prostate gland. If urinary reconstruction is required, urinary diversion can be continent (continent reservoir) or incontinent (ileal loop). Urine diversion can result in metabolic issues as well as renal issues that are outlined below in the neurogenic bladder dysfunction section.

13.2.19 Post-treatment sequelae of chemotherapy

The long-term effects of the chemotherapy are agent-specific and outlined above in the treatment of upper tract malignancy.

13.2.20 Post-treatment sequelae of radiation therapy

Radiation can impact fertility by causing primary gonadal failure as discussed above. In addition, radiation to the bony pelvis and spine can result in osseous deformities such as scoliosis, especially if the radiation therapy is asymmetric. Short stature can also be a result of radiation therapy to the bony pelvis and spine. Radiation to the bladder can increase the risk of bladder dysfunction. However, in the Intergroup Rhabdomyosarcoma Study I and II, 50% of survivors retained their bladder and 73% of those patients retained satisfactory bladder function. The risk of a secondary malignancy is also a concern for these patients. In the National Wilms' Tumor Study, the number of secondary malignancies was 8.5-times the expected value, which represented a cumulative 10-year risk of 1%. The Intergroup Rhabdomyosarcoma Study reported a 10-year risk of 1.7% (4).

13.2.21 Non-malignant lower tract and genital-associated pediatric urologic disease

Similar to non-malignant diseases of the upper urinary tract, most non-malignant diseases of the lower urinary tract and genitalia that require intervention will be definitively managed or effectively corrected within the pediatric setting. However, several abnormalities of the upper tracts may not require intervention or may not be discovered until adulthood. Conversely, most abnormalities of the lower tract and genitalia will require early intervention and may necessitate long-term follow-up and management (especially if urinary reconstruction is involved). Delineated below are some of the disorders of the lower tract and genitalia that have potential effects on the adolescent and adult patient.

13.2.22 Posterior urethral valves

Posterior urethral valves (PUVs) are obstructive membranes of tissue within the proximal urethra found in boys. They are one-way "valves" that do not allow antegrade flow of urine from the bladder through the urethra. They can lead to severe perinatal and lifelong damage to the urinary tract in infants who survive to term or do not pass from pulmonary hypoplasia (Potter's syndrome) in early life, as may be seen with several urinary obstructive phenomena. PUVs may occur as frequently as 1 in ~10,000 live births (36) and may be much more common than that observed on prenatal ultrasonography. In fact, most PUVs are now diagnosed by prenatal ultrasonography (37). Some boys are not diagnosed until a few years after birth and usually present with voiding dysfunction and UTIs. The concomitant damage to the urinary tract is usually not as severe (38).

For patients that survive the perinatal period and are diagnosed or have a suspected diagnosis of PUVs, immediate drainage of the urinary bladder is in order. This is usually accomplished by catheter drainage or cutaneous vesicostomy. Definitive treatment for PUVs usually involves endoscopic ablation and obliteration of the valves. Even after appropriate treatment, most PUV patients will have irreversible damage to the urinary system proximal to the obstruction, and may even continue to develop further damage for a period of time (38).

Proximal damage within the urinary system begins with the bladder and proximal urethra and extends in a retrograde fashion through the ureters to the kidneys. The bladder may suffer the worst of the damage but the common associated presence of reflux can lead to a significant amount of renal damage. PUVs may result in pulmonary hypoplasia and potentially death, low bladder compliance with associated hypercontractility and incontinence, ureteric dilation and defunctionalization, and progressive hydronephrosis with associated renal damage (dysplasia *in utero*) and renal insufficiency that may ultimately lead to hypertension, growth inhibition, and renal failure.

PUV patients require lifelong monitoring of renal function regardless of the severity of damage during childhood and, if renal damage/dysplasia is severe, require management for renal insufficiency (including hemodialysis and RTx). PUVs are also one of (if not the most) common reasons for RTx in children (38, 39). When it comes to the bladder, most patients suffering from a history of PUVs in childhood will have some form of lifelong voiding dysfunction and incontinence; one term used for this situation is "valve bladder syndrome. " Voiding dysfunction even after successful valve treatment is common. Dysfunction may be in the form of detrusor hyperreflexia (a severely overactive bladder), detrusor failure with associated urinary retention and overflow incontinence, and/or a small-capacity bladder with poor compliance (lower urine volumes raise the intravesical pressure to abnormal levels, resulting in proximal reflux and hydronephrosis). Each entity is treated appropriately with anti-cholinergic medications generally indicated for detrusor hyperreflexia, scheduled voiding and clean intermittent catheterization for detrusor failure, and anti-cholinergic medications with or without augmentation cystoplasty to enlarge a small-capacity bladder (38).

Regardless of the severity, adolescent and adult patients with a history of posterior urethral valves require long-term close follow-up to evaluate renal and excretory function. Some decline in renal and bladder function is expected with time, but the patient's continued adherence to management principles may delay functional decline. Any acute change in renal function or voiding function should prompt immediate evaluation by the patient's Physician to ensure that necessary changes in management are undertaken quickly.

13.2.23 Hypospadias

Hypospadias is an abnormal opening or ending of the urethra into a meatus located on the ventral aspect of the penis, scrotum, or perineum. Failure of fusion of the urethral folds leads to the abnormal position of the urethral meatus. There is debate on the exact mechanism from which the final uretha forms, the deficiencies that lead to incomplete fusion of the urethra, and the abnormal curvature of the penis ("chordee") that sometimes develops with hypospadias (40). Hypospadias is quite common, being present in one in a few hundred live male births. It is usually a solitary finding but has association with some uncommon congenital developmental and intersex disorders. Cryptochordism and inguinal hernias are also found in a small but significant percentage of boys presenting with hypospadias (41).

Hypospadias is generally treated successfully with surgical correction in children. There are a wide variety of surgical techniques employed depending upon the location (proximal versus distal), associated chordee, severity, and surgeon preference. Occasionally, surgical correction may fail or the patients may develop some form of complication such as an urethrocutaneous fistula or stricture/stenosis of the urethra or meatus. These usually develop within a relatively short time after the intial repair and are managed during childhood (40).

As far as adolescent and adult patients with a history of hypospadias are concerned, no significant long-term impairment or considerations are necessary. There is potential for an undiagnosed or treated hypospadias to persist into adulthood (especially if distal), but most men have no interruption in sexual function or voiding dysfunction. Men who have undergone successful repair in the past tend to have no significant dysfunction or fail to report it (40, 42). Assuming successful repair that is not fraught with complications and multiple redo procedures during childhood, most adult treatment consists of psychosocial counseling secondary to a perceived or real variation in normal penile appearance which may lead to a decrease in the number of sexual encounters and partners (42).

13.2.24 Undescended testicles

Cryptorchidism, or undescended testicle(s), is abnormal positioning of the testes anywhere from the abdominal cavity to just outside of the scrotum at birth. It is relatively common, occurring in ~1–3% of term births (bilaterally in ~25–50% as many) and in a substantially higher number of pre-term births (43, 44). Around three-quarters of undescended testicles descend spontaneously, most by 3–6 months of age (43). If by 1 year one or both testes have not descended into the scrotum, then surgical orchidopexy is indicated. This may be accomplished by various laparoscopic and open approaches depending upon the position of the undescended testicle.

Historically, surgical fixation of undescended testes at 1 year of age (or anytime thereafter) was done for two reasons: to bring the testes into the scrotum to make it readily available for palpation and examination for testicular neoplasms in the future; and (ii) to improve fertility rates. There is insufficient evidence to indicate that orchidopexy decreases the risk of testicular neoplasia, but there may be support for the idea that pre-pubertal fixation may decrease the overall risk (43, 44). Regardless, any male with a history of an undescended testicle is thought to have a relative risk 40-times greater than the general population to develop a testicular neoplasm within his lifetime, and regular testicular self-examinations should be heavily encouraged in this population and supplemented by clinical examinations with a high index of suspicion. There is also an increased incidence of testicular malignancy in the contralateral testes in the case of unilateral cryptorchidism (43).

The effect of cryptorchidism on fertility may be significant. The presence of one or both testicles within the temperatures and pressures of the abdominal cavity in early life can significantly and permanently damage spermatopoietic germ cell lines. Many cryptorchid patients may have a decrease in total sperm counts and an overall decrease in fertility. Some evidence goes so far as to demonstrate that untreated bilateral cryptorchidism always results in a decrease in fertility (45). Originally, most evidence suggested that early and pre-pubertal orchidopexy improved fertility rates and could be an indication for surgery alone, but newer data suggest that fertility indices do not change after orchidopexy (43). The need for manual and easier ultrasonographic examination of the testicles within the scrotum of a population at a much greater risk for testicular neoplasia in the future is a solid indication for operative fixation itself. Other evidence that suggests pre-pubertal orchidopexy may be beneficial for improvement of fertility rates, which only buffers a solid indication for surgery.

13.2.25 Non-neuropathic bladder voiding dysfunction

Non-neuropathic and neuropathic voiding dysfunction of children encompasses a broad spectrum of disease. Their specific nomenclature, disease pathogenesis, and treatments are well beyond the scope of this chapter. A brief mention of some of these disorders will be made below, but the intent is to describe most of the treatment options and how these will affect later care for the unfortunate individuals suffering from these disorders.

"Non-neuropathic voiding dysfunction" is used to describe several disturbances in physiologically normal voiding patterns and physiology or socially unacceptable voiding habits that do not have a known underlying neurologic lesion. These disorders range from nocturnal enuresis and dysfunctional elimination syndrome to conditions such as Hinman's syndrome (a constellation of incontinence, recurrent UTIs, and incomplete empyting usually associated with constipation and other fecal disturbances) that have no known neurologic lesion but manifest similar urologic disturbances (46).

Non-neuropathic voiding dysfunction is associated with or may lead to incontinence, UTI, and VUR. If inappropriately managed, these can potentially progress to permanent bladder dysfunction and progressive hydronephrosis, pyelonephritis, and renal scarring in the cases where incomplete emptying and increased intravesical pressures are seen. Most non-neuropathic voiding dysfunction is treated (usually successfully) with conservative and non-surgical interventions during childhood. These include: behavioral modification and voiding schedules, biofeedback and physical therapy, neuromodulation with Transcutaneous Electrical Nerve Stimulation (TENS) units, bowel management, anti-cholinergics for hyperreflexic and overactive bladders, alpha-blockers for bladder outlet obstruction, imipramine and 1-deamino-8-D-arginine vasopressin (DDAVP) for nocturnal enuresis, and clean intermittent catheterization for incomplete emptying (46).

Conservative management is usually successful and will eventually be discontinued. However, it may persist into early adolescence and adulthood and will primarily be managed by Urologists, Physical Therapists, and other specialists. Unless the patient has permanent renal or bladder dysfunction from late, inapprpriate, or poor response to therapy, a general knowledge of these conditions and their treatment options will suffice for long-term follow-up and care from a general practice standpoint.

In some cases, non-neuropathic voiding dysfunction may fail conservative therapies or be so severe as to warrant surgical intervention. This is primarily done for conditions resulting in decreased bladder capacity, defunctionalization of the bladder, or disturbances that are similar to neuropathic bladder dysfunction. Many neuropathic bladder voiding syndromes may ultimately require surgical intervention or urologic reconstruction, so the types of surgery, their complications, and management are discussed.

13.2.26 Neuropathic bladder voiding dysfunction and urinary reconstruction

Neuropathic voiding dysfunction and neurogenic bladder disorders of children are associated with a known neurologic lesion. Most of these are secondary to spinal dysraphisms such as myelomeningoceleand meningocele (otherwise known as spina bifida). Neurologic lesions of any etiology of childhood vary (according to level of the lesion) and evolve throughout early life but the general findings include detrusor hyperreflexia/hyporeflexia with or without sphincter dyssynergia (inappropriate relaxation or constriction of the sphincter in coordination with the bladder muscle).

Most neuropathic bladder dysfunction leads to small and/or non-compliant bladders for life. These may be managed conservatively at first or for life with anti-cholinergics and clean intermittent catheterization to combat increase bladder pressures and urinary system damage as well as to help with incontinence. Prophylactic antibiotics are also sometimes employed.

There is also a small but significant association of neuropathic voiding dysfunction with VUR. The VUR is generally treated via the management guidelines for VUR not associated with a neuropathic bladder. However, adequate drainage of the bladder via conservative or surgical therapies must be ensured to protect the upper tracts (46).

Surgical intervention may be warranted for neuropathic bladder dysfunction if conservative therapy fails to manage symptoms (incontinence) or if urinary tract deterioration persists without more aggressive intervention. Surgery may be done later in life (adolescence and adulthood) in some instances. Physicians should be aware that their patients have the option to visit and discuss surgical options with Urologists specializing in urinary system reconstruction if consistent urinary leak and wetting occurs (which may lead to awkward social situations or infection and deterioration of the perineum and surrounding areas) or if worsening renal/urinary function occurs. The same surgical and non-surgical options for urinary system reconstruction and management are employed for acquired neurologic disease, such as in spinal cord injury or stroke.

Permanent urinary reconstruction and/or diversion for any reason (neuropathic disease or after extirpative therapy for malignancy) usually employs a few basic principles. These are the use of a GI segment to augment (i.e., enlarge the capacity of) the bladder or form a new reservoir other than the bladder to store urine, and formation of a stoma or outlet that drains freely into a bag or which may be buttressed to form a valve-type mechanism that is continent and is catheterized at regular intervals (e.g., a continent catheterizable stoma) (47, 48). In some cases, the native bladder outlet may be obstructed or closed to combat incontinence through the native urethra (47).

Most urinary reconstruction for pediatric neuropathic voiding dysfunction consists of formation of a continent catheterizable stoma with or without augmentation of the native bladder to increase storage capacity and, sometimes, augmentation for the bladder alone. The augmented or non-augmented bladder is then drained at regular intervals via catheterization of the stoma to maintain continence and assure decompression of the bladder and proximal tracts.

These types of urinary reconstructions may lead to complications and problems. Stomal stenosis, parastomal hernia, stomal retraction, and failure of continence of the bowel segment mechanism may occur. Stenosis of the stoma may be managed by more frequent catheterization, stomal dilation and, sometimes, surgical revision of the stoma. Parastomal hernia and stomal retraction are usually managed conservatively unless they are symptomatic in the form of pain, inability to catheterize adequately or, in the case of non-continent stomas, inadequate adhesion or fitting of a stomal appliance (47, 48).

More serious complications such as perforation of the augment or stoma, secondary malignancy, and electrolyte disturbances may also occur. Perforation is uncommon and warrants immediate evaluation with imaging and/or exploratory laparotomy (47, 49). Secondary malignancy is not common in augmented bladders, but may occur in 1–5% of cases and present with gross hematuria, hydronephrosis, and systemic signs of metastatic disease. It is usually in the form of adenocarcinoma and some advocate annual bladder/renal ultrasonography (with annual/semi-annual urinalysis for significant amounts of blood) with or without cystoscopy of the augmented bladder (49). Potential electrolyte disturbances are dependent upon the segment of bowel used to augment the bladder or to form a diversion and the underlying renal and hepatic function of the patient. If intestinal segments are substituted or added to normalize the urinary system they tend to reabsorb electrolytes, acids, and bases that are excreted in the urine. Normal renal and hepatic function and regular drainage of the urinary system to limit contact time of the solutes with the bowel segment minimize this problem. Use of the stomach may lead to hypochloremic hypokalemic alkalosis; use of the jejunum may lead to hyponatremic hypochloremic hyperkalemic acidosis; and use of the distal small bowel and colon may lead to hyperchloremic acidosis. The jejunum seems to be the most likely to lead to electrolyte disturbances (potentially > 20% of patients) and is seldom used. The stomach is less frequently used than the distal small bowel and colon at some institutions secondary to a hematuria–dysuria syndrome related to the acidic secretions of the stomach causing painful urination and sloughing of bladder cells and bleeding. This is usually managed conservatively with histamine receptor-2 blockers (47).

One additional helpful piece of information for physicians taking care of patients with urinary reconstructions and diversions is the usefulness of a temporizing catheter if a Urologist is not available for immediate consultation. If a catheterizable stoma or augmented bladder is not draining appropriately secondary to stenosis or loss of the continence mechanism, the patient has not been catheterized regularly and the reconstructed bladder is over-distended, or the patient is having an electrolyte disturbance, placement of an indwelling catheter into the bladder or conduit diversion will remove the urine from the system, leading to decompression and reducing contact time with the GI mucosa (47, 48). Caution should be used before placing a catheter if a perforation is suspected, and catheters with a balloon should be placed carefully so as not to inflate the balloon within the stoma or at the continence mechanism. They are usually inserted safely as long as the balloon is inflated within the native or augmented bladder. If in doubt, use of a straight Robinson ("red rubber") catheter without a balloon and securing it externally with a stitch or tape is a good temporizing measure.

13.2.27 Prune belly syndrome, bladder exstrophy–epispadias complex, urachal cyst/patent urachus and congenital urethral strictures

Several rare malformations and syndromes associated with genitourinary conditions may occur. If they are only partially penetrant or incompletely manifest then pediatric medical and surgical management may lead to the absence of their effect on adult life. The syndromes and abnormalities described below will be relevant in later life only if they are associated with the abnormalities mentioned above.

Prune belly syndrome is a conglomerate syndrome associated with multiple genitourinary and extra-genitourinary anomalies. It is rare, occurring in ~1 in 30,000–40,000 live births and almost exclusively occurs in boys. It classically includes the development of abnormal abdominal musculature (leading to a prune-shaped belly), genitourinary abnormalities, and intra-abdominal testes. Genitourinary abnormalities include VUR (75%), renal dysplasia, a dilated or atretic urethra, enlarged bladders with or without urachal abnormalities, and tortuous ureters. It is also associated with a wide range of midline cardiopulmonary, GI, and musculoskeletal defects (50). Each abnormality is treated appropriately depending on the severity, such as orchiopexy for undescended testicles and urachal remnant excision for a patent urachus.

Bladder exstrophy–epispadias complex is another rare entity occurring in near the same frequency as prune belly syndrome, and is also seen more in males (3 to 4:1). For those children that survive with bladder exstrophy and epispadias (dorsal non-anatomic opening of the urethra), staged reconstruction of the bladder, anterior abdominal wall, and anterior pelvic ring is undertaken. Bladder exstrophy may also be associated with cloacal exstrophy and is associated with a higher mortality and more difficult course (51). Children with bladder exstrophy closure are at a higher risk of developing adenocarcinoma of the bladder later in life, and may require urinary diversion if repair fails (52). Types of urinary diversion and their sequelae are mentioned above.

Urachal remnants of the child include patent urachus, urachal sinus, urachal cyst, and vesicourachal diverticulum. The exact mechanism of their persistence and formation is not known, but they are non-obliterated tissue of the tract of the urachus from the bladder to the umbilicus, which was formerly the allantois. The overwhelming majority of these will be noticed in the perinatal period or first few years of life secondary to urine leak from the naval or cord, a swollen or misshapen cord stump, or infection and abscess formation. The recommendation for urachal remnants is surgical excision if found due to the greatly increased possibility of adenocarcinoma formation of the bladder/urachus in later life, and due to the fact that they may become chronically infected. Urachal cysts and vesicourachal diverticuli are the two entities more likely to be diagnosed later in life because they usually do not have a communication with the anterior abdominal wall (53). A urachal cyst may present with abscess formation deep to the umbilicus, and is best diagnosed with ultrasonography. A vesicourachal diverticulum may never be noticed unless cystoscopy or cystography is done and tends to be less problematic with respect to cancer or infection.

A congenital urethral stricture is a rare entity with effects similar to PUVs and immediate surgical management follows that for PUVs. Gradual dilation after immediate drainage is usually very successful (54).

13.3 Abnormalities of sexual differentation

There are a host of major and minor alterations in the number and integrity of chromosomes, function and sensitivity of hormone receptors, and hormone production that can lead to varying degrees of abnormal sexual differentiation and variations between a patient's genotypic and phenotypic sex. These include TS, Klinefelter syndrome, CAH, androgen receptor insensitivity, and mixed gonadal dysgenesis. The details of each of these and their resultant sexual characteristic, or lack thereof, is well beyond the scope of this chapter.

The key concept in dealing with adult or adolescent patients with a history of abnormal sexual differentiation or "ambiguous genitalia" at birth is to treat them in a manner consistent with their gender assignment as a child or their phenotypic presentation of sexual characteristics as they see fit to pursue their lives.

The two most common types of abnormalities/ambiguousity are CAH and mixed gonadal dysgenesis. CAH usually results in a masculinized female (female pseudohermaphroditism) due to deficient corticosterone production by the adrenals leading to increased ACTH production and increased androgen production by the same gland. Corticosteroid supplementation and, sometimes, feminizing genitoplasty as an infant, will usually produce genotypic and phenotypic females. Mixed gonadal dysgenesiscan be considered as one-half of the genitourinary tract forming male-type structures and one-half forming female-type structures, with an intra-abdominal testes on one side, a streaked gonad on the other, and a mixture of phallic enlargement with labioscrotal fusion. This is not "true" hermaphrodism and is usually associated with a 45X or 46XY phenotype. Mixed gonadal dysgenesis is managed by appropriate gonadectomy, gender assignment for life, and screening during childhood for Wilms' tumor. Around two-thirds of children are raised as female depending upon the original degree of masculinization. The amount of masculinization originally may be associated with a greater degree of androgen imprinting and a more difficult time coping with induced feminization later in life (55).

References

1. Neville, H., Ritchey, M. (2000) Wilms' tumor: overview of National Wilms' Tumor Study Group Results. Urol. Clin. North Am. 27:435–442.
2. Alexander, F. (2000) Neuroblastoma. Urol. Clin. North Am. 27:383–392.
3. Sklar, C., LaQuaglia, M. (2000) The long-term complications of chemotherapy in childhood genitourinary tumors. Urol. Clin. North Am. 27:563–568.
4. Ludin, A, Macklis R. (2000) Radiotherapy for pediatric genitourinary tumors: Its role and long-term consequences. Urol. Clin. North Am. 27:553–562.
5. Khoury, A., Bagli, D. J. (2007) Reflux and megaureter. In: Wein, A. J., Kavoussi, L. R., Novick, A. C., Partin, A. W., Peters, C. A., eds. Campbell-Walsh Urology, 9th ed. Philadelphia, USA: Saunders Elsevier, pp. 3428–3429.
6. Lebowitz, R. L., Olbing, H., Parkkulainen, K. V., et al. (1985) International system of radiographic grading of vesicoureteric reflux. International Reflux Study in Children. Pediatr. Radiol. 15:105–109.
7. Khoury, A., Bagli, D. J. (2007) Reflux and megaureter. In: Wein, A. J., Kavoussi, L. R., Novick, A. C., Partin, A. W., Peters, C. A., eds. Campbell-Walsh Urology, 9th ed. Philadelphia, USA: Saunders Elsevier, pp. 3462–3467.
8. Elder, J. S., Peters, C. A., Arant, B. S. Jr. et al. (1997) Pediatric vesicoureteral reflux guidelines panel summary report on the management of primary vesicoureteral reflux in children. J. Urol. 157:1846–1851.
9. Arant, B. S. Jr. (1987) Medical management of mild and moderate vesicoureteral reflux: follow-up studies of infants and young children. A preliminary report of the Southwest Pediatric Nephrology Study Group. BMJ 295:237–241.
10. Dave, S., Khoury, A. E. (2007) The current evidence based medical management of vesicoureteral reflux: the Sick Kids protocol. Indian J. Urol. 23:403–413.
11. Kissane, J. M., Smith, M. G. (1975) Pathology of infancy and childhood, 2nd ed. St. Louis, USA: Mosby, p. 587.
12. Cole, B. R., Conley, S. B., Stapleton, F. B. (1987) Polycystic kidney disease in the first year of life. J. Pediatr. 111:693.
13. Glassberg, K. I. (2007) Renal dysgenesis and cystic disease of the kidney. In: Wein, A. J., Kavoussi, L. R., Novick, A. C., Partin, A. W., Peters, C. A., eds. Campbell-Walsh Urology, 9th ed. Philadelphia, USA: Saunders Elsevier, pp. 3318–3325.

14. Frydenberg, M., Malek, R., Zincke, H. (1993) Conservative renal surgery for renal cell carcinoma in von Hippel-Lindau disease. J. Urol. 149:461.
15. Glassberg, K. I., Filmer, R. B. (1992) Renal dysplasia, renal hypoplasia and cystic disease of the kidney. In: Belman, A. B., King, L. R., Kramer, S. A., eds. Clinical Pediatric Urology, 3rd ed. Philadelphia, USA: W. B. Saunders.
16. Glassberg, K. I. (2007) Renal dysgenesis and cystic disease of the kidney. In: Wein, A. J., Kavoussi, L. R., Novick, A. C., Partin, A. W., Peters, C. A., eds. Campbell-Walsh Urology, 9th ed. Philadelphia, USA: Saunders Elsevier, pp. 3334–3338.
17. Glassberg K. I. (2007) Renal dysgenesis and cystic disease of the kidney. In: Wein AJ, Kavoussi LR, Novick AC, Partin AW, Peters CA, eds. Campbell-Walsh urology, 9th ed. Philadelphia, PA: Saunders Elsevier, pp. 3348–50.
18. Schlussel, R. N., Retik, A. B. (2007) Ectopic ureter, ureterocele, and other anomalies of the ureter. In: Wein, A. J., Kavoussi, L. R., Novick, A. C., Partin, A. W., Peters, C. A., eds. Campbell-Walsh Urology, 9th ed. Philadelphia, USA: Saunders Elsevier, p. 3413.
19. Atwell, J. D., Cook, P. L., Howell, C. J., et al. (1974) Familial incidence of bifid and double ureters. Arch. Dis. Child. 49:390.
20. Lebowitz, R. L., Blickman, J. G. (1983) The coexistence of ureteropelvic junction obstruction and reflux. Am. J. Roentgenol. 140:231–238.
21. Williams, D. I., Karlaftis, C. M. (1966) Hydronephrosis due to pelviureteric obstruction in the newborn. Br. J. Urol. 38:138–144.
22. Carr, M. C., El-Ghoneimi, A. (2007) Anomalies and surgery of the ureteropelvic junction in children. In: Wein, A. J., Kavoussi, L. R., Novick, A. C., Partin, A. W., Peters C. A., eds. Campbell-Walsh Urology, 9th ed. Philadelphia, USA: Saunders Elsevier, 3362.
23. Carr, M. C., El-Ghoneimi, A. (2007) Anomalies and surgery of the ureteropelvic junction in children. In: Wein, A. J., Kavoussi, L. R., Novick, A. C., Partin, A. W., Peters C. A., eds. Campbell-Walsh Urology, 9th ed. Philadelphia, USA: Saunders Elsevier, pp. 3370–3380.
24. Dairiki Shortliffe, L. M. (2007) Infection and inflammation of the pediatric genitourinary tract. In: Wein, A. J., Kavoussi, L. R., Novick, A. C., Partin, A. W., Peters, C. A., eds. Campbell-Walsh Urology, 9th ed. Philadelphia, USA: Saunders Elsevier, 3256–3260.
25. Jacobson, S. H., Eklöf, O., Eriksson, C. G. et al. (1989) Development of hypertension and uraemia after pyelonephritis in childhood: 27 year follow up. BMJ 299:703–706.
26. Cascio, S., Paran, S., Puri, P. (1999) Associated urological anomalies in children with unilateral renal agenesis. J. Urol. 162:1081–1083.
27. Bauer, S. B. (2007) Anomalies of number of the upper urinary tract. In: Wein, A. J., Kavoussi, L. R., Novick, A. C., Partin, A. W., Peters, C. A., eds. Campbell-Walsh Urology, 9th ed. Philadelphia, USA: Saunders Elsevier, 3269–3290.
28. Campbell, M. F. (1970) Anomalies of the Kidney. Urology, vol 2, 3rd ed. Philadelphia, USA: W. B. Saunders, 1447–1452.
29. Khoury, A., Bagli, D. J. (1970) Reflux and megaureter. In: Campbell, M. F. (1970) Anomalies of the Kidney. Urology, vol 2, 3rd ed. Philadelphia, USA: W. B. Saunders, 1447–1452.
30. Coplen, D. E., Duckett, J. W. (1995) The modern approach to ureteroceles. J. Urol. 153:166.
31. Schlussel, R. N., Retik, A. B. (1970) Ectopic ureter, ureterocele, and other anomalies of the ureter. In: Campbell, M. F. (1970) Anomalies of the Kidney. Urology, vol 2, 3rd ed. Philadelphia, USA: W. B. Saunders, pp. 1447–1452.
32. Acien, P., Susarte, F., Romero, J. et al. (2004) Complex genital malformation: ectopic ureter ending in a supposed mesonephric duct in a woman with renal agenesis and ipsilateral blind hemivagina. Eur. J. Obstet. Gynecol. Reprod. Biol. 117:105–108.
33. Diard, F., Eklöf, O., Leibowitz, R., Maurseth, K. (1981) Urethral obstruction in boys caused by prolapse of simple ureterocele. Pediatr. Radiol. 11:139.
34. Grady, R. (2000) Current management of prepubertal yolk sac tumors of the testis. Urol. Clin. North Am. 27:503–508.

35. Kaefer, M., Rink, R. (2000) Genitourinary rhabdomyosarcoma: treatment options. Urol. Clin. North Am. 27:471–487.
36. Thomas, D. F., Gordon, A. C. (1989) Management of prenatally diagnosed uropathies. Arch. Dis. Child. 64:58.
37. Gunn, T. R., Mora, J. D., Pease, P. (1995) Antenatal diagnosis of urinary tract abnormalities by ultrasonography after 28 weeks gestation: Incidence and outcome. Am. J. Obstet. Gynecol. 172:479.
38. Casale, A. J. (1970) Posterior urethral valves and other urethral anomalies. In: Campbell MF. Anomalies of the Kidney. Urology, vol 2, 3rd ed. Philadelphia: W. B. Saunders, 1447–1452.
39. Sheldon, C. A., Churchill, B. M., McLorie, G. A., et al. (1992) Evaluation of factors contributing to mortality in pediatric renal transplant recipients. J. Pediatr. Surg. 27:629.
40. Borer, J. G., Retik, A. B. (1970) Hypospadias. In: Campbell, M. F. Anomalies of the Kidney. Urology, vol 2, 3rd ed. Philadelphia, USA: W. B. Saunders, 1447–1452.
41. Wu, W. H., Chuang, J. H., Ting, Y. C., et al. (2002) Developmental anomalies and disabilities associated with hypospadias. J. Urol. 168:229–232.
42. Mieusset, R., Soulie, M. (2005) Hypospadias: psychosocial, sexual, and reproductive consequences in adult life. J. Androl. 26:163–168.
43. Schneck, F. X., Bellinger, M. F. (1970) Abnormalities of the testes and scrotum and their surgical management. In: Campbell, M. F. (1970) Anomalies of the Kidney. Urology, vol 2, 3rd ed. Philadelphia, USA: W. B. Saunders, 1447–1452.
44. Taran, I., Elder, J. S. (2006) Results of orchiopexy for the undescended testis. World J. Urol. 24:231–239.
45. Chilvers, C., Dudley, N. E., Gough, M. H., et al. (1986) Undescended testis: the effect of treatment on subsequent risk of subfertility and malignancy. J. Pediatr. Surg. 21:691.
46. Yeung, C. K., Sihoe, J. D. Y., Bauer, S. B. (1970)Voiding dysfunction in children: non-neurogenic and neurogenic. In: Campbell, M. F. (1970) Anomalies of the Kidney. Urology, vol 2, 3rd ed. Philadelphia, USA: W. B. Saunders, 1447–1452.
47. Adams MC, Joseph DB. Urinary tract reconstruction in children. In: Campbell MF. Anomalies of the kidney. Urology, Vol 2, 3rd ed. Philadelphia, PA: WB Saunders, 1447–1452.
48. Crispen, P. L., Blute, M. L. (2009) Catheterizable stoma problems. The 5-minute urology consult.
49. Kurzrock, E. A. (2009) Pediatric enterocystoplasty: long-term complications and controversies. World J. Urol. 27:69–73.
50. Caldamone, A. A., Woodard, J. R. (1970) Prune belly syndrome. In: Campbell, M. F. Anomalies of the Kidney. Urology, vol 2, 3rd ed. Philadelphia, USA: W. B. Saunders, 1447–1452.
51. Gearhart, J. P., Mathews, R. (1970) Exstrophy-epispadias complex. In: Campbell, M. F. Anomalies of the Kidney. Urology, vol 2, 3rd ed. Philadelphia, USA: W. B. Saunders, 1447–1452.
52. Woodhouse, C. R. J., Ransley, P. G., Williams, D. I. (1983) The patient with exstrophy in adult life. BJU 55:632–635.
53. Frimberger, D., Kropp, B. P. (1970) Bladder anomalies in children. In: Campbell, M. F. (1970) Anomalies of the Kidney. Urology, vol 2, 3rd ed. Philadelphia, USA: W. B. Saunders, 1447–1452.
54. Passerini-Glazel, G., Araguna, F., Chiozza, L., et al. (1988) The PADUA (progressive augmentation by dilating the urethra anterior) procedure for the treatment of severe urethral hypoplasia. J. Urol. 140:124–127.
55. Diamond, D. A. (1970) Sexual differentiation: normal and abnormal. In: Campbell, M. F. Anomalies of the Kidney. Urology, vol 2, 3rd ed. Philadelphia: W. B. Saunders, 1447–1452.

14 Adult patients with childhood anemias

Vlad C. Radulescu and Jeffrey A. Moscow

The chronic, lifelong anemias diagnosed in childhood and extending into adult life are due to genetic defects that affect the production and maturation of RBCs or that shorten the lifespan of the red blood cell and promote chronic hemolysis. This review will discuss various anemias and management from childhood into adulthood.

14.1 Introduction

The chronic, lifelong anemias diagnosed in childhood and extending into adult life are due to genetic defects that affect the production and maturation of RBCs or that shorten the lifespan of the RBC and promote chronic hemolysis.

14.2 Anemias through decreased production of RBCs

Fanconi anemia is an autosomal recessive disorder caused by mutations in specific genes which are important for DNA repair. It manifests with birth defects (café-au-lait spots, short stature, thumb and radius abnormalities, abnormal head, eyes, ears, kidneys), hematologic abnormalities (anemia, thrombocytopenia, neutropenia, bone-marrow failure) and a high risk of myelodysplastic syndrome, leukemia, as well as solid tumors.

The curative treatment for bone-marrow failure, myelodysplastic syndrome and leukemia is a bone-marrow transplant. Adult patients with Fanconi anemia who had a bone-marrow transplant continue to be at a high risk for solid tumors, including head, neck, esophagus and gynecologic carcinomas, as well as liver tumors.

All adult patients should be closely monitored for cancer. Non-transplanted patients should be monitored with CBC several times a year and bone-marrow aspiration at least yearly. All patients should have an annual screening examination for head and neck cancer (mouth, tongue, pharynx, larynx, esophagus). All women with Fanconi anemia should have an annual gynecologic examination, a Papanicolaou smear and testing for human papilloma virus (1).

Diamond–Blackfan anemia (DBA) is a constitutional form of pure red cell aplasia. It represents an intrinsic disorder of hematopoiesis secondary to structural mutation in *genes coding* for ribosome proteins. The inheritance is autosomal dominant; many cases are due to new mutations.

Most patients are diagnosed in the first year of life. The clinical picture includes severe anemia, short stature, and various birth defects: dysmorphic facies, webbed neck, abnormal thumbs. The anemia is normocytic or macrocytic, with low reticulocyte count, high percentage of hemoglobin F, elevated erythrocyte adenosine deaminase, and maturational arrest of the erythrocyte precursors on the bone-marrow aspirate. A mutation in the RPS19 gene can be identified in ~25% of patients.

Therapy includes corticosteroids and/or RBC transfusions. About 20% of patients will enter remission; the others will require lifelong therapy. Bone-marrow transplant has been used in a limited number of cases.

Adults with DBA have an increased risk of hematologic and non-hematologic malignancies. The long-term outlook is also influenced by the complications of therapy (corticosteroids, transfusions, bone-marrow transplant). The overall survival beyond the age of 40 years is ~75% (2).

Shwachman–Diamond Anemia (SDA) is an autosomal recessive disorder due to a mutation in the SBDS gene that affects ribosome biogenesis. Clinical manifestations include impaired hematopoiesis with neutropenia, anemia, thrombocytopenia, pancreatic insufficiency, and skeletal abnormalities. Patients with SDA have a high risk of developing leukemia or myelodysplastic syndrome. The treatment is supportive: granulocyte-colony stimulating factor for neutropenia, transfusions for anemia, thrombocytopenia, and pancreatic enzyme replacement for pancreatic insufficiency. Bone-marrow transplant has been used for profound cytopenias, myelodysplastic syndrome or leukemia transformation. The results of bone-marrow transplant when compared to supportive therapy have been inconclusive (3).

Paroxysmal nocturnal hemoglobinuria (PNH) is an acquired disease due to a somatic mutation of the PIGA gene occurring in hematopoietic stem cells. PIGA-mutated cells lack certain surface proteins; in the case of RBCs this makes them vulnerable to complement-mediated lysis. The main manifestations of the disease are hemolytic anemia, hemoglobinuria and thromboembolic events. Patients with PNH have a high risk of bone-marrow failure and leukemic transformation.

Treatment for PNH includes management of anemia and thrombosis. Ecluzimab, a monoclonal antibody that binds the C5 complement, has been effective in improving anemia and reducing transfusion requirements, and may reduce the risk of thromboembolic events (4). The only curative therapy is bone-marrow transplant.

14.3 Anemias through abnormal maturation of RBCs: thalassemia syndromes

Thalassemias are disorders of impaired hemoglobin production and abnormal maturation of RBCs. They are the result of mutations in the alpha- or beta-globin genes, leading to imbalanced production of alpha- and beta-globin, ineffective erythropoiesis and anemia. The compensatory expansion of the erythroid precursors may lead to bone changes, hepatomegaly and splenomegaly.

Thalassemias are more commonly encountered in populations from the Mediterranean basin of Europe and North Africa, Middle East and South and South-East Asia, areas were malaria had been endemic until recently. It is presumed that thalassemia confers a certain resistance to severe forms of malaria.

The thalassemias are classified based on the genetic defect: alpha- and beta-thalassemias and based on symptom severity. Thalassemia trait is manifested by borderline anemia and microcytosis; thalassemia intermedia is moderate anemia; and thalassemia major is severe anemia requiring chronic transfusions. Illness severity is directly related to the number of genes affected: there are four alpha- and two beta-globin genes.

The classical manifestation of thalassemia major –severe anemia, growth retardation, organomegaly and bone remodeling due to marrow expansion –are rarely encountered in industrialized countries due to early therapy.

Treatment consists of chronic transfusions and iron chelation. Bone-marrow transplant is curative but is limited by the availability of a matched related donor. Matched unrelated SCT as well as cord blood transplant have been done in a limited number of patients and are considered to be investigational. The probability of thalassemia-free survival after a bone-marrow transplant is 80–87% depending on disease severity (5).

Adults with thalassemia major who have received chronic transfusions since childhood may develop complications of this therapy: iron overload, transmission of viral infection, alloimunization. Some are survivors of an allogeneic bone-marrow transplant, others underwent splenectomy for massive splenomegaly or for hypersplenism. The complications of these therapeutic interventions are discussed at the end of the chapter.

The outlook for thalassemia has improved significantly over the past several decades as a result of improved safety of the blood supply, more efficient iron chelation, and improved bone-marrow transplant results. In a series of 977 patients from Italy, born since 1960, 68% were alive at 35 years. Most of the deaths were due to cardiac hemosiderosis. The patients born between 1980 and 1984 and 1985–1997 had significantly improved survival, and the probability of death from cardiac hemosiderosis was much lower (one cardiac death in the 1980–1984 cohort and none afterwards) (6).

14.4 Anemias through increased destruction of RBCs

As a group, these anemias are due to a genetic defect that leads to a shortened lifespan of the RBCs due to a membrane defect, an enzymatic defect, or anabnormal hemoglobin. Patients typically have anemia (which may be chronic or acute) and are at risk of developing cholelithiasis.

14.5 Sickle cell disease

Sickle cell disease is a genetic disorder due to a mutation in the beta-globin gene. The consequence of the mutation is a one amino-acid substitution in the structure of the beta-globin, resulting in the production of abnormal hemoglobin: hemoglobin S. The latter has reduced solubility and may polymerize in hypoxic conditions. The polymer containing RBCs frequently assume a sickle shape, are more rigid and likely to obstruct the microvasculature. This leads to painful episodes and ischemic damage to various organs. Sickle cells have a shortened lifespan due to their premature destruction in the spleen and liver, leading to manifestations of chronic hemolytic anemia.

Sickle cell disease is more frequently encountered in people residing in, or having ancestors in, Sub-Saharan Africa, the Mediterranean area of North Africa and Southern Europe, the Arabic Peninsula and South Asia. It is hypothesized that sickle cell disease confers protection against severe malaria, thus offering a genetic advantage in areas of the world were malaria was endemic. The genotypes that make up sickle cell disease are: SS, SC, and sickle beta-thalassemia. The common feature of these genotypes is that the patients have > 50% hemoglobin S (Hgb SS and HbS beta-thalassemia) or a combination of hemoglobin S and C. In hemoglobin S trait (genotype SA), patients have < 50% hemoglobin S, and are largely asymptomatic.

The clinical manifestations of sickle cell disease are a consequence of recurrent vaso-occlusive events involving the microcirculation and chronic hemolysis. Patients become symptomatic during the first year of life as the hemoglobin production transitions from the fetal pattern – with predominance of the hemoglobin F – to the adult pattern. There are wide individual variations in the clinical manifestations of sickle cell disease within a certain genotype as well as between genotypes. The persistence of hemoglobin F, as well as coexistence with alpha thalassemia trait, is associated with a milder form of disease. Patients with hemoglobin SC are less likely to develop stroke, less likely to have severe anemia, the frequency of painful episodes is lower, and the life expectancy is higher.

Acute painful episodes represent a new, rapidly developing pain usually involving the bones. It is believed that the mechanism is represented by vaso-occlusion of the bone-marrow vasculature causing bone infraction and subsequent local inflammation. The pain episodes represent the most frequent manifestation of sickle cell disease. One-third ofpatients rarely experience pain, one-third require 2–6 hospitalizations per year, and one-third require > 6 hospitalizations; their frequency peaks in the third and fourth decade of life Episodes are triggered by exposure to cold, dehydration, menstruation, stress or alcohol consumption. The pain may involve any area of the body, most commonly the back, chest and extremities. Episodes last for several days. Frequent pain episodes interfere with daily activities and may lead to apathy or depression. The diagnosis is based on the history and physical examination. There is no laboratory or imaging test that is specific enough to be useful in the diagnosis. Management of the acute painful episode starts with the identification of pain triggers (cold, infection, dehydration) and of other conditions that require specific intervention (acute chest syndrome). The pain is treated with non-steroidal anti-inflammatory drugs (NSAIDS, e.g., ketorolac), acetaminophen and opioids. It is important that the patient is well hydrated, carries out incentive spirometry periodically, and spends time out of bed.

Infections are a major cause of morbidity and mortality in sickle cell disease. By the age of 5 years, most patients with sickle cell disease are functionally asplenic due to recurrent splenic microinfarcts. This increases their susceptibility to severe infections with *Streptococcuspneumoniae* and *Haemophillusinfluenzae* type b. Pneumococcus and Haemophilus vaccinations and penicillin prophylaxis have reduced the risk of severe infections. Penicillin prophylaxis has the greatest impact in reducing the risk of pneumococcal sepsis in children aged < 5 years (7). The benefit of penicillin prophylaxis beyond this age is debatable, with the exception of patients who had an episode of pneumococcal sepsis or those who were splenectomized; these patients should stay on penicillin prophylaxis indefinitely due to their increased risk of sepsis. Infections with *Salmonella* species (including osteomyelitis and sepsis) are more common in sickle cell disease, probably as a result of infection of infracted bone. UTIs are more common in patients with sickle cell disease than in the general population. The increased frequency and prolonged course of UTIs may be related to papillary necrosis. Infections with parvovirus B19 induce a more severe anemia in the form of aplastic episodes in patients with sickle cell disease than in the general population due to the shorter lifespan of sickle red cells.

Chronic anemia is a common manifestation of sickle cell disease. It is due to chronic hemolysis of RBCs containing sickle hemoglobin. Patients with severe anemia are more likely to develop strokes and have sickle nephropathy (glomerular dysfunction) and less likely to develop acute chest syndrome and pain crises (after the age of 20 years). The anemia may be exacerbated at times due to decreased production of RBCs caused by infections (parvovirus B 19, Epstein–Barr virus, *Streptococcus pneumoniae*), folate or B12 deficiency, acute sequestration of RBCs in the spleen or liver, or increased hemolysis.

Neurologic events include transient ischemic attacks, cerebral infarction, cerebral hemorrhage, seizures and unexplained coma. Cerebral infarction with or without symptoms has a peak incidence in childhood (2–9 years) followed by a second peak after the age of 20 years. The lifetime risk of developing a silent or overt cerebral infarction is 30–44% depending on the diagnostic methods employed. The main risk factors include: increased cerebral blood flow velocity, history of cerebrovascular accident or transient ischemic attack, nocturnal hypoxemia with or without sleep apnea, hemoglobin SS genotype (the risk of stroke is lower in Hgb SC and Hgb S beta-thalassemia), severe anemia, and high reticulocyte count. Mortality after an initial event is ~20%, and the risk of recurrence at 3 years is ~70%. Clinical presentation may include overt hemiparesis, hemisensory loss, or more subtle manifestations such as weakness of one arm, uneven gait, or cognitive dysfunction.

Cerebral hemorrhage has a peak incidence around the age of 30 years. Signs include the neurologic deficits encountered in infarction along with nuchal rigidity, photophobia, severe headaches, and vomiting, and altered levels of consciousness. A common presentation is coma and seizures without hemiparesis. The mortality is ≤50%, but the morbidity among survivors is low.

Patients with sickle cell disease have a high prevalence(≤30%) of major cerebral vessel stenosis with development of collaterals. These friable collateral vessels appear as "puffs of smoke" on angiography (moyamoya disease). Moyamoya disease predisposes to thrombotic and hemorrhagic strokes.

Patients with signs and symptoms of cerebrovascular accidents should be evaluated with CT or MRI to differentiate between transient ischemic accident, ischemic infarction or hemorrhage.

In the pediatric population with sickle cell disease, the ischemic stroke is treated with supportive measures and exchange transfusion with the goal of reducing the Hgb S to < 30% of total hemoglobin. Given the high risk of recurrence, this is followed by a chronic transfusion regimen for ≥5 years or until the age of 18 years.

Adults with sickle cell disease have a high prevalence of stroke; the interaction between the risk factors associated with sickle cell disease and independent of sickle cell disease is not clearly understood. The treatment of ischemic stroke in adults with sickle cell disease is based on the recommendations for treatment of patients without sickle cell disease, with tissue plasminogen activator. Secondary prophylaxis is achieved with antiplatelet agents (aspirin, dipyridamole, clopidogrel) or anti-coagulants (warfarin). The role of exchange transfusion followed by chronic transfusion in the adult population is not clearly defined (8).

14.5.1 Pulmonary complications

Acute chest syndrome is a complication of sickle cell disease manifested through chest pain, dyspnea, fevers, hypoxia, decrease in the hemoglobin level, leukocytosis, as well as pulmonary infiltrates on chest radiography. It is caused by vaso-occlusion, infection, pulmonary embolization (distant thrombus or fat embolus from infarcted bone marrow). As a consequence of the initial vaso-occlusive event, the patient may develop ventilation/ perfusion mismatch and hypoxemia, which may lead to further sickling, vaso-occlusion and multi-organ failure. The infectious agents associated with pneumonia/acute chest include *Streptococcuspneumoniae, Haemophilus, Mycoplasma, Chlamydia, Legionella* and various viruses. Treatment includes antibiotics, supportive therapy (oxygen, mechanical ventilation, extracorporeal membrane oxygenation) and partial exchange transfusion. Adults have a lower prevalence but mortality approaches 10%.

Pulmonary hypertension is a complication that usually occurs in adults; the prevalence is ~4%. The etiology is unclear; sickle vasculopathy, chronic hypoxia, sleep hypoventilation, and recurrent acute chest syndrome may play a part. Pulmonary hypertension increases the risk of cardiac failure, pulmonary thrombosis, and chronic hypoxia. There is no proven therapy for sickle cell-associated pulmonary hypertension.

14.5.2 Hepatobilliary complications

Cholelithiasis is common in children and adults with sickle cell disease, affecting ≤70% of patients. It is a consequence of the increased prevalence of hemolysis and hyperbilirubinemia.

Acute hepatic syndromes include: acute hepatic crisis (tender hepatomegaly, fever, elevated bilirubin and liver enzymes), hepatic sequestration (hepatomegaly, declining hemoglobin) and sickle cell intrahepatic cholestasis (asymptomatic severe hyperbilirubinemia).

14.5.3 Renal complications

Hematuria may result from thromboses in the peritubular vessels or form papillary necrosis. Treatment includes increased fluid intake to increase diuresis, urine alkalinization (using bicarbonate infusions, acetazolamide), and bed rest.

Proteinuria is encountered in about one-quarter of adults with sickle cell disease; it may progress to nephrotic syndrome. ACE inhibitors may reduce the degree of proteinuria; it is unclear if they slow the progression towards nephrotic syndrome and renal failure.

Hyposthenuria is a common occurrence in sickle cell disease and sickle cell trait. Hyposthenuria is due to recurrent episodes of sickling and infarction in the medullary area of the kidneys (vasa recta) with subsequent decreased ability to concentrate the urine. If the patient becomes water-deprived he/she is more likely to become dehydrated and hypovolemic.

Priapism is a condition characterized by a sustained, unwanted erection that does not resolve after a sexual act. The process probably starts with a physiologic erection; the relative stasis of the blood in the erect penis may lead to deoxygenation, acidosis, sickling of RBCs and venous occlusion. The primary complication is impotence; the longer the duration of priapism the higher the risk of impotence.

Treatment starts with hydration and pain medications if there is no resolution in 12 h. It continues with exchange transfusion; if unsuccessful, urologic procedures may be considered: intracavernosal injection of alpha adrenergic agents, irrigation with normal saline, and vascular bypass procedures.

14.5.4 Ocular complications

The most important ocular complication is sickle cell retinopathy. It is manifested through retinal hemorrhages, development of iridescent spots, retinal neovascularization, and retinal detachment. It is more common in Hgb SC and Hgb-beta thalassemia than in Hgb SS. Peripheral sickle cell retinopathy may require laser therapy.

14.5.5 Bone complications

Patients with sickle cell disease may develop bone changes secondary to expansion of the hematopoietic marrow and thinning of cortical bone (frontal bossing, fishmouth vertebrae) and/or due to repeated bone infarctions (aseptic necrosis of the femoral and humeral heads). Aseptic necrosis of the femoral head commonly leads to joint destruction that requires surgery: core decompression surgery in the early stages or joint replacement in more advanced stages.

14.5.6 Dermatologic complications

Leg ulcers are a common complication in adults, affecting ≥25% of patients. They most commonly occur on the lower legs, over the malleoli. They may occur spontaneously or secondary to trauma, and may become infected. They are secondary to vaso-occlusive events in the skin vasculature. Treatment includes debridement, wet-to-dry dressings, topical zinc oxide cream and antibiotics. The healing process takes weeksto months.

14.5.7 Management

Sickle cell disease is a chronic, lifelong disorder with episodes of acute exacerbations and progressive end-organ damage. There is no curative therapy with the exception of bone-marrow transplant. The goal of the therapy is to prevent and treat the acute exacerbation and to delay end-organ damage. Similarly to other chronic disorders, these patients benefit from routine medical visits, preferably in centers experienced in the management of sickle cell disease. The goal of these visits is to: evaluate illness severity; establish baseline physical findings and laboratory values; educate the patient in the recognition, prevention and management of various complications of the illness; offer support for the lifestyle changes needed.

14.5.8 Transfusion therapy

The goals of transfusion therapy in sickle cell disease vary according to the indication. Simple transfusion is used for correction of severe anemia in aplastic episodes, or splenic sequestration. Simple transfusion is also used preoperatively in patients with

Hgb SS disease, with the goal to increase the hemoglobin level up to 10 g/dL and to reduce the risk of complications.

Exchange transfusion is used to reduce the percentage of sickle hemoglobin below the level at which vaso-oclusive episodes may occur (< 30% hemoglobin S). It is indicated for acute, severe events such as acute chest syndrome, stroke, and priapism.

Chronicmonthly transfusions are aimed at keeping the hemoglobin S below 30–50%. Chronic transfusions are typically used for primary and secondary prophylaxis for stroke in populations at risk.

14.5.9 Hydroxyurea

Hydroxyurea is a cytotoxic agent that can elevate the level of hemoglobin F. Increased level of hemoglobin F decreases hemoglobin S polymerization. In adults, hydroxyurea has been shown to decrease the: severity of painful episodes; frequency of hospitalizations; number of blood transfusions; incidence of acute chest syndrome. The effects of hydroxyurea on end-organ damage (spleen, kidney, brain) have not been evaluated. The short-term side effects of hydroxyurea include anemia, leukopenia, thrombocytopenia (they are dose-dependent and temporary), reversible decrease in sperm production, and skin hyperpigmentation. The long-term effects of hydroxyurea include the risk of birth defects (proven in laboratory animals, suspected in pregnant women). There is no evidence that hydroxyurea, if used in sickle cell disease, increases the risk of leukemia (9).

14.5.10 SCT

SCT represents the only curative therapy for sickle cell disease. It is currently used for severely symptomatic patients with good organ function who have a HLA-matched related donor. Transplant associated mortality approaches 10%, and the long-term side effects in survivors are significant.

14.5.11 Prognosis

Life expectancy has improved significantly over the past three decades, mainly due to decreased incidence of invasive infections. According to Platt et al., in 1994 the median age of death was in the forties for patients with Hgb SS disease and in the sixties for patients with Hgb SC (10). The main risk factors for a severe course and early death are Hgb SS phenotype, low hemoglobin levels, low hemoglobin F levels, high leukocyte count, and frequent pain episodes (11).

14.6 Anemias due to membrane defects: hereditary spherocytosis

Hereditary spherocytosis is the most common disorder of the RBC membrane. It is inherited in an autosomal dominant or in a autosomal recessive pattern. It occurs in all ethnic groups but is more common in people of North European descent. The molecular defect resides in one of the genes that encode for membrane proteins (most commonly band 3, spectrin or ankyrin). The consequence of these abnormalities is the loss of membrane surface with a change in the shape of the RBC from discoid to spherical. The spherical RBCs (spherocytes) are trapped in the spleen and destroyed, leading to anemia with high reticulocyte count, splenomegaly and increased incidence of cholelithiasis. The disease has different degrees of severity. The mild forms, manifesting with anemia or borderline hemoglobin levels, increase reticulocyte count, low mean corpuscular volume (MCV) increased mean corpuscular hemoglobin concentration (MCHC), mild splenomegaly may not be recognized until adulthood.

Common complications include cholelithiasis due to the chronic hyperbilirubinemia and aplastic episodes – precipitous drops in hemoglobin levels during viral infections – especially parvovirus B19 infection.

Treatment is supportive: RBC transfusion for anemia exacerbations, splenectomy for persistent, severe anemia, and cholecystectomy for cholelithiasis. Given the high RBC turnover, folic acid supplements may be useful to prevent folate-deficient anemia.

14.7 Anemias due to enzyme deficiencies in RBCs

The most common red cell enzyme deficiencies leading to chronic anemia are glucose 6 phosphate dehydrogenase deficiency (G6PD) and pyruvate-kinase (PK) deficiency.

G6PD is an X-linked disorder caused by a mutation in the G6PD gene. G6PD is an enzyme that catalyzes the first reaction in the pentose phosphate pathway; this pathway is important for the production of the reduced form of nicotinamide adenine dinucleotide phosphate (NADPH) and protection of the cell from oxidative stress. RBCs deficient in G6PD tend to hemolyze when exposed to oxidative drugs, infection or substances derived from ingested fava beans. Some of the drugs that trigger hemolysis include anti-malarials (primaquine, pamaquine), sulphonamides, nitrofurantoin, and nalidixic acid. These individuals typically have a normal lifespan and a good QoL. Rarely G6PD manifests as a chronic non-spherocytic hemolytic anemia. These patients may require blood transfusions, and have an increased risk of developing cholelithiasis (12).

PK is an enzyme of the glycolytic pathway. PK deficiency is transmitted as an autosomal recessive trait. Clinical manifestations are highly variable, ranging from asymptomatic, compensated hemolysis to severe hemolysis requiring blood transfusions. Splenomegaly is common. Patients are at increased risk of developing gallstones. Splenectomy is beneficial in severe cases because it reduces hemolysis and improves anemia.

14.8 Long-term consequences of therapies used for various anemias

Patients with chronic anemias share certain common therapeutic interventions such as splenectomy, chronic transfusions or bone-marrow transplant. Patients who underwent those interventions will have certain complications or limitations in their lifestyle not necessarily related to the underlying illness but to the therapy.

14.8.1 Splenectomy

Removal of the spleen may be done as an open or laparoscopic procedure. The main indications in a patient with chronic anemia are listed below.

- Hypersplenism: A moderate-to-severely enlarged spleen will increase the destruction of platelets and RBCs. Patients on chronic transfusion for sickle cell disease, thalassemia or DBA who have splenomegaly and hypersplenism may expect a lower transfusion requirement after splenectomy.
- Massive splenomegaly: The spleen may become severely enlarged in thalassemia and sickle cell disease (especially Hgb SC), causing abdominal discomfort and posing a risk of rupture with moderate trauma and severe internal hemorrhage.
- Severe hemolysis: The spleen, along with the liver, represents the main site of destruction of RBCs. Splenectomy has been shown to improve the baseline hemoglobin level in chronic hemolytic anemias such as hereditary spherocytosis or PK deficiency.
- Splenic sequestration: Due to the nature of the splenic vasculature, the cellular elements of the blood become increasingly concentrated as the blood passes through the spleen which, in patients with sickle cell disease, creates conditions for sickling of RBCs. Obstruction of the splenic vessels by sickled RBCs leads to sequestration of large amounts of blood in the spleen with subsequent life-threatening acute anemia and hypovolemia. Splenectomy is thus indicated after the first or second episode of splenic sequestration to prevent recurrence of a dangerous complication.

The main risk of splenectomy is the subsequent lifetime risk of post-splenectomy sepsis. Asplenic patients have an increased risk of invasive infections with encapsulated microorganisms such as *Streptococcus pneumoniae, Neisseria meningitides* and *Haemophilus influenza* type B. Vaccination against these organisms prior to splenectomy and at recommended intervals post-splenectomy is indicated.

Although children aged < 5 years are at the highest risk of post-splenectomy sepsis, and although the risk is highest in the first 2 years post-splenectomy and gradually decreases afterwards, the risk continues to be significant for the entire life of the individual. The overwhelming infections that occur post-splenectomy have a high mortality (~50%) and a fulminant course: 68% of deaths occur within 24 h and 80% within 48 h (13). Therefore, asplenic adults should be instructed to seek immediate medical attention if they are febrile. Primary care providers and Emergency Department Physicians should always evaluate the febrile asplenic patient with a blood culture and CBC with a differential diagnosis, and should at a minimum administer a parenteral broad-spectrum antibiotic such as ceftriaxone. Patients who appear ill, or who show high white blood cell counts, should be admitted for aggressive hydration and antibiotic therapy.

14.8.2 Chronic transfusion therapy

Chronic RBC transfusion has been used as replacement therapy in severe anemias (e.g., thalassemia, DBA) or as a means of suppressing the endogenous erythropoiesis and substituting the sickle cell-containing RBCs with normal ones (e.g., in sickle cell disease complicated by stroke). Chronic transfusion therapy has several risks: transmission of infections, iron overload, and alloimmunization.

The risk of infection transmission through transfused blood has been progressively lowered by screening donors and checking donated blood with serologic, antigenic and nucleic acid amplification testing. The risk of transmission of the human immunodeficiency virus (HIV) and hepatitis C virus (HCV) is ~1: 2 million units; the risk of transmission of hepatitis B is 1:400.000 units (14).

With respect to the risk of iron overload, in health, iron homeostasis is controlled by intestinal absorption; the physiologic iron losses are negligible. Each RBC transfusion introduces 200–250 mg ironinto the body. Once the normal iron-storing capacity of transferrin is exceeded, iron is deposited in the monocyte–macrophage system and then in parenchymal organs: the heart, liver, and endocrine glands. Iron deposition leads to fibrosis and irreversible damage.

Iron overload may be accurately assessed through the liver iron content determined on a liver biopsy. Magnetic susceptibility measurement is another reliable method of estimating iron content. Serum ferritin is a less precise but simple and cheap test. MRI is an emerging, non-invasive method for this type of measurement.

Transfusional iron overload is treated with chelation therapy. Chelation is typically started when the patient receives 10–20 transfusions (~100 cm^3/kg) and/or the ferritin level reaches 1000 µg/L (15). Two products are currently available in the USA: deferoxamine (Desferal) is an injectable agent administered as 12-h subcutaneous infusion. Deferasirox (Exjade) is a new oral agent which seems to have comparable efficacy.

RBC alloimmunization is the development of antibodies against some antigens of the transfused RBCs. It is more common in patients with sickle cell disease given the fact that the donor pool is mostly Caucasian while the recipients are predominantly African. The consequences of alloimmunization include decreased availability of compatible units, delayed hemolytic reactions, and autoantibody formation. The incidence of alloimmunizatiion may be reduced by transfusing blood matched not only in the major blood groups, but also in some of the minor blood groups as well as by increasing the pool of African–American donors (16).

References

1. Owen, J., Frohnmayer, L., Eiler, M. E., eds. (2003) Fanconi anemia. Standards for care, 2nd ed. Eugene, USA: Fanconi Anemia Research Fund.
2. Lipton, J. M., Ellis, S. R. (2009) Diamond blackfan anemia: diagnosis, treatment and molecular pathogenesis. Hematol. Oncol. Clin. North Am. 23:261–282.
3. Burroughs, L., Woolfrey, A., Shimamura, A. (2009) Shawchaman-Diamond syndrome: a review of the clinical presentation, molecular pathogenesis, diagnosis and treatment. Hematol. Oncol. Clin. North Am. 23:233–248.
4. Parker, C. J. (2009) Bone marrow failure syndromes: paroxysmal nocturnal hemoglobinuria. Hematol. Oncol. Clin. North Am. 23:333–346.
5. Lucarelli, G., Gaziev, J. (2008) Advances in the allogeneic transplantation for thalassemia. Blood Rev. 22:53–63.
6. Borgna-Pignatti, C., Rugolotto, S., De Stefano, P., Zhao, H., Capellini, M. D., DelVechio, G. C., et al. (2004) Survival and complications in patients with thalassemia major treated with transfusion and desferoxamine. Haematologica 89:1187–1193.
7. Falletta, J. M., Woods, G. M., Verter, J. I., Buchanan, G. R., Pegelow, C. H., Iyer, R. V., Miller, S. T., Holbrook, C. T., Kinney, T. R., Vichinsky, E. (1995) Discontinuing penicillin prophylaxis in children with sickle cell anemia. J. Pediatrics 127(5):685–690.

8. National Institutes of Health. (2002) The management of sickle cell disease. Washington, USA: Department of Health Human Services, National Institutes of Health, National Heart and Lung Blood Institute.
9. Brawley, O. W., Cornelius, L. J., Edwards, L. R., Gamble, V. N., Green, B. L., Inturrisi, C (2008) National Institutes of Health consensus development conference statement: hydroxyurea treatment for sickle cell disease. Ann. Intern. Med. 148:932–938.
10. Platt, O. S., Brambilla, D. J., Rosse, W. F., Milner, P. F., Castro, O., Steinberg, M. H., Klug, P. P. (1994) Mortality in sickle cell disease. Life expectancy and risk factors for early death. New Engl. J. Med. 330(23):1639–1644.
11. Buchanan, G. R., De Baun, M. R., Quinn, C. T., Steinberg, M. H. (2004) Sickle cell disease Hematology Am Soc Hematol Educ Program. 1:35–47.
12. Cappellini, M. D., Fiorelli, G. (2008) Glucose-6-phosphate dehydrogenase deficiency. Lancet 371:64–67.
13. Melles, D. C., de Marie, S. (2004) Prevention of infections in hyposplenic and asplenic patients: an update. Neth. J. Med. 62:45–52.
14. Stramer, S. L. (2007) Current risk of transfusion-transmitted agents. Arch. Pathol. Lab. Med. 131:702–707.
15. Angelucci, E., Barosi, G., Camaschella, C., Cappellini, M. D., Cazzola, M., Galanello, R., et al. (2008) Italian Society of Hematology practice guidelines for the management of iron overload in thalassemia major and related disorders. Haematologica 93:741–752.
16. Eder, A. F., Chambers, L. A. (2007) Noninfectious complications of blood transfusions. Arch. Pathol. Lab. Med. 131:708–718.

15 Transition from pediatric to adult care: Social and family issues

Jacqueline A. Noonan

Transition of the pediatric patient to an adult care provider is a challenge for patient and provider. Recognition of the family's role in the adult with a chronic illness can be of great value to the adult care provider. The initial visit on transition will be greatly helped if a parent accompanies their adult child to provide the important part medical history often long and complicated which the adult patient might be unable to provide. There are many challenges to successful transition which will be discussed.

15.1 Introduction

Transition of the pediatric patient to an adult care provider is a challenge for patient and provider (1). Children with chronic illnesses develop a strong bond with their pediatric care provider and may be reluctant to change to another doctor. Some children with rare disorders may need to have continued long-term follow-up by the current expert if an appropriate adult expert is not available. An adult provider is needed to provide ongoing primary care in collaboration with the specialist.

For children with chronic illness, management is a family affair, with the mother playing a prominent part in keepingmedical records. The adult care provider should seek help from the parents at the time of transition. The patient often will be unable to provide the history and the adult patient should be encouraged to give permission for the family to provide the medical history. It is common for a family member (usually the mother) to accompany adult children on their visit to a medical provider.

A young adult patient moved from another state in the USA and came to see me for continuing care. She was accompanied by her mother who was able to provide all the essential information regarding the complex cardiac lesion which had required multiple procedures and which had been accompanied by multiple complications. The patient would have been unable to answer her medical history from early childhood, and obtaining all the necessary medical records is difficult and time-consuming. Until the mother's death, she continued to accompany her now married daughter to all of her visits. They were a good team (1). A study published in 2004 (2) regarding adults attending a Cardiac Follow-up Clinic in a rural area revealed that, of 32 adults aged 18–53 years, 63% were accompanied by one or both parents.

15.2 Transition

Although transition from a pediatric to an adult care provider should ideally introduce the patient to the team of adult care providers, making sure the adolescent or young adult understands the chronic illness and the need for follow up, this seldom occurs. Transition occurs at an awkward time. Adolescents once they reach 18 years of age are legally independent and going to the doctor for follow-up is seldom a high priority. Even if there is a Transition Team in place and the patient is given appropriate education regarding his/her condition and need for follow-up, the results are disappointing. A study from Toronto (3) showed that, despite transition patient education and adequate medical insurance coverage, only 40% of patients with significant cardiac disease such as transposition of great arteries, tetralogy of Fallot or aortic stenosis kept an appointment in the Adult Congenital Clinic within 2–3 years. Patients requiring follow-up for cardiac problems are frequently asymptomatic and feel little need for follow-up. Unfortunately, the development of symptoms usually occurs after the heart has undergone significant or severe changes. For example, pulmonary valve insufficiency afterrepair for tetrolagy of Fallot causes no symptoms until a significant arrhythmia occurs or signs of heart failure develop. Pulmonary valve replacement at this late stage carries a higher surgical risk and the return to normal ventricular function less likely to occur. Likewise, a patient with a dilated aorta associated with a bicuspid aortic valve or MFS may have no symptoms until aortic dissection develops. Regular follow-up of the diameter of the ascending aorta can lead to surgical intervention before dissection occurs.

Some chronic conditions require daily intervention, such as insulin-dependent DM and CF. Children with these conditions become by necessity involved directly in their own care. The child with DM learns quickly what happens when his/her blood glucose level falls or if too little insulin results in ketoacidosis. Early on these children learn to give their own insulin shots, check their blood glucose levels and accept a good deal of responsibility for managing their DM. Likewise, patients with CF learn what happens if they fail to take their enzyme supplements or have their daily sessions of postural drainage and percussion. During adolescence, some become non-compliant, often with serious consequences. As adults they are likely to become more compliant but they may be quite demanding. Both of these conditions are usually treated at a Children's Hospital or an Academic Medical Center with a team of Nurses, Dieticians, Nutritionists, Social Workers and other HealthcareProviders working with pediatric specialists. Unfortunately, such a team may not be available to the adult specialists, leading to possible patient concern.

Unfortunately, children learn more from how a parent actually behaves rather than what the parent says. For example, I have seen several mothers with MFS who are very conscientious about follow-up visits for their affected child and see that the child is compliant with prescribed medications, but these same mothers may be non-compliant in their own follow-up visits and medication. A recent patient of mine is a good example. His mother was very conscientious in keeping all of her son's follow-up visits but she was non-compliant for her own health needs. When he became an adult, she continued to urge him to continue his yearly follow-up visits and take his medications. Unfortunately, her son, as a young adult, in spite of repeated scheduled follow-up visits, has not returned for > 2 years for his needed cardiac ultrasonography and follow-up care.

As a group, pediatric care providers understand the importance of successful transition from pediatric to adult care, but how to do this remains a problem. Many studies have shown that, even with an attempt at patient education, many adolescents have little understanding of their condition, their past procedures, and their prognosis or why they need follow-up when they feel well. Denial is common in young adults. A recent study from Canada (4) showed that young adults with moderate-to-complex congenital heart disease expect to live almost as long as their healthy peers.

15.3 Conclusions

The great medical progress which allows children with all kinds of previously untreatable conditions to survive to adulthood has not been accompanied by the same progress in psychological and social factors which will assure that as adults they truly understand their condition and the need for continued follow-up. Pediatric care providers need to temper their enthusiasm as they see infants and children survive what was once considered a "hopeless" situation and remember that in many the condition has been improved but not "cured. " They must be honest with parents regarding the risks, complications and long-term outcome of their child's condition. Children need to be educated and all questions must be answered truthfully so that as adults they can make informed life choices regarding education, careers and family. Primary Care Physicians are in a position to help facilitate transition and, in some circumstances, be part of the bridge between childhood and adult cases.

References

1. Reiss, J. G., Gibson, R. W., Walker, L. R. (2005) Health care transition: youth, family and provider perspectives. Pediatrics 115:112–120.
2. Jefferies, J. L., Noonan, J. A., Keller, B. B., Wilson, J. F., Griffith, C, III. (2004) Quality of life and social outcomes in patients with adult congenital heart disease. Am. J. Cardiol. 94:263–266.
3. Reid, G. J., Irvine, M. J., McCrindle, B. W., Sananes, R., et al. (2004) Prevalence and correlates of successful transfer from pediatric to adult health care among a cohort of young adults with complex congenital heart defects. Pediatrics 113:e197–e205.
4. Reid, G. J., Webb, G. D., Barzel, M., McCrindle, B. W., Irvine, M. J., Siu, S. C. (2006) Estimates of life expectancy by adolescents and young adults with congenital heart disease. J. Am. Coll. Cardiol. 48:349–355.

16 Disabled women and reproductive healthcare in the USA

Marlene B. Huff

There are few articles about disability and women's needs during the childbearing cycle. Studies are primarily anecdotal and derived from the clinical experiences of practitioners. Medical providers in primary care settings can respond to the concerns of pregnant, disabled women by providing information, providing care in facilities that are physically accessible and psychologically supportive, and by putting in place an interdisciplinary plan of care based on a thorough assessment of physical and psychosocial needs. All women should have access to pre-conception, pre-natal, and post-natal care. Women with disabilities are increasingly making the choice of motherhood, but little is known about their pregnancy experiences. Pregnant women with disabilities are a little-studied topic and are routinely included in national survey questionnaires. To improve our clinical understanding of the care that pregnant, disabled women need, more research is needed.

16.1 Introduction

Society, including women's and disability rights movements, has paid little attention to disabled women's right to freedom of sexual expression, reproductive freedom, and the ability to serve as "mothers" to children. Reproductive rights of women are limited by society's assumptions that women with disabilities are asexual beings and, therefore, are little more than their biological components. Within this societal context, it is little wonder that a lack of access to reproductive healthcare, contraception, and information about sexuality (including treatment options for sexually transmitted infections, abortion, *in-vitro* fertilizations, adoption, and surrogate motherhood) is more the norm than the exception (1). Whether the disability is characterized as being physical, developmental, cognitive, or associated with mental illness, women around the world continue to be at risk for a range of undesirable reproductive and pregnancy outcomes, including subtle coercive sterilization, abortion, and loss of child custody.

Pregnant disabled women are often associated with significant levels of disability and increased need for specialized services, including pre-conception, pre-natal and post-natal care. This review directly addresses many of the reproductive healthcare issues that females face when entering, and throughout their reproductive years in a primary care setting as well as the ways that healthcare providers can continue to enhance medical services available to this group of neglected women. Currently, a growing number of women with disabilities are becoming pregnant. Anecdotal evidence suggests that many pregnant, disabled women with disabilities encounter negative attitudes towards their pregnancies and report difficulty receiving comprehensive prenatal care (2).

16.2 Health disparities for females with disabilities

According to the American Public Health Association, some health disparities (3) are unavoidable (those associated with genetically-based disabilities) whereas other disparities are the result of the disability state and are avoidable. According to the National Study of Women with Physical Disabilities (4), women with disabilities are often denied reproductive and other types of healthcare, or given substandard care compared with women with uncomplicated healthcare needs. Issues such as lack of health insurance, poverty, and architectural barriers increase the level of healthcare disparity for females with disabilities despite the fact that people with disabilities tend to make greater use of healthcare services than the general population.

16.2.1 Demographics

According to the 2000 USA Census, of the 132 million non-institutionalized, civilian women in the population, 19.1% (25,306,717) had some type of disability (5). This number included sensory, physical, mental, or self-care limitations plus limitations in going outside the home and engaging in gainful employment activities. The number of women living in nursing homes is 1 million or 5.3% of the population of women over the age of 65 years (6). Hence, 24.4% of women in the USA have a disability, and comprise a formidable group of medical care consumers of reproductive care (▶ Tab. 16.1).

16.3 Women with physical disabilities

Traditionally, disabled females have been primarily referred to specialists in physical medicine and rehabilitation instead of specialists in primary care (7). Women with disabilities have, however, advocated for their inclusion into primary care settings for many decades. These female activists have claimed that the gaps between services provided in physical medicine and rehabilitation clinics and primary care settings has created significant gaps in healthcare for women, particularly in the area of reproductive health. Some of the reproductive healthcare issues that limit services to this group of patients in primary care are discussed below.

Tab. 16.1: Disability types.

Age (years)	Disability type (mutually exclusive)						
	All	Sensory	Physical	Mental	Self-care	Going outside the home	Employment disability
5–15	4.3%	0.9%	0.9%	3.1%	0.8%	–	–
16–64	17.6%	1.9%	6.4%	3.7%	1.9%	6.4%	10.9%
65+	43.0%	13.2%	30.7%	11.4%	11.0%	23.0%	–

16.3.1 Access to services

Females with physical disabilities have limited access to all healthcare services, including reproductive healthcare and information. Most rural communities, for example, may not have suitable transportation (accessible mass transit, use of a wheelchair-accessible automobile) available for disabled females to use for medical appointments and procedures. The entrances of clinic facilities may be accessible to females with physical disabilities but the interior of the clinic may not be arranged in such a way that encourages access for females that use wheelchairs, crutches, canes, or for those whose gait may be disturbed. A lack of examination tables that raise and lower or uninformed clinic staff who can transfer the female safely to the examination area discourages females from seeking reproductive healthcare. Small examination rooms that will not allow the door to close when a wheelchair enters the room limits confidentiality significantly. To summarize, many females choose not to struggle to find a reproductive healthcare provider that can provide the same level of care women without disabilities receive.

In some ways, physical barriers to the provision of adequate reproductive healthcare are one of the easier issues to address. Issues involving staff and medical provider education are more difficult to alter in a systemic way. Techniques and strategies for providing annual Papanicolaou smears for women with cognitive and physical disabilities, a staple of appropriate reproductive healthcare, continues to be neglected by most medical school curricula. This lack of education is not limited to Medical Schools. For example, simple transfer techniques for patients require only a small mention in many nursing education curricula (8).

16.3.2 Sexuality

In general, females with disabilities are seen as asexual beings that are not biologically capable of carrying children and, therefore, their reproductive health may go unchecked and uncared for. Many healthcare providers fail to ask females with disabilities about their sexual lives, conduct full pelvic examinations, or screen for sexually transmitted infections because it is assumed that these women do not have sex (or that they should not have sex). According to the Center for Research on Women with Disabilities at the Baylor College of Medicine (9), gynecologists are significantly less likely to ask women with functional limitations or obvious physical deformities about the use of contraceptives and their sexual health when compared to women without disabilities.

16.3.3 Specific reproductive issues

Contraception

Very little information is available on the risks and benefits of various forms of contraception for females with disabilities. This lack of research about safe and effective birth control for females with disabilities may involve a mistaken belief that few women with disabilities are sexually active and, therefore, do not use birth control. When making decisions about birth control, many medical providers do not take into account disabilities such as limited hand use to insert a diaphragm or other barrier methods, increased risk of blood clots, and the additional urge to use hormones to manage menstrual periods (8). Many primary care physicians will suggest the use of birth control for hormonal control without considering issues of sexual health.

Menstruation

There has been little research on how various disabilities affect menstrual cycles and menstrual flow, and most of these have focused on spinal cord injury. Some disabilities affect menstruation more than others. Females with cerebral palsy (CP), for example, whose spasticity is a primary characteristic of their disability, may experience worsened menstrual cycles, whereas the completeness of a spinal cord injury does not affect menstruation at all. Menstruation hygiene and the use of menstruation products is a major issue for females with disabilities and, yet, rarely discussed during a reproductive health examination. Recommendations for enhancing reproductive care visits include assessing the adequacy of personal assistance to manage the use of hygiene products, management of skin breakdown, odor, leakage, interference with catheterization, as well as the management of increased rates of vaginal infections and urinary tract infections (UTI's) across the lifespan should be targeted topics during such health-provider visits.

Sexual activity

A national survey conducted by the Center for Research on Women with Disabilities revealed that most females with disabilities have had sexual experience at some point in their lives, and nearly half were sexually active at the time of the survey. However, they were significantly less likely to be sexually active currently and within the last month than similar women without disabilities.

Sexually transmitted infections

The prevalence of sexually transmitted infections (STIs) is the same for females with disabilities and non-disabled women. However, STIs often go undetected and undiagnosed, and result in preventable pelvic inflammatory disease and infertility. Those women who do not receive adequate reproductive health information cannot detect the difference between UTIs and symptoms related to STIs. Females with disabilities many not choose to undergo screening for STIs because of difficulty transferring onto the examination table or questioning the ability of the medical provider to manage issues such as spasticity, imbalance, and autonomic dysreflexia.

Pregnancy and delivery

In national studies in the USA, disabled females reported negative experiences with pregnancy and childbirth because they had difficulty finding healthcare providers and hospitals that had experience managing pregnancy and childbirth in women with disabilities, and "settled" for primary care services from inexperienced providers (9). Typically overlooked difficulties by medical providers include: greater limitations in physical functioning that increase the need for assistance from others during and directly after pregnancy; increased problems with bladder function (including infections, bladder spasms and leakage); increased difficulties surrounding catheter usage which may require a change in the bladder management program; the increase in probability of skin problems during pregnancy; breathing difficulties and the risk of pneumonia and autonomic dysreflexia; as well as the progression of increased risk of blood clots during pregnancy.

16.3.4 Reproductive health and mental illness

Mental health issues

Inadequate treatment of female mental health issues can have direct repercussions on reproductive and endocrine health. A recent study by Harlow et al. (10) indicated that a lifetime history of major depression may be associated with an early decline in ovarian function. Rhodes et al. (11) suggested that mental health disorders play a part in many reproductive illnesses and conditions, and recommended that particular attention during reproductive health visits be paid to pre-menstrual dysphoric disorder, anxiety disorders, and depression. Research indicates that depression is the most common mental health issue to be addressed by reproductive health specialists and that several biological changes occur in depression, including increased cortisol levels that may explain the association between depression and decreased bone mineral density (BMD) in women (12). Not to minimize the importance of such mental health issues as depression, many females live with serious, lifelong mental illness that have even more far-reaching effects upon reproductive health.

Seriously mental ill women

Matevosyan (13) conducted an extensive review of original studies published from 1971 to 2008 to determine if serious mental illness interferes with reproductive health. This meta-analysis revealed that women with serious mental illness have more lifetime sex partners, low contraceptive usage, higher rates of unwanted pregnancies, and are at high risk ofSTIs. Matevosyan's (13) review article revealed little in the data about the awareness, knowledge, and attitudes in medical settings about women with serious mental illness. Findings of such studies stress the importance of integration of the reproductive health issues into not only medical and nursing school curricula but also collaborating with psychosocial rehabilitation programs (especially during and directly after pregnancy).

Little research is available about the reproductive health issues of females with mental illness. Some limited evidence about females with schizophrenia suggests a higher number of lifetime sexual partners and unwanted pregnancies (14). The extent to which access to reproductive health services would affect these research findings is unclear.

According to one of the few studies available about women with significant mental illness (14), the proportion of pregnant women who did not have a live birth was significantly higher in the group with mental illness. Miller and colleagues (14–16) did not find significant differences between the two groups of women in reported age at the time of first sexual intercourse or first live birth, or in the proportion who had ever taken birth-control pills.

Reduced numbers of pregnancies and successful childbearing may be related to extraneous psychosocial factors, including fewer marriages, usage of and side effects related to psychotropic drugs, and/or the symptoms of psychiatric illness (15). Whether the reduced pregnancy numbers were due to therapeutic abortions or spontaneous miscarriages is not known. The major point to be taken from such studies is that, when considering women with mental illness and reproductive healthcare needs, physicians should pay particular attention to the sexual and reproductive health needs of persons with mental illness.

16.3.5 Pre-conception counseling

Though many of the qualities associated with pregnancy among women without disabilities are held in common with disabled women, pre-conception counseling is necessary to address the medical, psychological, and social impacts of pregnancy (17) as well as the level of stability of the woman's social support systems for those with disabilities that choose to become pregnant. Pre-conception care is directly associated with improved pregnancy outcomes for all women but is absolutely essential for women with disabilities. This remains true for women with physical, cognitive, and/or mental disabilities. When caring for pregnant, disabled women, an interdisciplinary approach is most effective. The team may be composed of the primary care physicians, obstetricians, anesthesiologists, neurologists, psychiatrists, and allied health professionals including Occupational Therapists and Physical Therapists (18–22). Most gynecologists and obstetricians do not routinely serve women with disabilities of childbearing age. Hence, an interdisciplinary approach to care can reassure the patient that the care received is state-of-the-art and not limited by areas of medical specialization.

16.3.6 Medications

A detailed discussion of the potential effects of the many medications used by women with various types of disabilities is beyond the scope of this chapter. Clearly, however, questions about medications will be raised by pregnant, disabled women. Hence, it is important that primary care providers discuss the potential maternal and fetal effects of medications with all disabled patients of childbearing age.

16.4 Conclusions

The few articles about women's needs during the childbearing cycle are primarily anecdotal and derived from the clinical experiences of practitioners. Medical providers in primary care settings can respond to the concerns of pregnant, disabled women by providing information, providing care in facilities that are physically accessible and psychologically supportive, and by putting in place an interdisciplinary plan of care based on a thorough assessment of physical and psychosocial needs.

All women should have access to pre-conception, pre-natal, and post-natal care. Women with disabilities are increasingly making the choice of motherhood, but little is known about their pregnancy experiences. Pregnant women with disabilities are a little-studied topic and are routinely included in national survey questionnaires. To improve our clinical understanding of the care that pregnant, disabled women need, more research is needed.

References

1. Chevarley, F. M., Thierry, J. M., Gill, C. J., Ryerson, A. B., Nosek, M. A. Health and well-being for women with disabilities. Unpublished data.
2. Rogers, J. (2005) The disabled woman's guide to pregnancy and birth. New York, USA: Demos.
3. American Public Health Association, National Public Health Week. Eliminating Health Disparities: Communities Moving from Statistics to Solutions, 5–11April2004.

4. Nosek, M. A. (1996) National study of women with physical disabilities. Houston, USA: Center for Research of Women Disabilities, Departmentof Physicaland Medical Rehabilitation, Baylor College of Medicine.
5. US Census Bureau, Census 2000. Characteristics of the Civilian Non institutionalized Population by Age, Disability Status, and Type of Disability: 2000, Summary File 3, P042. Available from:http://factfinder. census. gov/servlet/DTTable?_bm=y&-geo_id=04000US03&-ds_name=DEC_2000_SF3_U&-redoLog=false&-mt_name=DEC_2000_SF3_U_P042&-format=&-CONTEXT=dt. Accessed 12 May 2010.
6. Lethbridge-Cejku, M., Schiller, J. S., Bernadel, L. (2004) Summary health statistics for US adults: National Health Interview Survey, 2002. Washington, USA: National Center for Health Statistics, Vital Health Stat10(222): Table 31.
7. Wong, A. (2000) The work of disabled women seeking reproductive healthcare. Sex Disabil. 18:301–306.
8. Welner, S. L. (1999) A provider's guide for the care of women with physical disabilities and chronic medical conditions. North Carolina, USA: Office Disability and Health.
9. Health care: Access to reproductive health care. Houston, USA: Center for Research in Women Disability. Available from:http://www. bcm. edu/crowd/?pmid=1436. Accessed 14 Mar 2010.
10. Harlow, B. L., Wise, L. A., Otto, M. W., Soares, C. N., Cohen, L. S. (2003) Depression and its influence on reproductive endocrine and menstrual cycle markers associated with perimenopause: The Harvard Study of Moods and Cycles. Arch. Gen. Psychiatry 60:29–36.
11. Rhodes, J. C., Kjerulff, K. H., Langenberg, P. W., Guzinski, G. M. (1999) Hysterectomy and sexual functioning. JAMA 282:1934–1941.
12. Michelson, D., Stratakis, C., Hill, L., Reynolds, J., Galliven, E., Chrousos, G. (1996) Bone mineral density in women with depression. N. Engl. J. Med. 335:1176–1181.
13. Matevosyan, N. R. (2009) Reproductive health in women with serious mental illnesses: a review. Sex. Disabil. 27:109–118.
14. Miller, L. J., Finnerty, M. (1996) Sexuality, pregnancy, and childrearing among women with schizophrenia-spectrum disorders. Psychiatr. Serv. 47:502–506.
15. Nimgaonkar, V. L., Ward, S. E., Agarde, H., Weston, N., Ganguli, R. (2007) Fertility in schizophrenia: results from a contemporary US cohort. Acta Psychiatr. Scand. 95:364–369.
16. Haukka, J., Suvisaari, J., Lonnqvist, J. (2002) Fertility of patients with schizophrenia, their siblings, and the general population: a cohort study from 1950 to 1959 in Finland. Am. J. Psychiatry 160:460–463.
17. Demsio, K., Magriples, U. (1999) Pregnancy complicated by maternal paraplegia or tetraplegia as a result of spinal cord injury and spinal bifida. Sex. Disabil. 17:223–232.
18. Rogers, J., Matsumura, M. (1996) The disabled woman's guide to pregnancy and birth. New York, USA: Demos Medical Publishers.
19. American Congress of Obstetricians and Gynecologists. 2004. [cited 2010, June 1]. Available from URL: https://www. acog. org/navbar/current/publications.cfm.
20. Welner, S. (2000) Pregnancy in women with disabilities. In: Cohen, W. R., ed. Complications of pregnancy, 5th ed. Philadelphia, USA: Lippincott Williams Wilkins.
21. Baschat, A. A., Weinter, C. P. (2004) Chronic neurologic diseases and disabling conditions in pregnancy. In: Welner, S. L., Haseltine. F., eds. Welner's Guide to the Care of Women with Disabilities. Philadelphia, USA: Lippincott Williams Wilkins.
22. Weiner, C. P., Buhimschi, C., eds. (2004) Drugs for pregnant and lactating women. London, UK: Churchill Livingstone.

17 Adults with congenital bleeding disorders

Susan M. Peterson, Vlad C. Radulescu and Jeffrey A. Moscow

Patients suffering from hemophilia have been affected by two recent major events. First, the advent of lyophilized factor concentrates during the 1960–70s greatly lessened the morbidity of moderate and severe disease. Hemophilia patients were freed from frequent trips to Emergency Rooms, prolonged hospitalizations, anddependence upon transfusions of blood products. Their QoL improved and Hemophilia Treatment Centers were established throughout the USA to provide comprehensive medical and psychosocial care. Second, members of the hemophilia community who had now hoped for a more normal life began to experience the opportunistic infections that were ultimately understood as the sentinel signs of acquired immune deficiency syndrome (AIDS). When scientists identified HIV, its mode of transmission via plasma-derived clotting factor concentrates became evident. By 1984, 50% of all persons with hemophilia had become infected with HIV. In 1980, life expectancy of people with hemophilia was almost 68 years of age, but declined to 49 years in the late 1980s. An entire generation of adult hemophilia patients became affected by the HIV epidemic and also HCV. A growing number of young adults with hemophilia have been born after 1990, where hemophilia factor replacement therapy was proved to be safe. The risk of acquiring an infection through the use of these factors is extremely low; the last documented concentrate-mediated HIV transmission occurred in 1987. The challenge remains to prevent the crippling effects of hemophilia while paying attention to the health and wellness of these individuals.

17.1 Introduction

The past 50 years of hemophilia care have been punctuated by two major events. First, the advent of lyophilized factor concentrates during the late 1960s and early 1970s greatly lessened the morbidity of moderate and severe disease. Hemophilia patients were freed not only from frequent trips to Emergency Rooms and prolonged hospitalizations, but also from dependence on transfusions ofblood products including whole blood, fresh frozen plasma and eventually, cryoprecipitate that contained missing blood clotting proteins. Patients were taught to infuse these concentrates at home. Their QoL improved dramatically when pain was reduced with early treatment of bleeding episodes, and activities such as school, travel and regular employment became possible. Hemophilia Treatment Centers were established throughout the USA to provide comprehensive medical and psychosocial care and education programs aimed at reducing the complications associated with hemophilia.

Second, within a decade of these concentrates becoming available, members of the hemophilia community who had hoped for a more normal life began to experience the opportunistic infections that were ultimately understood as the sentinel signs of

AIDS (1). When scientists identified HIV, its mode of transmission via plasma-derived clotting factor concentrates became evident. By 1984, 50% of all persons with hemophilia had become infected with HIV (2). In 1980, the life expectancy of a man with hemophilia was almost 68 years of age, but had declined to 49 years during the late 1980s (3).

Thus, an entire generation of adult hemophilia patients and their families were gravely affected by the HIV epidemic, as well as by another virus transmitted through plasma concentrates: HCV. Spouses and children of persons with hemophilia were at risk of contracting HIV through sexual and peri-natal transmission. Advances in therapies for HIV disease and opportunistic infections along with HCV treatment have enabled some persons with bleeding disorders to survive with these comorbidities well into the 21st century. The fact that even the youngest persons who became infected with HIV virus in the late 1970s and 1980s are now in their thirties and forties, respectively, means that these adults will be in need of primary care and preventive healthcare for many years.

There is now a growing number of young adults with hemophilia who were born after 1990 for whom hemophilia factor replacement therapy has proven to be safe. Factor concentrates used in the treatment of hemophilia today are virally inactivated plasma-derived products or are made from recombinant technology. The risk of acquiring an infection through the use of these factors is extremely low; the last documented concentrate-mediated HIV transmission occurred in 1987 (4). The challenge remains to prevent the crippling effects of hemophilia while paying attention to the health and wellness of these individuals.

17.2 Hemophilia A and B

Hemophilia A, classical hemophilia, or factor VIII deficiency is the more common form, occurring in one of every 5, 000–7, 000 live male births worldwide. The absence of the factor VIII protein results in defective or weak blood clot formation and prolonged bleeding at the site of vessel injury. The genetic defect is located on the X chromosome and transmitted to sons by carrier mothers. The male fetus of a carrier has a 50% chance of inheriting the affected X chromosome and manifesting the symptoms of hemophilia. All daughters of a man with hemophilia are obligate carriers and do not require carrier detection testing. The daughter of a hemophilia carrier has a 50% chance of inheriting the carrier state with an affected X chromosome. The vast majority of female carriers are asymptomatic. Carrier women with skewed chromosome X inactivation (extreme lyonization) may have low factor VIII levels and exhibit bleeding manifestations. There are very few cases of homozygous or compound heterozygous factor VIII mutations (the daughter of a man with hemophilia and a mother who is a carrier of the same disorder) (5) or of hemophilia occurring in patients with TS (45XO). Women who have these rare conditions will have a bleeding diathesis similar to men with hemophilia and require factor concentrate infusions to prevent prolonged bleeding. Although many persons with hemophilia have a family history of the disorder, ~30% of cases arise from new mutations (6, 7).

Factor VIII deficiency can be mild, moderately severe, or severe with corresponding factor VIII levels of > 5%, 1–5% or < 1% of normal, respectively. The probability and extent of prolonged internal bleeding into tissues, organs and joints varies with the severity of the inherited disorder, and the role of factor replacement therapy also varies by severity of disease. Factor replacement is administered only episodically for trauma or surgery in the case of mild hemophilia. In contrast, prophylactic infusions are often given several times/week to prevent spontaneous hemorrhage in children with severe hemophilia (6).

Treatment for bleeding in patients with hemophilia A include intravenous factor VIII concentrates, intravenous or intranasal DDAVP or desmopressin for mild hemophilia, oral anti-fibrinolytic agents such as aminocaproic acid or tranexamic acid, and topical agents such as fibrin glue. A combination of these therapies is often indicated. Additional measures including ice, rest or immobilization, elevation and compression are also beneficial.

Management of pain associated with bleeding or common causes is complicated by the fact that aspirin and traditional NSAIDs interfere with platelet aggregation and disrupt primary hemostatic mechanisms in addition to the defect in coagulation, the factor VIII deficiency. Irritation to the gastric mucosa associated with NSAIDs is a concern with respect toGI bleeding. Celecoxib is useful and recommended for otherwise appropriate patients (8). Acetaminophen may be used, but with caution in hemophilia patients with HCV liver disease.

Complications of hemophilia A treatment include the development of an allo-antibody or inhibitor to exogenous factor VIII. The risk of inhibitors is higher in patients with severe hemophilia, in patients with certain mutations in the factor VIII gene as well as in African–Americans. Other possible risk factors include first exposure to factor VIII early in life, intensive exposure in infancy, and association of factor VIII exposure with inflammatory conditions (infection, surgery, immunization) (9). High doses of factor VIII can be used to overcome the effects of the low-titer inhibitor (Bethesda unit titer < 10). Agents that bypass factor VIII (recombinant factor VIIa or plasma-derived activated prothrombin complex concentrate) are used to control bleeding in patients with higher titers. Immune tolerance regimens are undertaken to eradicate inhibitors early in life because of the serious consequences of episodes of uncontrollable bleeding (6).

Hemophilia B (Christmas disease) or factor IX deficiency occurs in 1 of 25,000–30,000 male births. The role of factor IX in the blood clotting cascade is associated with activation of factor X and ultimately the conversion of PT to thrombin (6). The result of factor IX deficiency is delayed blood clotting. Hemophilia B has the same X-linked inheritance pattern as hemophilia A. Carriers may have low factor IX activity levels based on skewed X inactivation, and may require factor IX infusion support.

Degrees of severity of hemophilia B are classified as mild, moderate or severe in the same way as those for hemophilia A. Clinical features are also the same. DDAVP has no role in factor IX deficiency therapy. Anti-fibrinolytic therapy may be used with the recombinant factor IX concentrates and the current monoclonal or high-purity plasma-derived factor IX concentrates only (10).

The development of allo-antibody inhibitors to factor IX occurs in ~3% of patients with severe factor IX deficiency. However, it can be associated with anaphylactic reaction to factor IX administration and the development of nephrotic syndrome. If a patient with hemophilia B develops inhibition and the titer is > 10 Bethesda units, bleeding episodes should be treated with recombinant factor VIIa (6).

17.3 Von Willebrand disease

Von Willebrand disease (vWD) is the most common bleeding disorder, with an incidence of ~1 in 1,000 births. Most forms of the disease have an autosomal dominant mode of inheritance, thereby affecting males and females equally. Circulating von Willebrand factor (vWF) is a multimeric protein that carries factor VIII in the circulation and which is involved in appropriate functioning of platelets in primary hemostasis (11).

Von Willebrand disease is classified under three types according to whether a qualitative or quantitative defect is involved. There are also subtypes which are important for correct treatment options. Type 1 is a quantitative defect due to decreased production of functional vWF. Type 2 is considered to be the qualitative or functional defect category. Type 3 is characterized by the absence or extremely low level of vWF resulting in bleeding similar to that experienced in moderate-to-severe hemophilia (12). Type-3 von Willebrand disease is rare, with an incidence ranging from 1 in 250,000 to 1 in 1,000,000.

With the exception of hemarthoses in type-3 VWD, the bleeding experienced by persons with vWD is mostly mucocutaneous. Excessive bruising, prolonged epistaxis and menorrhagia and post-partum bleeding in women are typical (11).

Treatment for bleeding in vWDtype 1 is DDAVP or desmopressin intravenous infusion or Stimate™ (the more concentrated form of DDAVP nasal spray). Depending on the subtype, DDAVP can also be used in some of the subtypes of type-2 VWD as well. DDAVP is not effective in type-3 disease.

It is also appropriate to use anti-fibrinolytic therapy for mucosal bleeding and dental procedures. Estrogen therapy is often utilized in the form of oral contraceptive pills for increasing vWF levels and decreasing menstrual bleeding. The benefits of systemic hormonal therapy have to be weighed against the risks (13). Hormonal therapy delivered through an intrauterine device is a new, emerging method of treatment of vWD-related menorrhagia (14). Anti-fibrinolytic agents (especially tranexamic acid) are helpful during menstruation along with oral contraceptive pills (14).

Plasma-derived factor concentrates that contain von Willebrand protein are used for replacement of dysfunctional and low levels of vWF. These concentrates have been virally inactivated to remove infectious agents such as HIV and HCV (15).

17.4 Hemophilia Treatment Centers

Ideally, the adults that would be seeking care in primary care practices would be "graduates" of a pediatric program at a Hemophilia Treatment Center. Transition programs at the centers prepare teenagers and their parents to become appropriately less dependent on the Hemophilia Treatment Center for primary care, and more integrated into a Family Practice or Internal Medicine Clinic. The young man with hemophilia or the young woman with vWD should be well versed in the management of their bleeding disorder, and know when to seek Hemophilia Treatment Centerinput for dental procedures, surgical or invasive procedures, and in emergency situations.

The network of Hemophilia Treatment Center contacts in the USA can be accessed on the Centers for Disease Control Internet website under the Blood Disorders section.

Personnel at the Center are willing to give advice regarding the appropriate treatment for injury or invasive procedure (including dental surgery). Often, collaboration between the Hemophilia Treatment Center and local provider allows the patient to have a procedure closer to home. Most Hemophilia Treatment Centersprefer that they be called prior to a patient going to an Emergency Room so that a phone call is then made provider-to-provider and there is less anxiety for everyone. Local providers should question the patient about Hemophilia Treatment Center care and contact the latter if there is a question about treatment. These specialized centers have often known the patient for many years, and can provide valuable information.

17.5 Emergency care

In case of injury, persons with bleeding disorders should be seen immediately upon arrival in the Emergency Room even if there is no obvious bleeding. If a hemophilia patient presents with a history of trauma, they should be given their major dose of factor concentrate prior to any diagnostic procedure. Trauma to the head, neck, chest or abdomen could be life-threatening. Hence, the sooner the dose of factor concentrate is administered the better the outcome that can be expected. Often, patients carry emergency cards or a computer flash drive that identifies the disorder and explains the amount of clotting factor the individual should receive. The initial dosing for factor replacement in the Emergency Department setting is as follows:

- Factor VIII can be dosed at 50 units/kg to achieve 100% level
- Factor IX can be given at 96 units/kg for a 80% level with recombinant factor IX and a 96% level for plasma-derived factor IX concentrates
- vWF containing concentrates can be dosed at 50VWF units/kg for a patient with low levels or type 3 and a life-threatening injury.

In case of serious injury, the patient should contact the Hemophilia Treatment Center as soon as possible for recommendations for follow-up dosing and/or transport to the tertiary care facility.

If the injury is mild and can be treated locally, it is preferable to give the intravenous factor concentrate first and then evaluate sprains, fractures, and lacerations. Immobilization of the injured area will help the clot remain in place as well as prevent re-injury.

17.6 Orthopedic complications of hemophilia

Chronic arthropathy from repetitive bleeding in joint spaces is a major cause of morbidity and disability in adults with hemophilia. Two processes occurring simultaneously contribute to hemarthropathy. The iron from blood destroys chondrocytes in cartilage and simultaneously stimulates inflammation and proliferation of synovial membranes (16). These processes begin with the first joint hemorrhage in the young child with hemophilia.

In recent years, primary hemophilia factor prophylaxis regimens have been adopted for the treatment of children with severe hemophilia to decrease the number of joint bleeds and the resultant complications of premature adult hemarthropathy. Unfortunately, present-day adult patients were not beneficiaries of primary prophylaxis regimens. Many young adults with severe hemophilia present with severe arthropathy, especially in the knees, ankles and elbows. These are painful joints with decreased range of motion that affect the ability of the young person to work on a regular basis, as well as disrupting many other aspects of QoL(including the ability to have intimate relationships).

Orthopedic surgical procedures such as total knee replacement, ankle arthrodesis, and radial head excisions may be needed at a much earlier age. Patients are often referred to Pain Clinics for the management of chronic pain.

Occupational and physical therapy may be needed to assess the older patient for fall risk and to provide appropriate assistive devices. Negotiating stairs in the home may necessitate a move to a different residence. Maintaining ideal body weight will minimize stress on weight-bearing joints. Collaboration between the primary care provider and the Hemophilia Treatment Center regarding the orthopedic complications of hemophilia is vital.

17.7 Dental care

Adult hemophilia patients may have avoided dental treatment when they were young because of the risk of bleeding and issues with the administration of factor concentrates (17). Consequently, many adults with hemophilia may have poor dentition, and lack an understanding of good dental health and its relationship to overall wellness. In addition to the obvious need to use factor for invasive dental treatment, poor dental hygiene now places patients at risk for joint sepsis through bacterial infection from the oral route. Education about frequent brushing and flossing to prevent gum bleeding is important. With loss of permanent teeth at an early age, appropriate support of dentures becomes an issue due to bone reabsorption. This affects the ability to have a proper diet. Many Hemophilia Treatment Centers have a Dentist as part of their comprehensive team to educate and recommend treatment for optimal oral health.

17.8 Cardiovascular disease

As persons with hemophilia and vWD age, their risk of developing atherosclerosis and associated heart disease increases. There is evidence that hemophilia patients have higher levels of risk factors for cardiovascular disease, including smoking, obesity and lack of exercise, DM and hypertension (18). It is essential that primary care providers reach these men and women with prevention education and medications when necessary.

If anti-coagulant medications are indicated, they can be administered while the patient is being replaced with the missing clotting factor. Long-term anti-coagulation is dangerous and this therapy requires close collaboration with hemophilia specialists. Cardiac surgery and catheterization can be done with a continuous infusion of clotting factor and monitoring of factor activity level (18).

17.9 Renal disease

Patients with hemophilia commonly develop hematuria. Several retrospective studies showed conflicting results with respect to the association between hematuria and CKD (19). Although anti-fibrinolytic medications are often used to control bleeding complications in hemophilia, they should not be used if hematuria is present because of the risk of clotting with subsequent obstructive uropathy.

HIV-infected patients with hemophilia have various renal problems, including glomerulonephritis, interstitial nephritis, and HIV-induced nephropathy. These manifestations are a direct consequence of the HIV infection as well as a side effect of the antimicrobial treatments for HIV (or for opportunistic infections).

17.10 Cancer

Screening procedures and therapies for various cancers are complicated by bleeding disorders. Routine colonoscopy, for instance, must be done only after administration of factor concentrate. Biopsies and surgery must be coordinated with hemophilia professionals. Thrombocytopenia from chemotherapy and skin effects from radiation therapy can cause bleeding that requires treatment with factor concentrates. Often, because bleeding is a symptom of malignancy that may be dismissed in a patient with hemophilia, the presence of certain malignancies (e.g., GI cancers) may be missed (20). Thus, vigilance is required on the part of the primary care provider into the investigation of any bleeding episode.

17.11 Immunizations

There are several new vaccines for adults such as the pneumococcal pneumonia vaccine, the herpes zoster virus vaccine, influenza vaccine, and pertussis vaccine. Persons with bleeding disorders should have access to all of these, but the route of administration requires planning. Some vaccinations can be given by the intramuscular or subcutaneous routes. Due to the possibility of muscle hemorrhage associated with intramuscular injections, subcutaneous administration is preferred unless contraindicated by the manufacturer. A dose of clotting factor calculated to raise the level to ≥50% activity may be considered prior to the intramuscular injection. Local pressure with an icepack may reduce the risk of intramuscular bleeding. Live influenza virus vaccines are acceptable for persons with bleeding disorders as long as the person is not immunocompromised.

17.12 Pregnancy

Women who are carriers of the hemophilia X chromosome and women who have vWD may have issues with prolonged bleeding that require treatment to prevent iron deficiency or anemia from acute blood loss. How this bleeding relates to menstruation has been discussed above. There are changes in factor levels as well as precautions that must be taken during pregnancy to ensure a safe outcome for mother and baby.

When a woman presents with a family history of a bleeding disorder, it should be determined whether or not she is a carrier of hemophilia or has vWD. If the history involves hemophilia, there is a good chance that the Hemophilia Treatment Center has identified the mutation in the family and could assist with identifying the carrier status of the woman. Genetic testing and pre-conception counseling should be offered to all carriers of hemophilia.

Factor VIII levels go up during pregnancy. By term, the hemophilia carrier mother may have levels of factor VIII in the normal range. It is important to measure the factor level prior to pregnancy so that everyone knows what to expect when the level drops after delivery. The factor VIII level should be measured again prior to any invasive procedure during the pregnancy and also during the third trimester to determine if factor support for anesthesia or delivery will be required (21). DDAVP can also be used if the mother has had a previous trial and had an adequate response.

In the case of a carrier of factor IX deficiency, the factor IX level does not increase during pregnancy. The baseline and ante partum level is used to determine the level of factor support needed during and after delivery (21).

If the woman has vWD, she should understand the risk for herself during pregnancy and the risk of transmission of the disorder to her baby. Type-1 and type 2 vWD are inherited by the autosomal dominant pattern. Type-3 vWD has an autosomal recessive inheritance risk.

Von Willebrand protein levels and corresponding factor VIII levels increase during pregnancy in type-1 vWD. In type-2 vWD (i.e., the qualitative variety), levels of factor VIII and vWF antigen increase, but the activity of the dysfunctional ristocetin cofactor does not. Depending on the baseline and ante partum levels, support during delivery made be required and vWF-containing concentrates or DDAVP would be used. It is uncertain when vWF levels fall after delivery. one recommendation proposes factor support for 3 days in case of a vaginal delivery and 5 days if a caesarian section isundertaken (21). Anti-fibrinolytic therapy may also be useful for controlling post-partum bleeding.

17.13 Conclusion

Adults with congenital bleeding disorders have primary care and preventive health needs that are appropriately delivered by specialists in these areas. The unique needs of this population require collaboration with specialized Hemophilia Treatment Centers for safe outcomes if there is a potential for bleeding to occur.

References

1. Stehr-Green, J. K., Holman, R. C., Jason, J. M., Evatt, B. L. (1988) Hemophilia-associated AIDS in the United States, 1981–September 1987. Am. J. Public Health 78:439–442.
2. Evatt, B. L. (2006) The tragic history of AIDS in the hemophilia population, 1982–1984. J. Thromb. Haemost. 4:2295–2301.
3. Jones, P. K., Ratnoff, O. D. (1991) The changing prognosis of classic hemophilia (factor VIII deficiency). Ann. Int. Med. 114:641–648.
4. Kasper, K. C. (2002) Concentrate safety and efficacy. Haemophilia 8:161–165.

5. Pavlova, A., Brondke, H., Müsebeck, J., Pollmann, H., Srivastava, A., Oldenburg, J. (2009) Molecular mechanisms underlying hemophilia A phenotype in seven females. J. Thromb. Haemost. 7:976–982.
6. Roberts, H. R., Escobar, M., White, II, G. C. (2006) Hemophilia A and Hemophilia B. In: Lichtman, M. A. et al. eds. Williams Hematology, 7th ed. New York, USA: McGraw-Hill, 1867–1886.
7. Tuddenham, E. (2009) Genetic and laboratory diagnosis. In: Lee, C. A., Kadir, R. A., Kouides, P. A. (2009) Inherited Bleeding Disorders in Women. Sussex, UK: Wiley-Blackwell, 90–98.
8. Rattray, B., Nugent, D. J., Young, G. (2006) Celecoxib in the treatment of haemophilia synovitis, target joints, and pain in adults and children with haemophilia. Haemophilia 12:514–517.
9. DiMichele, D. M., Hoots, W. K., Pipe, S. W., Rivard, G. E., Santagostino, E. (2007) International workshop on immune tolerance induction: consensus recommendations. Haemophilia 13(Suppl. 1):1–22.
10. Djulbegovic, B., Hannan, M. M., Bergman, G. E. (1995) Concomitant treatment with factor IX concentrate and antifibrinolytics in hemophilia B. Acta Haematol. 94(Suppl. 1):43–48.
11. Johnsen, J., Ginsburg, D. (2006) Von Willebrand disease. In: Lichtman, M. A., et al. eds. Williams Hematology, 7th ed. New York, USA: McGraw-Hill, 1929–1945.
12. Metjian, A. D., et al. (2009) Bleeding symptoms and laboratory correlation in patients with severe von Willebrand disease. Haemophilia 15:918–925.
13. Kadir, R. A., Chi, C. (2006) Women and von Willebrand disease: controversies in diagnosis and management. Semin. Thromb. Hemost. 32:605–615.
14. Kouides, P. A. (2006) Current understanding of von Willebrand's disease in women –some answers, more questions. Haemophilia 12(Suppl. 3):143–151.
15. National Heart, Lung and Blood Institute. (2007) The diagnosis, evaluation and management of von Willebrand disease. Washington, USA: National Institutes of Health.
16. Lafeber, F. P. J. G., Moissec, P., Valentino, L. A. (2008) Physiopathology of haemophilic arthropathy. Haemophilia 14(Suppl. 4):3–9.
17. Harrington, B. (2004) Primary dental care of patients with hemophilia. Revised ed. Treatment of Hemophilia Series. Montréal, Québec, Canada: World Federation of Hemophilia, 3.
18. Street, A., Hill, K., Sussex, B., Warner, M., Scully, M-F. (2006) Haemophilia and ageing. Haemophilia 12(Suppl. 3):8–12.
19. Kulkarni, R., Soucie, J. M., Evatt, B., Hemophilia Surveillance System Project Investigators. (2003) Renal disease among males with haemophilia. Haemophilia 9:703–710.
20. Franchini, M., et al. (2009) Hemophilia and cancer: a new challenge for hemophilia centers. Cancer Treat. Rev. 35:374–377.
21. Chi, C., Kadir, R. (2009) Obstetric management. In: Lee CA, Kadir, R. A., Kouides, P. A. Inherited Bleeding Disorders in Women. Sussex, USA: Wiley-Blackwell, pp. 124–150.

18 Children with allergic disease as adults

Maria C. Veling, Abbas Younes and Richard C. Haydon

In children, allergic rhinitis is considered the most common chronic disease, affecting as many as 40% of the USA population, a rising trend in prevalence seen for many allergies and is a very common encounter in everyday practice. We believe that through appropriate recognition and intervention, QoL for the patient can be influenced by the clinician, which will result in improved outcomes in health and function. Children with allergic disease as adults deserve the time and effort necessary to improve and preserve the often overlooked impaired physical and mental functions associated with IgE-mediated disease. Appropriate history-taking, testing, and therapeutic intervention can go a long way in improving outcomes in these patients and, in nearly all cases, patients will very much appreciate your efforts.

18.1 Introduction

For the practicing pediatrician and Primary Care Physician, allergies involving the ear, nose, throat, and related structures are rising in prevalence, and are a very common encounter in everyday practice. In fact, in children allergic rhinitis is considered the most common chronic disease, affecting as many as 40% of the USA population (1). Although a rather broad term, most allergies are well characterized under the mechanism of the IgE-mediated response. Under this mechanism, the sequence of immunologic events that follow repeated exposure to environmental antigens often lead to impaired functional and physical status. It is believed that through appropriate recognition and intervention, these sequences can be influenced by the clinician, which will result in improved outcomes in health and function.

Allergens can present to the body in four ways: airborne, ingestion, skin and mucosal contact, and injection. From here, the protein epitopes on the allergen surface are engulfed by macrophages (referred to as "antigen-processing cells"). They are then packaged, and, in genetically predisposed patients, will be presented to thymus-derived lymphocyte receptors, resulting in the creation of epitope memory and pro-inflammatory cytokines and antigen-specific IgE. If enough repeated stimulation continues, a large allergic cascade of acute and chronic inflammation ensues, mediated by these cytokines, histamine, leukotrienes, IgE, and eosinophilic cellular infiltration. This inflammation causes the typical symptoms of itching, increased secretions, edema, and neuronal stimulation and, over time, is often associated with worsening psychosocial and physical function.

The hygiene hypothesis (2) has been advanced as one explanation for what appears to be a worldwide increase in allergies over the past 30 years, especially in industrialized nations. Factors stressed in this theory are blamed for what appears to be a shift toward the immunological expression of these pro-inflammatory cytokines, mediated by

Th2 lymphocytes. Some of these factors include an increase in the measurable allergens in the indoor environment, early sensitization to these allergens, less Th1 immunological stimulation due to "cleaner, healthier living" because of a decrease in family size, generous vaccinations and antibiotics, urbanization, less ventilation, and higher ambient room temperatures. Thus, our charge in the global management of allergies should be to: (i) identify and control factors affecting prevalence, (ii) identify susceptible persons, and (iii) identify and control allergic mediators and their receptors.

From a clinical standpoint, this exposure to environmental allergens, which necessarily begins in early childhood, will manifest at an early age. Typically this may begin as dermatitis, GI upset, bronchial hyper-reactivity, and nasal drainage and obstruction. The "allergic march" – the progression from atopic dermatitis and food allergy in the first years of life, with subsequent development of asthma, environmental allergies, and allergic rhinitis – is well described in children susceptible to IgE-mediated allergic stimulation (3). To what degree this progression continues rests on multiple, unknown, and sometimes controversial interventions, including further environmental exposure versus avoidance, pharmacotherapy, and immunotherapy.

18.2 Allergy intervention during childhood

Because allergic disease and theallergic march have potential repercussions throughout a patient's life, they should be aggressively managed as early as possible. Populations at risk need to be identified, and steps should be taken to minimize the expression of genetic factors. Controlling environmental exposures, including allergic mediators and their receptors, is especially important in patients with known genetic predisposition, and indoor allergen and food-specific IgE sensitization, especially if this is coupled with a wheezing history as well as atopic dermatitis or rhinitis at an early age.

18.3 Management of allergies after childhood

In children, there has been a lot of attention paid to the impact of allergies on school performance. However, in adults, the impact has been measured in work productivity and QoL. Several studies on allergic rhinitis have indicated the existence of a substantial disease burden in the adult population in the areas of attention and reaction times, energy level, sleep, and work productivity. In addition, untreated allergic rhinitis has been shown to negatively impact cognitive function in the areas of sustained attention over time, working memory, psychomotor speed, reasoning/computation, and divided attention.

Allergic rhinitis patients also report lower energy levels, increased bodily tiredness, and mental fatigue. Also, symptoms of nasal congestion, frequently associated with allergic rhinitis, can often disrupt sleep and lead to daytime somnolence, which can affect productivity at work and/or school (4–8). Nasal allergy sufferers also experience feelings of being miserable, irritable, depressed and embarrassed. While at work, allergy sufferers who are at the peak of their symptoms rate their productivity to be significantly impaired (9).

From the work and cost perspective, the annual costs in the USA for prescriptions and outpatient visits are in the billions of dollars (10). Work-loss days (defined as more than a half day loss due to illness or injury) are in the range of $3–4 million per year, resulting in losses of about $0.5 billion (11). Additionally, among all disease states, allergic rhinitis has been shown to be one of the leading, if not the leading cause, of absenteeism and "presenteeism" while in the work place. "Presenteeism" describes a worker who reports to work but is impaired due to the impact of a disease and thus exhibits a loss in productivity while on the job (8, 12). The ability to concentrate, work without mistakes, and handle workload has also been reported by allergic rhinitis sufferers to be worse than for their healthy counterparts (13).

The approach to the adult patient who experienced allergies in younger life involves a combination of steps, including confirmation of disease, assessment of severity, and intervention. Many patients with allergies do not seek professional care, and to what degree healthcare providers and vendors should pursue services and products for these patients is debatable. What seems less debatable, however, is the need to help patients who seek advice and verbalize dissatisfaction with associated unfavorable health and functional status. Once this is determined, then it becomes necessary to confirm or validate their allergies and to provide evidenced-based intervention that lead to improvement.

Confirmation of IgE-mediated allergies should begin with history-taking. The clinician should attempt to elicit positive symptoms associated with the usually affected target organs (eye, middle ear, nose, sinus, throat, larynx, cutaneous, GI tract) that are acute (itching, tickling, clear hypersecretions, swelling, wheezing, urticaria, angioedema) or chronic (obstruction, congestion, drainage, wheezing, GI hypermotility). Genetic predisposition signals the importance of inquiring about family history. Although symptom severity may be mild, they can be severe, rapidly progressing, and associated with life-threatening anaphylaxis, especially in the case of food triggers. Physical examination should follow these same organ systems looking for acute and chronic inflammation of the skin, respiratory and pharyngeal mucosa (including the middle ear). Attempts should also be made to connect these findings to suspect food and inhalant triggers in the home, during seasons, time of day, and humidity changes.

18.4 Testing methods

During the care of patients with suspected allergies, there are various time points at which it is appropriate to initiate formal testing so as to confirm the presence of IgE-mediated disease, especially if attempts to control symptoms have fallen short. Some tests can confirm the presence and level of sensitization to specific allergens, which will widen treatment options for the patient and may offer a more tailored approach to symptom control and improved outcomes (14).

Antigens that are typically chosen for inclusion in a test panel include airborne outdoor (tree, grass, weed pollens, mold spores), indoor (dust mite, cat dander, cockroach, mold spores), and foods (in the case of suspected food allergies). In young children, the most common foods causing IgE-mediated allergies include milk, eggs, peanuts, tree nuts, soybeans, and wheat. In adults, tree nuts and peanuts are common

IgE mediated allergens, along with fruits and vegetables; also with the increased popularity of seafood, crustaceans (shellfish, i.e., shrimp, crab, crawfish, lobster) and mollusks (snails, mussels, oysters) are commonly involved.

18.4.1 Skin testing

Skin testing remains the most widely practiced method for several good reasons. Mast cells are the key effector cells in the IgE-mediated reaction and reside in the subepithelial layer of nearly all epithelial organs, including the respiratory tract and the skin.

Intracutaneous (intradermal) testing by injection of an appropriately diluted liquid allergen extract into the dermal layer of the skin is one of the most reliable and proven skin testing techniques. However, it is reserved for testing of inhalant allergens only, not foods. Injecting food extracts into the dermis carries a high potential for anaphylaxis and false-positive reactions.

Akin to a tuberculin test, a 4-mm intracutaneous wheal is created by injecting a small amount of antigen (usually 0.01–0.02 mL) using a one-piece syringe and 27-G needle. This allows for contact of antigen with subepithelial mast cells. If IgE-mediated sensitivity is present and the patient has been previously sensitized to the test allergen, the allergen-specific IgE proteins coating the mast cells will become crosslinked with the antigen, causing mast cell degranulation and eventual growth/expansion of the wheal. Within 10–20 min the wheal is then re-measured; if there has been growth to ≥7mm, the test is positive. An accompanying erythematous urticarial reaction surrounding the positive wheal, termed the "flare reaction", offers further confirmation.

Unfortunately, there are factors besides allergy that can affect skin whealing responses, making interpretation sometimes challenging. Clinical factors that inhibit the whealing response include antihistamines, tricyclic anti-depressants, and systemic beta agonists. Also, pediatric and geriatric patients can be less reactive. Factors that enhance the whealing response include dermatopathologies (dermatographism, eczema, urticaria), and beta antagonists (beta blockers). Therefore, before proceeding with skin testing, the clinician needs to take a good history and undertake positive and negative control skin tests. If these control tests do not yield appropriate results, skin testing should be aborted because the results will most probably be unreliable.

Intracutaneous (intradermal) testing using only one single dilution of an antigen has been practiced for many decades. However, testing with only one dilution does not give the quantitative or relational information that would be validated by testing responses to additional dilutions of different strengths. Nevertheless, some clinicians will quantify sensitivity based on the size of the wheal growth from that one single dilution.

Intracutaneous testing using multiple serial dilutions of the same antigen ("intradermal dilutional testing" or IDT) has also been practiced for many decades. Assessing test accuracy over a range of antigen strengths serves to confirm allergy as well as to quantify the intensity of the response. Proponents of this technique point out that patients vary in sensitivity to individual antigens and therefore vary in tolerance to initial antigen doses when starting immunotherapy. In addition, the premise that some patients' allergies are less sensitive than others implies that some patients may not always test positive to single dilution tests containing weaker dilutions or prick puncture tests. Thus, they may be labeled as false-negative.

Epicutaneous tests were also one of the earliest methods used for the diagnosis of inhalant allergy. Scratch tests were probably the earliest and involved the placement of antigen onto the abraded surface of the superficial epidermis. However, scratch tests possessed multiple disadvantages and have been largely replaced by prick/puncture techniques. Patch tests are done by applying allergen to the skin. Patch testing looks at skin responses 48 h after application of the patch and is primarily used for chemical contact and drug sensitivity.

Prick/puncture testing has become the most popular skin test for the diagnosis of respiratory and food IgE-dependent allergy. The prick/puncture technique involves the introduction of antigen extract through the epidermis through a superficial prick/puncture with a sharp instrument (scalpel, needle, plastic). The penetrating end of the instrument may be single, bifurcated, or multi-pronged. Single antigen testing devices are useful if isolated tests are desired. Multiple-antigen testing devices enable simultaneous testing for multiple antigens and controls. The clinician interprets the prick/puncture tests by comparing measured wheal responses to positive and negative controls after 20 min.

Prick/puncture testing is quick, easy, and safe, even for highly sensitive patients. It is commonly used without other supplemental testing for the diagnosis of allergy and the provision of immunotherapy. It is also appropriate and safe for evaluation of IgE-mediated food allergies. However, skin testing should be avoided in patients with known serious reactions from previous testing or allergen exposure, and the clinician must always be prepared to treat anaphylaxis (14).

18.4.2 *In-vitro* testing

In-vitro testing of serum samples for the presence of antigen-specific IgE antibody has been available to many clinicians since the 1980s. This is a passive test that does not provoke or challenge the patient with antigen (as do skin and end-organ provocation tests). This test is based upon the presumption of the production of antigen-specific IgE antibodies in genetically predisposed patients who have been sensitized from antigen exposure. Because there is correlation between skin test reactivity and the presence of measurable serum antigen-specific antibodies, it is assumed that the presence of these serum antibodies correlate with the presence of these same antibodies when affixed to the surface of mast cells in the skin. Not only is there a qualitative relationship, there is a quantitative one between measured titers of antigen-specific antibodies and the intensity of skin reactivity. Thus, these tests can be used to tailor starting doses for immunotherapy for individual antigens based upon these measured serum titers. In fact, *in-vitro* IgE levels are relied upon to appropriately dose patients for insect venom immunotherapy as well as anti-IgE monoclonal antibody therapy in asthmatics.

The benefits of *in-vitro* testing include convenience (one venipuncture), no affect of medications or skin conditions that contraindicate testing (as can occur with skin testing), no risk of reactions from testing, it is useful for women known to be pregnant, and less need for patient cooperation (e.g., in children).

The RAST was among the first tests designed to measure IgE antibodies. This became possible after the development of IgG antibodies that would complex with the antigen-specific IgE antibodies present in a patient's serum. Initially, these anti-IgE (IgG) antibodies were labeled with radioactive isotopes that were then measured.

Over time, the original RAST techniques have undergone many refinements. Techniques for labeling the anti-IgE antibody have diversified by using enzyme and flouroscein labels that can be measured using spectrophotometers and luminometers without the need for use of radioisotopes and Geiger counters (14).

The reporting of *in-vitro* scores for antigen-specific IgE antibody is fairly straightforward because it reflects a fairly linear continuum from class 0 to class 5 based upon the intensity of the measurements of the labeled anti-IgE IgG–IgE antibody complexes in the patient's serum. Class 0 and1/0 are negative and equivocal (respectively), whereas classes 1–5 are associated with a linear increase in measurable antibody.

Interpretation of *in-vitro* scores is straightforward. A reported *in-vitro* class score correlates with the amount of serum antibody titers, which is an objective measure of allergic sensitivity of the patient to that specific antigen. It also approximately correlates to the amount of skin reactivity that would be present during skin tests. However, akin to skin tests, *in-vitro* tests by themselves do not necessarily reflect symptom severity or presence of clinically significant allergy.

For IgE-mediated food allergies, skin prick and *in-vitro* assays are acceptable test methods. However, as is the case with inhalant testing, these tests merely detect the presence of antibodies, which imply that sensitization has taken place, but do not by themselves diagnose clinically relevant allergy. A notable example of this is in the preschool child (3–5 years) who very commonly will exhibit sensitivity to egg, milk, wheat and soy. These may or may not be clinically relevant, and they may remain positive for some time even after clinical reactivity, if present, has resolved. This is in contrast to sensitivity to peanut, tree nut, and seafood, which tend to persist throughout one's lifetime (15).

In general, the sensitivity of skin prick and *in-vitro* tests are reliable. In other words, the likelihood of a test that is negative being associated with no reaction when the patient is challenged with said allergen is high. However, as already alluded to, the specificity of skin prick and *in-vitro* tests are not as reliable. In other words, the likelihood of a test that is positive being associated with a clinically relevant reaction when the patient is challenged with said allergen is not as predictable unless the *in-vitro* titer is in the high range or the skin wheal is in the large range in comparison with negative controls. Therefore, the interpretation of these tests and final diagnoses should be coupled with information from history-taking, physical examination, and possibly additional challenge or elimination testing.

18.4.3 Positive and negative challenge testing

Under many circumstances, instead of formal testing, it is not unreasonable to subject patients to a trial of pharmacotherapy designed to achieve symptom control and build evidence in favor of an allergic mechanism. Environmental avoidance of inhalant antigens or suspect foods is another example of negative challenge testing, which carries the advantages of decreased testing expense, time-saving, and simultaneous therapy. By the same token, to challenge a patient to a suspect food may also be reasonable but must be done in a setting prepared to treat anaphylaxis (in fact, the clinician is cautioned against challenging a patient who gives a history of anaphylaxis to that food). Formal single and double-blind challenges to the nose, eyes, bronchi, and digestive tract are best done in the research environment.

18.5 Allergy therapy

To impact the allergic march in early childhood, it makes sense to practice more aggressive allergy intervention. However, as the allergic child reaches adulthood, the decision to treat or not to treat rests first with the patient and is usually dependent upon the impact of symptoms on the overall functional status and QoL. The purpose of allergy therapy is to control allergic mediators and their receptors, thereby having an impact at multiple points of the allergic cascade, thus controlling symptoms and perhaps altering disease course. Methods available to the clinician involve avoidance of allergenic triggers, pharmacotherapy and immunotherapy.

18.5.1 Environmental avoidance

Environmental avoidance of food and inhalant allergens is easy in theory but frequently difficult in practice. There is clear evidence that avoidance of allergenic foods is efficacious and is the best approach to food allergies. With inhalants, however, the avoidance methods presently practiced are not as well proven. Nevertheless, some of the more popular approaches to environmental interventions for control of inhalant allergens are discussed below.

Dust mites thrive on human skin scales, so the patient should concentrate on the bedroom and bed linens by considering the following: enclosing the mattress, pillow, and comforter in impervious covers; placing an electric blanket on surface of mattress on high setting for 8 h; washing bedding and treating carpets with benzylbenzoate every 1–2 weeks; using chlorine bleach; tumble-drying bedding at 140°F for 6 h; and freezing infested items for 1–2 days. Molds thrive in humid conditions, so the following should be considered: maintaining relative humidity < 50%; increasing ventilation; removing sources of water accumulation; washing or replacing bathroom rugs frequently; and cleaning moldy surfaces with bleach or fungicides. Cat dander is sticky and seems to be nearly everywhere. To combat cat allergens, the patient should keep pets out of the bedroom and residence, wash pets, and keep female rather than male cats. Cockroach allergens, often blamed for asthma, are also in all households but have a propensity for urban environments, older dwellings, storage areas, and they enjoy food and dark conditions. The best approach is to remove food sources before nightfall and get rid of stored boxes and paper bags (16).

Air-filtration devices are theoretically and psychologically beneficial but they are largely unstudied in placebo-controlled research. Although there is an array of devices that are available, including those with fiberglass, electrical attraction or activated charcoal filters, only those equipped with high-efficiency particulate air filtershave shown impact on allergen counts (probably due to their ability to remove very small particles from the air). Unfortunately, they have not by themselves improved patient outcomes (17).

18.5.2 Pharmacotherapy

Pharmacotherapy gives the clinician various tools in which to control inflammatory mediators and their receptors. Topical and systemic options are available, and the use of combinations from different classes can frequently offer greater success in patient outcomes.

The use of topical hypertonic nasal saline irrigation in the treatment of allergic rhinitis is extremely underestimated in its utility. Saline irrigation mechanically rinses nasal secretions and inflammatory mediators contained within. It improves mucociliary clearance and reduces reliance on other allergy medications (18).

Histamine is an extremely important allergic mediator that is released during mast cell degranulation, causing most of the symptoms verbalized by patients relating to vasodilation, increased vascular permeability, and sensory nerve irritation (19). Histamine receptors, not surprisingly, are located on peripheral blood vessels and nerves, as well as in the frontal and temporal cortex. Antihistamines antagonize the actions of histamine by stabilizing H1 receptors. They enjoy a long track record having been in clinical use for > 60 years (20, 21).

A well-known characteristic of the classical first-generation systemic antihistamines is their ability to penetrate the blood–brain barrier and, because they are lipid-soluble and molecularly small, they can enter and influence the CNS. Thus, in addition to their ability to block peripheral receptors, first-generation antihistamines show central pharmacologic activity in serotonergic, α-adrenergic, dopaminergic, and muscarinic–cholinergic pathways (22), causing most notably drowsiness, fatigue, and an inability to concentrate, aggravating an already impaired patient. Understandably, they also impair psychomotor reflexes, cognition, driving skills, and interact dangerously with alcohol and tranquilizers (23). Because of these central effects, first-generation antihistamines have been abused and misused by the general public (including teenagers) and, in young children, over-dosage has been associated with seizures and death (20).

For the reasons stated above, second-generation antihistamines are a better choice. A well-known characteristic of these newer, molecularly larger second-generation systemic antihistamines, which are less lipid-soluble, is their lesser ability to penetrate the blood–brain barrier and thus influence the CNS (20). In fact, learning tests in children depict a performance hierarchy, with healthy patients turning in the top scores, patients with allergies treated with second-generation antihistamines or placebo achieving scores in the middle range, and patients with allergies treated with first-generation antihistamines scoring in the lower range (24).

Topical antihistamines are available for use in the nose and the eyes. As with any topical therapy, the onset of action is faster than with oral medications. Also, higher tissue levels, and efficacy can be achieved without as many systemic side effects. If the symptoms are primarily affecting the nose or the eye, and the most rapid symptom relief is sought, then topical antihistamines may be a better choice compared with their systemic counterparts.

Systemic decongestants (alpha-adrenergic receptor agonists) are most effective for the one symptom of congestion. However, associated insomnia, tachycardia and hypertension restrict their use and efficacy. Topical decongestants are available for the eyes and the nose and have a much quicker onset of action and potency in comparison with their systemic counterparts. If used too frequently, however, the congestion that was being successfully treated topically becomes aggravated, and efficacy diminishes (rhinitis medicamentosa). However, these adverse effects should not manifest if used only for 3–7 days or < 10 times per month (25).

Leukotrienes are important inflammatory allergic mediators. They are produced by mast cells, eosinophils, basophils, macrophages, and monocytes. At the time of mast cell degranulation, leukotrienes are synthesized from their phospholipid-rich outer membrane. Leukotriene receptors are widely distributed in the nose and lungs on the secretory epithelium, inflammatory cells, and vascular endothelial cells (26). Receptor engagement by leukotrienes causes increased vascular permeability, edema, increased mucus secretion, and smooth muscle contraction. Another important effect of leukotrienes relates to their influence on eosinophil chemotaxis and accumulation. Eosinophils are a major component in the late-phase allergic reaction, during which cytiokines and leukotrienes cause them to migrate to the site of allergic inflammation and where they cause tissue injury and chronic eosinophilic airway inflammation (24, 28). The leukotriene receptor antagonist montelukast is approved for treatment of allergic rhinitis; zafirlukast (another antagonist) and zileuton (an inhibitor of the leukotriene synthesis enzyme 5-lipoxygenase inhibitor) are approved for the treatment of asthma.

Ipratropium, a synthetic quaternary ammonium compound derived from atropine, reduces allergic rhinitis-induced rhinorrhea if given through the intranasal route. The nasal mucosa is innervated by parasympathetic nerves, and muscarinic receptors in the respiratory tract are responsive to the neurotransmitter acetylcholine. Parasympathetic stimulation will augment mucous secretion volume, water content, and mucociliary beat frequency, all of which can be reduced to baseline with topical ipratropium bromide (29).

Mast cell stabilizers such as cromolyn are topically used and work by inhibition of mast cell degranulation. Theoretically this mechanism sounds promising, but experience has shown this class of medications to be less effective than most other topical medication choices. They have been shown to inhibit infiltration of eosinophils and neutrophils, which are a part of the late phase of the allergic reaction, and are effective in rhinorrhea when due to allergies. They are available for the nose and the eye, but frequent dosing is usually required.

Topical and even sometimes systemic glucocorticoids (corticosteroids) are useful in the management of allergies because they can impact the allergic cascade at several levels. Due to their lipophilicity, corticosteroids penetrate through the outer cellular membrane with relative ease. They then engage glucocorticoid receptors within the cell, which prevent the transcription of enzymes that are necessary for the synthesis of inflammatory cytokines. This in turn inhibits the attraction of inflammatory cells, most notably eosinophils. Corticosteroids also stabilize mucous-producing glands so that they are less likely to secrete mucous, and they also increase sympathetic vascular tone, leading to constriction and decreased vascular permeability.

The topically administered corticosteroids for use in the nose take advantage of the higher tissue levels that can be achieved without as many systemic side effects as with their systemic counterparts. Furthermore, congestion is better controlled by corticosteroids than all other drug classes, except topical decongestants. In addition, meta-analyses have shown the topical corticosteroid class to do the best overall job of controlling all of the allergic rhinitis symptoms, including those associated with histamine-mediation (sneezing, rhinorrhea, itching). However, these medications must be used on a regular basis and for several days to achieve and maintain desired efficacy, and regular compliance with nasal sprays can be a deterrent to success. Although it appears that the systemic side effects are minimal, the possibility of reduction of growth velocity in children must also be considered if used for prolonged periods.

Corticosteroids administered systemically are effective and can be used, but with caution. Systemic corticosteroids should not be administered in children except under extreme circumstances and only in adults on a very selective basis, with appropriate education to patients and parents about side effects (including potential growth disturbance in children).

18.5.3 Immunotherapy

Immunotherapy as it applies to allergy is a form of vaccination or immunization. It is used to treat IgE-mediated inhalant allergy causing rhinoconjunctivitis, asthma or insect-venom anaphylaxis. It is generally reserved for the patient in whom symptoms are present for long periods of time each year, and pharmacotherapy and environmental avoidance have been insufficient. To use immunotherapy requires a positive allergen-specific IgE test.

Immunotherapy is potentially life-threatening because it can provoke anaphalyxis, usually within 30 min of an injection but perhaps as long as 24 h, and thus it should not be undertaken haphazardly. Therefore, on the day of treatment, patients should be observed for 30 min and should carry auto-injectable epinephrine and antihistamines, and know how to and when to administer them.

Immunotherapy is accomplished by intentional exposure to regular, progressive doses of the same specific aeroallergens that are presumed to be responsible for producing symptoms and should be continued for 2–5 years. It results in down-regulation of the immunologic response and control of symptoms associated with usual levels of environmental exposure to the treated allergens. It is usually administered by subcutaneous injection (subcutaneous immunotherapy, SCIT), although other routes, including oral, sublingual (sublingual immunotherapy, SLIT), nasal, conjunctival, and bronchial, are possible. To control symptoms, the goal of immunotherapy is to escalate antigen dose to the point of highest tolerated dose or to a pre-determined antigen dose range but without causing unacceptable local or systemic reactions (30).

Appropriately administered immunotherapy results in several changes in the immune system. There is a shift away from the expression of the pro-inflammatory cytokines, mediated by Th2 lymphocytes, which are characteristic of IgE-mediated disease. There is also a reduction in number, activity and migration of eosinophils, a reduction in mast cells, and an elevation of the threshold for mast cell degranulation. There is an increase in the levels of allergen-specific IgG4, frequently referred to as "blocking antibody. " These antibody levels are correlated with symptom improvement but, with discontinuance of immunotherapy, IgG4 falls gradually over several years (30).

Many well-designed double-blinded clinical trials have shown efficacy. After an adequate course of therapy, allergen immunotherapy typically reduces the frequency and duration of allergy symptoms, improves QoL, reduces the need for adjunctive medication, and reduces allergen-specific IgE and IgG as well as skin, nasal, conjunctival, and bronchial reactivity (31). Immunotherapy also diminishes the incidence of sensitivities to new allergens (32). Immunotherapy has also been shown to impact the allergic march by decreasing the development of asthma in children (33). For insect-venom sensitivity, immunotherapy has been shown to reduce the rate of re-sting reactions to 5% in comparison with 60% in placebo patients (34).

SLIT has been in use for many years, especially in Europe, and allows for a sublingual route of administration of antigen extracts. This involves the placement of antigen under the tongue for one to several minutes, allowing for systemic absorption through the sublingual mucosal barrier. This carries the potential advantage of increased patient compliance and safety. The problem is that there are less data validating the SLIT technique. However, the European data, which includes 46 doubled-blind placebo-controlled studies, strongly support safety and efficacy. Dosing is generally higher than with SCIT. Nevertheless, there is a lot of heterogeneity among these trials, and there are no completed trials in the USA that support efficacy. Therefore, SLIT has yet to be approved by the Food and Drug Administration even though its use in the USA continues (35, 36).

18.5.4 Monoclonal antibody therapy for asthma

Monoclonal antibody therapy, like *in-vitro* IgE testing, is based on the development of murine anti-IgE IgG antibodies. However, in addition, these therapeutic antibodies have been "humanized" by genetic alteration so as to be used safely in humans. These antibodies have been designed to combine with all IgE antibodies; if they interact with the correct IgE receptor, the IgE antibody is disabled from attaching to mast cells and other inflammatory cells.

Omalizumab, which is the generic name for this antibody, has for several years been commercially available for the treatment of asthma. There are ample trials supporting its safety and efficacy for asthma and allergic rhinitis. However, it is indicated for asthma only in patients ≥12 years. Eligible patients must have a positive skin test or *in-vitro* reactivity to a perennial aeroallergen and must have symptoms that are inadequately controlled with inhaled corticosteroids. Furthermore, they must have a positive total IgE *in-vitro* test to validate use and to calculate dose. It is administered via injection every 2–4 weeks. Anaphylaxis has been reported with this therapy, and malignancy prevalence is twice as common as compared with the general population (0.05% versus 0.2%) (37). This is currently an expensive treatment option.

18.6 Conclusion

Children with allergic disease as adults deserve the time and effort necessary to improve and preserve the often overlooked impaired physical and mental function associated with IgE-mediated disease. Appropriate history-taking, testing, and therapeutic intervention can go a long way in improving outcomes in these patients and, in nearly all cases, patients will very much appreciate your efforts.

References

1. Mahr, T. A., Sheth, K. (2005) Update on allergic rhinitis. Pediatr. Rev. 26:284–289.
2. Kay, A. B. (2001) Allergy and allergic diseases. N. Engl. J. Med. 344:30–37.
3. Wright, A. L., Holberg, C. J., Martinez, F. D., Halonen, M., Morgan, W., Taussig, L. M. (1994) Epidemiologyof physician-diagnosed allergic rhinitis in childhood. Pediatrics 94:895–901.
4. Wilken, J. A., Berkowitz, R., Kane, R. (2002) Decrements in vigilance and cognitive functioning associated with ragweed-induced allergic rhinitis. Ann. Allergy Asthma Immunol. 89:372–380.

5. Marshall, P. S., O'Hara, C., Steinberg, P. (2002) Effects of seasonal allergic rhinitis on fatigue levels and mood. Psychosom. Med. 64:684–691.
6. Bousquet, J., Neukirch, F., Bousquet, P. J., Gehano, P., Klossek, J. M., Le Gal, M., Allaf, B. (2006) Severity and impairment of allergic rhinitis in patients consulting in primary care. J. Allergy Clin. Immunol. 117:158–162.
7. Léger, D., Annesi-Maesano, I., Carat, F., Rugina, M., Chanal, I., Pribil, C., et al. (2006)Allergic rhinitis and its consequences on quality of sleep: an unexplored area. Arch. Intern. Med. 166:1744–1748.
8. Lamb, C. E., Ratner, P. H., Johnson, C. E., Ambegaonkar, A. J., Joshi, A. V., Day, D., et al. (2006) Economic impact of workplace productivity losses due to allergic rhinitis compared with select medical conditions in the United States from an employer perspective. Curr. Med. Res. Opin. 22:1203–1210.
9. Allergies in America? A landmark survey of nasal allergy sufferers (executive summary). http:// www. myallergiesinamerica. com. Accessed 15 October 2009.
10. Law, A. W., Reed, S. D., Sundy, J. S., Schulman, K. A. (2003) Direct costs of allergic rhinitis in the United States: estimates from the 1996 Medical Expenditure Panel Survey. J. Allergy. Clin. Immunol. 111(2):296–300.
11. Crystal-Peters, J., Crown, W. H., Goetzel, R. Z., Schutt, D. C. (2000) The cost of productivity losses associated with allergic rhinitis. Am. J. Manag. Care 6:373–378.
12. Goetzel, R. Z., Long, S. R., Ozminkowski, R. J., Hawkins, K., Wang, S., Lynch, W. (2004) Health, absence, disability, and presenteeism cost estimates of certain physical and mental health conditions affecting U.S. employers. J. Occup. Environ. Med. 46:398–412.
13. Bunn, W. B. 3rd, Pikelny, D. B., Paralkar, S., Slavion, T., Borden, S. 4th, Allen, H. M. Jr. (2003) The burden of allergies – and the capacity of medications to reduce this burden – in a heavy manufacturing environment. J. Occup. Environ. Med. 45:941–955.
14. Haydon, R. C. (2008) Current approaches to skin and in-vitro testing. Otolaryngol. Clin. North Am. 41:331–346.
15. American College of Allergy, Asthma, & Immunology. (2006) Food allergy: a practice parameter. Ann. Allergy Asthma Immunol. 96:S1–S68.
16. Haydon, R. C. (2003) Addressing the prevalence of respiratory allergy in the home environment. Otolaryngol. Clin. North Am. 36:1–22.
17. Reisman, R. E. (2001) Do air cleaners make a difference in treating allergic disease in homes?Ann. Allergy Asthma Immunol. 87:S41–S43.
18. Rosenfeld, R. M., Andes, D., Bhattacharyya, N., Cheung, D., Eisenberg, S., Ganiats, T. G., et al. (2007) Clinical practice guideline: adult sinusitis. Otolaryngol. Head Neck Surg. 137:S1–S31.
19. Iriyoshi, N., Takeuchi, K., Yuta, A., Ukai, K., Sakakura, Y. (1996) Increased expression of histamine H1 receptor mRNA in allergic rhinitis. Clin. Exp. Allergy 26:379–385.
20. Haydon, R. C. (2001) Are second-generation antihistamines appropriate for most children and adults? Arch. Otolaryngol. Head Neck Surg. 127:1510–1513.
21. Li, H., Sha, Q., Zuo, K., Jiang, H., Cheng, L., Shi, J., Xu, G. (2009) Nasal saline irrigation facilitates control of allergic rhinitis by topical steroid in children. ORL J. Otorhinolaryngol. Relat. Spec. 71:50–55.
22. Gengo, F. M. (1996) Reduction of the central nervous system adverse effects associated with antihistamines in the management of allergic disorders: strategies and progress. J. Allergy Clin. Immunol. 98(Suppl. 6, Pt. 3):S319–S325.
23. Meltzer, E. O. (1990) Antihistamine- and decongestant-induced performance decrements. J. Occup. Med. 32:327–334.
24. Vuurman, E. F., vanVeggel, L. M., Uiterwijk, M. M., Leutner, D., O'Hanlon, J. F. (1993) Seasonal allergic rhinitis and antihistamine effects on children's learning. Ann. Allergy 71:121–126.
25. Bousquet, J., van Cauwenberge, P., Khaltaev, N. Aria Workshop Group, World Health Organization. (2001) Allergic rhinitis and its impact on asthma. J. Allergy Clin. Immunol. 108(Suppl. 5):S147–S334.

26. Shirasaki, H., Kanaizumi, E., Watanabe, K., Matsui, T., Sato, J., Narita, S., et al. (2002) Expression and localization of the cysteinyl leukotriene 1 receptor in human nasal mucosa. Clin. Exp. Allergy 32:1007–1012.
27. Lipworth, B. J. (2001) Emerging role of antileukotriene therapy in allergic rhinitis. Clin. Exp. Allergy 31:1813–1821.
28. Meltzer, E. O. (2000) Role for cysteinyl leukotriene receptor antagonist therapy in asthma and their potential role in allergic rhinitis based on the concept of "one linked airway disease". Ann. Allergy Asthma Immunol. 84:176–187.
29. Gallagher, J. T., Kent, P. W., Passatore, M., Phipps, R. J., Richardson, P. S. (1975) The composition of tracheal mucus and the nervous control of its secretion in the cat. Proc. R. Soc. Lond. B. Biol. Sci. 192:49–76.
30. Haydon, R. C., Gordon, B. (2001) Aerollergen injection immunotherapy. In: Gordon, B., Krouse, J., Derebery, J., Chadwick, S., eds. Allergy and Immunology: An Otolaryngic Approach. Philadelphia, USA: Lippincott Williams and Wilkins, pp. 151–182.
31. Calderon, M. A., Alves, B., Jacobson, M., Hurwitz, B., Sheikh, A., Durham, S. (2007) Allergen injection immunotherapy for seasonal allergic rhinitis. Cochrane Database Syst. Rev. (1):CD001936. [Comment in: Otolaryngol. Head Neck Surg. 2007;136:511–514].
32. Des Roches, A., Paradis, L., Menardo, J. L., Bouges, S., Daures, J. P., Bousquet, J. (1997) Immunotherapy with a standardized *Dermatophagoides pteronyssinus* extract, VI: specific immunotherapy prevents the onset of new sensitizations in children. J. Allergy Clin. Immunol. 99:450–453.
33. Lombardi, C., Passalacqua, G., Gargioni, S., Senna, G., Ciprandi, G., Scordamaglia, A., Canonica, G. W. (2001) The natural history of respiratory allergy: a follow-up study of 99 patients up to 10 years. Respir. Med. 95:9–12.
34. Yang, X. (2001) Does allergen immunotherapy alter the natural course of allergic disorders? Drugs 61:365–374.
35. Leatherman, B. D., Owen, S., Parker, M., Chadwick, S., Fornadley, J. A., Colson, D. et al. (2007) Sublingual immunotherapy: past, present, paradigm for the future? A review of the literature. Otolaryngol. Head Neck Surg. 136:S1–S20.
36. Nelson, H. S. (2008) Preparing and mixing allergen vaccines for subcutaneous immunotherapy. Clin. Allergy Immunol. 21:303–320.
37. Amiri, P., Haak-Frendscho, M., Robbins, K., McKerrow, J. H., Stewart, T., Jardieu, P. (1994) Anti-immunoglobulin E treatment decreases worm burden and egg production in *Schistosoma mansoni*-infected normal and interferon gamma knockout mice. J. Exp. Med. 180:43–51.

19 Aging with intellectual disability: Current health issues

Joav Merrick, Isack Kandel, Meir Lotan, Shoshana Aspler, Brian S. Fuchs and Mohammed Morad

Over the past decade, we have observed an increase in lifespan for people with intellectual disability, which can be seen as the consequence of progress in medical technology and improved social awareness in the twentieth century. In the past, most individuals with intellectual disability died at a young age due to their additional medical problems, congenital malformations and infections with the result that very few survived into adulthood or went through the aging process. This trend has resulted in not only pediatricians, but now also adult physicians becoming involved in the management of this population. Today we see the first generation of aging persons with intellectual disability, which is a challenge for service providers. Older people with intellectual disability have the same needs as other older people, and they are subject to the same age-related impairments and illnesses. Moreover, because many disabled individuals live together with their families, the burden is double because the family members are also aging and, with time, will not be able to continue their care-giving. Medical needs from pediatric to adult care can be met by enrollment in universal healthcare or programs. Periodic health assessments and healthcare should be normalized and provided as an overall system of supports when needed or as assistance provided for the adequate self-directed use of general or specialty health services. Risk assessments and health reviews should be part of the individual's life-plan and provided to detect diseases and conditions that could compromise longevity. This field of medicine also needs to evaluate the applicability of a new discipline of lifespan developmental medicine to lead in interdisciplinary care, healthcare education, service delivery and research for people with intellectual disability within an academic framework.

19.1 Introduction

In the 1930s, the mean age at death for people with intellectual disability was ~19 years, in the 1970s it was ~59 years, in the 1990s it was 66 years and today it is close to general life expectancy; whereas, for Down syndrome, the mean age at death was 9 years in the 1920s and is 56 years today (1). Such an increase in lifespan can be seen as the consequence of progress in medical technology and improved social awareness in the twentieth century. In the past, most individuals with intellectual disability died at a young age due to their additional medical problems, congenital malformations and infections with the result that very few went through the aging process. This trend has resulted in not only pediatricians, but now also adult physicians being involved in the management of this population. Today we see the first generation of aging persons with intellectual disability, which is a challenge for service providers.

Mental retardation or intellectual disability has, since 1908 (2), been defined and re-defined by the American Association of Intellectual and Developmental Disability with ~10 years apart in recent years with a new definition. The last revision (the tenth) took place in 2002 (2), whereby mental retardation/intellectual disability is defined as a disability characterized by significant limitations in intellectual functioning and adaptive behavior as expressed in conceptual, social and practical adaptive skills and originating before the age of 18 years. There are five assumptions essential to the application of this definition:

- Limitations in present functioning must be considered within the context of community environments typical of the individual's age peers and culture.
- Valid assessment considers cultural and linguistic diversity as well as differences in communication, sensory, motor and behavioral factors.
- Within an individual, limitations often coexist with strengths.
- An important purpose of describing limitations is to develop a profile of needed supports.
- With appropriate personalized supports over a sustained period, the life functioning of the person with mentalretardation/intellectual disability will generally improve.

This definition and standards are used worldwide. In Israel, the Division for Mental Retardation (DMR) of the Ministry of Social Affairs and Social Services has the responsibility for the assessment, treatment, rehabilitation and service for persons with intellectual disability. In Israel, with a population of ~7.5 million, the DMR is in contact with ~30,000 persons of all ages. Residential care is provided to ~7,000 persons in 60 residential centers all over the country; in about ~50 locations, residential care is provided to an additional 3,000 persons in hostels or in group homes in the community, whereas the remainder are served with Day-care Kindergartens, Day Treatment Centers, sheltered workshops, or integrated care in the community while living at home with their families (3).

The purpose of this review is to look at the trends of people with intellectual disability, as well as the aging and medical needsin this population.

19.2 Trends in the aging in the population of persons with intellectual disability in residential care centers in Israel

The Office of the Medical Director (OMD) of the DMR in Israel have, since 1998, conducted an annual national survey of all residential care centers for people with intellectual disability to monitor the health service for people with intellectual disability (4).

The most recent data available are from the 2008 National survey (5). The age distribution of 6, 988 persons with intellectual disability in residential centers from 2008 is presented in ▶Tab. 19.1 and the level of intellectual disability is presented in ▶Tab. 19.2. It can be observed that people with intellectual disability are now living into old age.

The trend toward longer living for persons with intellectual disability in residential care can be seen from ▶ Tab. 19.3 and ▶ Tab. 19.4, in which data have been extracted from the 1999–2008 national surveys. It is evident that this population is getting older.

Tab. 19.1: Population of persons with intellectual disability in residential care centers in Israel in 2008.

Age (years)	Males	Females	Total	Percentage
0–9	72	49	121	1.73
10–19	465	311	776	11.11
20–39	1, 649	1, 122	2, 771	39.65
40–49	782	600	1, 382	19.78
50–59	672	591	1, 263	18.07
>60	311	364	675	9.66
Total	**3, 951**	**3, 037**	**6, 988**	**100.00**
%	**56.54**	**43.46**	**100.00**	

Unfortunately, we do not have data from people with intellectual disability living in hostels, protected apartments, living at home with their family, or living alone.

In the past decade, it has been observed worldwide that there will be increased numbers of persons aged > 65 years. This larger number of older people worldwide will require a better and more effective health and social service because many will have chronic diseases in need of management and surveillance. This load will increase health, social and long-term care expenses, but also make public-health interventions important to sustain good health and a good QoL even in the face of chronic disease. It will also require a transition process from pediatric to adolescent care to adult healthcare providers, which so far have had little experience with adults with intellectual disability.

Tab. 19.2: Level of intellectual disability in the population of persons with intellectual disability in residential care in Israel in 2008. Mild intellectual disability was classified as an IQ of 55–70; moderate, IQ 35–54; severe, IQ 20–34; and profound, IQ <20. "Other" are 23 persons who historically were placed in institutions for other reasons and preferred to stay on because they regarded the institution as their home, or persons under observation or persons not yet assessed.

Age (years)	Mild	Moderate	Severe	Profound	Other	Total	Percentage
0–9	2	16	58	41	4	121	1.73
10–19	108	270	255	137	6	776	11.11
20–39	370	1, 021	963	378	39	2, 771	39.65
40–49	223	543	418	182	16	1, 382	19.78
50–59	182	589	347	137	8	1, 263	18.07
>60	86	378	160	45	6	675	9.66
Total	**972**	**2, 831**	**2, 190**	**916**	**79**	**6, 988**	**100.00**
Percentage	**13.91**	**40.51**	**31.34**	**13.11**	**1.13**	**100.00**	

Tab. 19.3: Population of persons with intellectual disability in residential care centers in Israel aged 40 years and older during 1999–2008 (given as percentage of total population).

Age (years)	1999	2000	2001	2002	2003	2004	2005	2006	2007	2008
40–49	21.69	21.81	21.73	22.23	21.32	20.49	20.30	20.77	20.20	19.78
50–59	11.52	12.36	13.22	14.15	15.32	16.05	16.95	17.14	18.22	18.07
>60	4.26	4.46	4.88	5.64	5.72	6.38	6.89	7.16	8.57	9.66
40 and older	**37.47**	**38.63**	**39.83**	**42.02**	**42.36**	**42.92**	**44.14**	**45.07**	**46.99**	**47.51**

This increase in the number of older people in the general population is also reflected in the population of persons with intellectual disability. Today the mean life expectancy of older adults with intellectual disability is 66.1 years and increasing (6). This population will present increasing challenges to the clinician and to the public health system (6, 7). This will be characterized by an increased prevalence of hearing and visual impairments, obesity, osteoporosis, dementia, and other chronic diseases with a need for more intensive medical surveillance and interventions (7).

19.3 Our study of > 2, 000 aging persons with intellectual disability

A total of 2, 283 adults with intellectual disability aged ≥40 years in residential care centers in Israel were studied to determine health status (8). Age was a significant factor in disease frequency, functional behavior, and age-related changes in organ system diseases. The frequency of all disease categories increased significantly with age, except for GI, hematological and infectious diseases. There were increases with age in both sexes for cardiovascular disease, cancer, and sensory impairments. Cardiovascular disease was less prevalent than in the general population, suggesting that under-diagnosis of some diseases may be more common than expected in this population.

This study was a replication of an American large-scale population-based survey of health status and health-service utilization in > 1, 300 adults aged ≥40 years with

Tab. 19.4: Population of persons with intellectual disability in residential care centers in Israel aged 40 years and older during 1999–2006 (given as numbers).

Age (years)	1999	2000	2001	2002	2003	2004	2005	2006	2007	2008
40–49	1, 328	1, 355	1, 384	1, 412	1, 386	1, 354	1, 370	1, 421	1, 388	1, 382
50–59	705	768	842	899	996	1, 061	1, 144	1, 172	1, 252	1, 263
>60	261	277	311	358	372	422	465	490	589	675
40 and older	**2, 294**	**2, 400**	**2, 537**	**2, 669**	**2, 754**	**2, 837**	**2, 979**	**3, 083**	**3, 229**	**3, 320**

intellectual disability living in small group, community-based residences in New York (USA) (9). The main questions for both studies were whether the trends reported in previous studies could be confirmed in a large sample, whether these trends were comparable to data on older persons without intellectual disability, and what factors may place persons with intellectual disability at higher risk for decline in health and functional status as they age.

For this Israeli study (8) the response rate was 95%. The study population had a mean age of 49.8 years, indicating that the residents were generally younger adults. Most (88%) were < 59 years of age. There were slightly more males (51%) than females (49%). The mean length of stay in current residence was 20.8 years (SD = 12.0) indicating a stable population. About 48% had severe or profound intellectual disability. Down syndrome was reported in 11% of the study population. Cerebral palsy as a coincident condition was reported for 14% of adults. The mean BMI of the Israeli cohort was 25.7 with 35% classified as overweight with a BMI > 27.

19.3.1 Functional behavior

About 25% of the cohort had impaired or limited vision. Impaired hearing was less prevalent because only 12% were reported to have impaired or no hearing. The prevalence of visual and hearing impairment significantly increased with age (p< 0.0001). Inferred frailty, stemming from poor activities of daily living (ADL) skills and general functioning, was observed, but appeared within expected ranges of this population. In terms of impaired function, 17% could not eat by themselves, 37% could not dress themselves, 28% could not toilet independently, and 55% could not wash and bathe without assistance. In addition, 31% lacked complete bowel and bladder control (continence). The ability to independently toilet (p=0.035), bathe (p=0.002), and control continence (p=0.003) all were significantly lower than in older age groupings.

19.3.2 General health and utilization/coordination of healthservices

Irrespective of age group, over half of the cohort were reported not to engage in any exercise. Very few adults experienced injuries. Nearly everyone saw a Physician annually and very few had been hospitalized or visited the Emergency Room in the last year. As would be expected, perception of health status declined and use of health services increased significantly with increasing age.

In general, diseases occurred at about the same frequencies for males and females. However, age-related changes in most organ system diseases differed by sex. The prevalence of cardiovascular disease, cancer, as well as impairments of vision and hearing increased with age groupings for both sexes. The only disease that did not significantly increase with age grouping in females or males was hematologic disease. Psychiatric disorders decreased with age in both sexes. Neurological disease decreased with age only in females, with most of the decrease occurring after age 70 years. The prevalence of neurological disease in this cohort was high (44% overall), but declined in older age groups, most probably reflecting early mortality among those adults who were most impaired. Epilepsy and cerebral palsy were the two most frequent neurological conditions (16% and 14%, respectively). The prevalence of cancer was generally low.

The prevalence for adults with dementia was ~3%. Depression, anxiety disorders, and schizophrenia were found in < 5% and bipolar disease in < 1%. However, ~30% of adults displayed some form of behavioral problems.

19.3.3 Cardiovascular diseaseand risk factors

The apparently low frequency of cardiovascular disease in this studyprompted further analyses of cardiovascular disease and risk factors. No specific cardiovascular diagnosis occurred at a prevalence of > 13%. The frequency of hyperlipidemia and T2DM increased with age in the cohort. The BMI remained constant with increasing age. This study population appeared to have lower frequencies of hyperlipidemia, hypertension, and DM than that found in the general Israeli population.

A decrease in the frequency of cardiovascular disease with increasing cognitive severity was observed. The percentage of those adults with known cardiovascular disease risk factors such as hyperlipidemia, BMI > 27 kg/m^2, Type 2 Diabetes Mellitus, lack of weekly exercise, and hypertension decreased with more severe intellectual disability. Older people, those with high BMI values, those with DM, and those with hyperlipidemia had greater frequencies of heart disease.

19.4 Health needs of older persons with intellectual disability

With more persons with intellectual disability living longer comes an increase in age-related health problems seen in the general population. These include heart disease, cardiovascular disease, cancer, as well as visual and hearing impairment. Many of the physicians and care staff involved with the health service of persons with intellectual disability came from the field of pediatrics. Hence, there will be a need to take a long-term view and involve the fields of family medicine and geriatrics in the care. The physician working in family medicine in the community has very little training or experience working with subjects with intellectual disability. This is despite the fact that more people with intellectual disability are living in the community compared with residential care.

In this review, we would like to share some of our experiences on health-related problems and needs of adult persons with intellectual disability relevant for family physicians or other allied professionals working with persons with intellectual disability in residential care or in the community.

19.4.1 Mild and moderate intellectual disability

In this population, the concerns will be the same as for the general aging population. However, due to communication problems, lack of service, lack of interest or commitment from the service providers, the diagnosis or treatment can be ignored, overlooked or delayed for this population (10). This is unfortunate because simple medical problems that could be solved will have adverse effects on the QoL for the person with intellectual disability.

The prevalence of cardiovascular disease was found to be less in persons with intellectual disability aged ≥65 years admitted to nursing homes than persons without intellectual disability (24.4% versus 56.5%) (11), but there are very few studies on the prevalence of heart disease in this population. A study from New York State (USA) (9) of 1,371 adult persons with intellectual disability living in the community showed that cardiovascular disease increased with increasing age and was more likely among adults who were more functional, in adults with seizures, and in those with the highest BMI.

The prevalence of death from cancer in the United Kingdom for persons with intellectual disability has been lower than for the general population (11.7–17.5% versus 26%), but the prevalence of cancer is now on the increase due to increased longevity (12, 13). In New York State, the prevalence of cancer increased significantly with age and was more likely to occur in females (8). The prevalence of GI cancer was proportionally higher than in the general population (48–58.5% versus 25% of cancer deaths in the United Kingdom) (12, 13). In a study of cancer and Down syndrome, a statistically significant increaseinthe prevalenceof leukemiawas found, as well as an increase in the prevalence of gastric cancer in institutionalized males (14).

Women with intellectual disability are much less likely to undergo cervical smear tests than the general population (19% versus 77%) (15). They are also less likely to have breast cancer examinations or receive mammography (16).

Visual and hearing impairment affect about half of the general population aged > 65 years and will also be seen in older persons with intellectual disability. Visual impairment was found to be seven-fold higher in adults with intellectual disabilitythan in the general population (17). Cataract, glaucoma, macular degeneration and diabetic retinopathy should be considered. Ocular and orbital abnormalities in persons with Down syndrome are numerous: blepharitis (2–47%), keratoconus (5–8%), glaucoma (< 1%), iris anomalies (38–90%), cataract (25–85%), retinal anomalies (0–38%), optic nerve anomalies (very few cases), strabismus (23–44%), amblyopia (10–26%), nystagmus (5–30%) and refractive errors (18–58%) (18). Deafness is also common in this population (19) and impairment increase with increasing age (19). Presbycusis (high-pitched tones become harder to hear) and hearing loss is also seen in this population as a result of impacted earwax (20).

Constipation is seen frequently in this population and can be a lifelongproblem, which increases with age due to decline in mobility and less bowel motility or movement. Medication can also be a factor in constipation. Caretakers need to be aware of this problem because of the dangers to accumulation and sometimes even intestinal perforation and death (21, 22).

In aging, the bladder capacity and muscle tone will decrease and cause urinary incontinence. In men, enlargement of the prostate gland can also restrict urinary flow.

Dental problems in surveys of this population have identified poor oral hygiene, a high prevalence of gingival disease and untreated dental caries with dental care difficult to implement (23).

19.4.2 Health concerns in severe and profound intellectual disability

Many persons with severe and profound intellectual disabilitywill have associated medical problems and disease. In our review of mortality in this population in Israel (24) for the 1991–97 period, 60% of 450 cases were deaths before the age of 41 years and 68% in the severe-profound group. Cardiovascular reasons accounted for 35%, respiratory disease for 25% and infectious diseases for 9% of the cases.

The group with severe and profound intellectual disability who survived into old age will therefore have musculoskeletal problems, respiratory disease, problems with swallowing, and some will need gastrostomy. Therefore a high service level will be required.

Osteoporosis and increased fractures should be kept in mind in this population (25) due to immobility, nutrition and lack of activity.

19.4.3 Health concerns in Down syndrome

In the 1920s, the life expectancy for persons with Down syndrome was only 9 years, but this has now increased to 56–60 years, which is still 20 years less than in the general population (1, 26).

Alzheimer's disease was first described by Professor Alois Alzheimer in Germany in 1906 (27). He reported the case of Auguste D, a 51-year old female patient he had followed at a Frankfurt hospital since 1901 up until her death on 8 April 1906. Even after her death he went on to study the neuropathological features of her illness. Shortly after her death, he presented her case at the 37th Conference of German Psychiatrists in Tubingen in 1906 in which he described her symptoms:

- Progressive cognitive impairment
- Focal symptoms
- Hallucinations
- Delusions
- Psychosocial incompetence
- Neurobiological changes found at autopsy: plaques, neurofibrillary tangles and artheriosclerotic changes

These symptoms are still the characteristics of Alzheimer's disease today, which is the most common cause of dementia in western countries. Alzheimer's disease most often presents with a subtle onset of memory loss followed by a slowly progressive dementia that has a course of several years. The duration of Alzheimer's disease can be 3–10 years from the diagnosis to death, and this progress is more rapid in persons with Down syndrome. Seizures usually present itself at the end stage. Epilepsy is seen in ~5% of persons with Down syndrome, but the combination of the latter and Alzheimer's disease will produce epileptic seizures in 85% of cases.

Besides Alzheimer's disease, persons with Down syndrome are prone to other medical problems when aging. A study from Holland (28) of 96 adults with Down syndrome from an institution were investigated systematically over the period 1991–95 with cytogenetic diagnosis, mental functioning, dementia, ophthalmological and audiological assessments and thyroid function. A total of 73% were aged > 40 years and only 4.3% were females. Three percent had mild intellectual disability, 82% had moderate and severe intellectual disability, and 15% had profound intellectual disability. Nineteen percent already had dementia, but this number increased to 42% in persons aged > 50 years of age.

Epilepsy was present in 16.7% of all subjects, but in those with dementia it was 50%. Vision problems were frequent, with only 17% with normal vision and the problems increased with increasing age. In the 50–59 year age group, 44.8% had moderate-to-severe vision loss. Seventy percent had moderate, severe or very severe hearing loss, which was undiagnosed before systematic hearing tests were done. Forty-nine percent had thyroid dysfunction.

Besides the above-mentioned health problems, persons with Down syndrome have increased obesity, premature aging of the immune system resulting in various diseases, increased sleep apnea and musculoskeletal problems (29).

19.4.4 Epilepsy and cerebral palsy

Persons with intellectual disability, epilepsy and seizures who receive anti-epileptic drugs over long periods will be at an increased risk for premature mortality, increased risk of osteoporosis, and increased risks of falls.

A study of risk factors for injuries and falls (30) among 268 adults with intellectual disability from 18 nursing homes in Chicago (USA) revealed that 11% (30 cases) had reported injuries 12 months prior to the follow-up study. Over 50% of the injuries were caused by falls. Persons with a higher frequency of seizures, more destructive behavior and usage of anti-psychotic drugs had the highest risk of injuries. Further analysis of the data revealed that persons aged > 70 years who were ambulatory and who had a higher frequency of seizures had the highest risk of injurious falls.

Studies of the effect of aging in persons with cerebral palsy are few (and studies with persons with intellectual disabilityand cerebral palsy are even less). Common sense would dictate that mobility would be decreased over the years, osteoporosis would increase, and there would be increased dependency on care over the years.

19.5 Intellectual disability and general practice

The number of persons with intellectual disability in general practice in Holland has been studied (31). A general practice database with 62,000 patients had 318 persons (or 0.65%) with intellectual disability which, together with persons in residential case, showed a total prevalence of 0.82%.

Barriers to treatment in general practice has been studied in Australia among 912 randomly selected general practitioners (32), where communication difficulties with patients and other health professionals, and problems in getting patient histories, were the most significant barriers. Other difficulties were lack of training and experience, poor patient compliance, consultation time limitations, difficulties in problem determination, examination difficulties, poor continuity of care and inadequate knowledge of services and resources.

Researchers in Cardiff in Wales have developed a health screening tool in general practice for persons with intellectual disability (33), which has also been used in general practice in New Zealand (34). Here the introduction of an annual health screen resulted in medical findings of 72.6% of the 1,311 persons screened, which afterward required follow-up interventions.

A survey conducted through all USA Family Practice Residency Directors (35) showed that 84% of the programs had provided residents with one or more experience about the healthcare needs of persons with intellectual disability and that 60% had instructed residents in that area. Holland in the year 2000 established a professorship in Intellectual Disability in the Department of Family Medicine at the University of Rotterdam, and started a three-year sub-specialty in intellectual disability (36), where the first class of specialists in intellectual disability graduated in November 2003. In 2010, a second professorship was established at the University Medical Centre in Nijmegen.

19.6 Conclusions

We have seen an increase in the population of persons with intellectual disability surviving into adulthood and now also older age over recent years. This has resulted in health problems emerging just like in the general population, but sometimes at a much earlier stage (e.g., Alzheimer's disease in Down syndrome). There is therefore a need to provide more evidence-based practice standards to enhance health status, longevity, functional capability and QoL in this population (37) and transition from pediatric to adult care.

Older people with intellectual disability have the same needs as those of other older people, and they are subject to the same age-related impairments and illnesses (9). Moreover, because many disabled individuals live together with their families, the burden is double because the family members are also aging and, with time, will not be able to continue their care-giving. As with older people in general, older people with intellectual disability also have the needs listed below (10).

- Social needs for people with intellectual disabilities should be met by making it possible for them to attend, use, and benefit from the social, recreational, and leisure resources and amenities that communities develop and operate for their elderly citizens.
- Housing needs can met by supporting families if they are the primary carer or by providing financial resources for rentals or ownership of property. Housing can also be providing by brokering co-living arrangements with other people or by providing for small group homes or self-catered apartments.
- Medical needs can be met by enrollment in universal healthcare or programs. Periodic health assessments and healthcare should be normalized and provided as an overall system of supports when needed or as assistance provided for the adequate self-directed use of general or specialty health services. Risk assessments and health reviews should be part of the individual's life-plan and provided to detect diseases and conditions that could compromise longevity.
- Activity or work is a normal part of life for everybody and should also be facilitated for this population because we have seen that continued activation is preventative for old-age-associated depression and other emotional problems.
- Special care needs for age-associated conditions, such as Alzheimer's disease and related dementias, increasing fragility, or conditions or diseases compromising independent functioning, should be addressed with the focus on care in community or family settings. Institutionalization of persons with intellectual disabilityshould not be based on old age alone.

For health professionals, efforts must be made to accomplish transition from pediatric to adult care and expertise, as listed below.

- Acquisition of additional clinical and epidemiological knowledge regarding specific syndromes with linkages to basic science research in biomolecular genetics and metabolism.
- Development of adapted diagnostic and therapeutic methods for people who have difficulties with cooperation or communication.
- Development and evaluation of interdisciplinary interventions for complicated conditions (e.g., sensory impairment, dysphagia, communication and functional decline).
- Development of clinical measures in several areas (functional capability, QoL, mental health, pain assessment and clinical diagnosis) that are sensitive and specific, easy to administer, and applicable to persons with a wide range of mental and physical capabilities.
- Evaluation of clinical guidelines (including referral protocols) to support community-based Primary Care Physicians within specific healthcare systems to care for people with intellectual disabilities.
- Evaluation of the applicability of a new discipline of lifespan developmental medicine to lead in interdisciplinary care, healthcare education, service delivery and research for people with intellectual disability within an academic framework.
- Development of the knowledge base regarding the health status and needs of people with intellectual disabilities living in less "developed" countries.

References

1. Janicki, M. P., Dalton, A. J., Henderson, C. M., Davidson, P. W. (1999) Mortality and morbidity among older adults with intellectual disability: Health services considerations. Disabil. Rehabil. 21:284–294.
2. Luckasson, R., Borthwick-Duffy, S., Buntinx, W. H. E., Coulter, D. L., Craig, E. M., Reeve, A., et al. (2002) Mental retardation. Definition, classification and systems of support, 10 ed. Washington, USA: American Association of Mental Retardation.
3. Merrick, J. (2007) Community based services for persons with intellectual disability in Israel, 2006. Jerusalem, Israel: Office of the Medical Directorate, Ministryof Social Affairs.
4. Merrick, J. (2005) National survey 1998 on medical services for persons with intellectual disability in residential care in Israel. Int. J. Disabil. Hum. Dev. 4:139–146.
5. Merrick, J. (2010) Survey of medical clinics, 2008. Jerusalem, Israel: Office of the Medical Directorate, Ministry of Social Affairs.
6. Centers for Disease Control and Prevention. (2003) Trends in aging – United States and worldwide. Morb. Mortal. Wkly. Rep. 52:101–106.
7. Fisher, K., Kettl, P. (2005) Aging with mental retardation: increasing population of older adults with MR require health interventions and prevention strategies. Geriatrics 60:26–29.
8. Merrick, J., Davidson, P. W., Morad, M., Janicki, M. P., Wexler, O., Henderson, C. M. (2004) Older adults with intellectual disability in residential care centers in Israel: health status and service utilization. Am. J. Ment. Retard. 109:413–420.
9. Janicki, M. P., Davidson, P. W., Henderson, C. M., McCallion, P., Taets, J. D., Force, L. T., et al. (2002) Health characteristics and health services utilization in older adults with intellectual disability living in community residences. J. Intellect. Disabil. Res. 46:287–298.
10. Kerr, A. M., McCulloch. D., Oliver. K., McLean. B., Coleman, E., Law, T. et al. (2003) Medical need of people with intellectual disability require regular reassessment and provision of client- and carer-held reports. J. Intellect. Disabil. Res. 47:134–145.

11. Anderson, D. J. (1993) Health issues. In: Sutton, E. Factar, A. R., Hawkins, B. A., Heller, T., Seltzer, G. B., eds. Older Adults with Developmental Disabilities. Baltimore, USA: Paul Brookes, pp. 29–48.
12. Cooke, L. B. (1997) Cancer and learning disability. J. Intellect. Disabil. Res. 41:312–316.
13. Duff, M., Hoghton, M., Scheepers, M., Cooper, M., Baddeley, P. (2001) *Helicobacterpylori*: has the killer escaped from the institution? A possible cause of increased stomach cancer in a population with intellectual disability. J. Intellect. Disabil. Res. 45:219–225.
14. Boker, L. K., Merrick, J. (2002) Cancer incidence in persons with Down syndrome in Israel. Down Syndr. Res. Pract. 8:31–36.
15. Djuretic, T., Laing-Morton, T., Guy, M., Gill. M. (1999) Concerted effort is needed to ensure the women use preventive services. BMJ 318:536.
16. Davies, N., Duff, M. (2001) Breast cancer screening for older women with intellectual disability living in community group homes. J. Intellect. Disabil. Res. 45:253–257.
17. Warburg, M. (1994) Visual impairment among people with developmental delay. J. Intellect. Disabil. Res. 38:423–432.
18. Merrick, J., Koslowe, K. (2001) Refractive errors and visual anomalies in Down syndrome. Down Syndr. Res. Pract. 6:131–133.
19. Evenhuis, H. M. (1995) Medical aspects of ageing in a population with intellectual disability: II. Hearing impairment. J. Intell. Disabil. Res. 39:27–33.
20. Crandell, C. C., Roesser, R. J. (1993) Incidence of excessive/impacted cerumen in individuals with mental retardation: A longitudinal investigation. Am. J. Ment. Retard. 97:568–574.
21. Bohmer, C. J. M., Taminiau, J. A. J. M., Klinkenberg-Knol, E. C., Meuwissen, S. G. M. (2001) The prevalence of constipation in institutionalized people with intellectual disability. J. Intellect. Disabil. Res. 45:212–218.
22. Morad, M., Nelson, N. P., Merrick, J., Davidson, P. W., Carmeli, E. (2007) Prevalence and risk factors of constipation in adults with intellectual disability in residential care centers in Israel. Res. Dev. Disabil. 28:580–586.
23. Walman, H. B., Perlman, S. P. (2002) Providing dental services for people with disabilities: why is it so difficult? Ment. Retard. 40:330–333.
24. Merrick, J. (2002) Mortality for persons with intellectual disability in residential care in Israel 1991–97. J. Intellect. Dev. Disabil. 27:265–272.
25. Center, J., Beange, H., McElduff, A. (1998) People with mental retardation have an increased prevalence of osteoporosis: a population study. Am. J. Ment. Retard. 103:19–28.
26. Merrick, J. (2000) Aspects of Down syndrome. Int. J. Adolesc. Med. Health 12:5–17.
27. Alzheimer, A. (1906) Uber einen eigenartigen schweren Erkrankungsprozess der Hirnrinde. Neurol. Centralblatt 23:1129–1136.
28. van Buggenhout, G. J. C. M., Trommelen, J. C. M., Schoenmaker, A., De Baal, C., Verbeek J. J. M. C., Smeets, D. F. C. M. et al. (1999) Down syndrome in a population of elderly mentally retarded patients: genetic–diagnostic survey and implications for medical care. Am. J. Med. Genet. 85:376–384.
29. Merrick, J., Ezra, E., Josef, B., Hendel, D., Steinberg, D. M., Wientroub, S. (2000) Musculoskeletal problems in Down syndrome. European Paediatric Orthopaedic Society Survey: the Israeli sample. J. Pediatr. Orthop. Pt. B 9:185–192.
30. Hsieh, K., Heller, T., Miller, A. B. (2001) Risk factors for injuries and falls among adults with developmental disabilities. J. Intellect. Disabil. Res. 45:76–82.
31. van Schrojenstein Lantman-de Valk, H. M. J., Metsemakers, J. F. M., Soomers-Turlings, M. J. M. S. J. G., Haveman, M. J., Crebolder, H. F. J. M. (1997) People with intellectual disability in general practice: case definition and case findings. J. Intellect. Disabil. Res. 41:373–379.
32. Lennox, N. G., Diggens, J. N., Ugoni, A. M. (1997) The general practice care of people with in tellectual disability: Barriers and solutions. J. Intellect. Disabil. Res. 41:380–390.
33. Jones, R. G., Kerr, M. P. (1997) A randomized control trial of an opportunistic health screening tool in primary care for people with intellectual disability. J. Intellect. Disabil. Res. 41:409–415.

34. Webb, O. J., Rogers, L. (1999) Health screening for people with intellectual disability: the New Zealand experience. J. Intellect. Disabil. Res. 43:497–503.
35. Tyler, C. V., Snyder, C. W., Zyzanski, S. J. (1999) Caring for adults with mental retardation: survey of family practice residency program directors. Ment. Retard. 37:347–352.
36. Evenhuis, H. M., van Praag, P. H., Wiersema, M. I., Huisman, S. (1998) Curriculum for the medical specialist training for physicians for people with intellectual disability. Amsterdam, The Netherlands: Dutch Society Physicians for People with Intellectual Disability.
37. Evenhuis, H. M., Henderson, C. M., Beange, H., Lennox, N., Chicoine, B. (2000) Healthy ageing in people with intellectual disability. Physical health issues. Geneva, Switzerland: World Health Organization.

20 Rett syndrome into adulthood

Meir Lotan, Joav Merrick, Mordechai Raskas and Mohammed Morad

Rett syndrome (RS) is a neurological disease affecting mainly females characterized by an arrest of brain development caused by an X-linked mutation. RS is the first human disease found to be caused by defects in a protein involved in regulating gene expression through its interaction with methylated DNA. The disease has been traced to a defective gene called MECP2. In this chapter we look into aging with RS as an example of a syndrome in childhood where persons live into adulthood. However, our review revealed very few studies, but the published casestudies showed that females with RS can live even to the age of 79 years. The existing knowledge suggests that individuals with RS present the therapist/physician with specific clinical challenges that require appropriate, long-lasting, intervention programs to be individually tailored for this population. The case studies presented here and recent findings showed that females with RS can also live into old age. Due to the observed longevity of individuals with RS, it is suggested that appropriate, long-term and intensive care should be provided at all ages in the hope to prevent (or at least reduce) the age-related deterioration that is typical in this population.

20.1 Introduction

Until recently, most individuals with intellectual disability lived much shorter lifespans in comparison with individuals without intellectual disability. Adults with intellectual disability are currently living to advanced age due to developments in medical care and technology, which have increased life expectancy of this population (1–3). An estimated 641,000 adults with intellectual disability at ages ≥60 years were residing in the USA in the year 2000, and official expectations are that this group will increase threefold by 2020 (4). Not only are adults with intellectual disability living longer and healthier lives and their life expectancy increased substantially over the last few decades, expectations are that this trend will continue (5). As persons with intellectual disability are living longer, geriatric healthcare providers need to learn about the characteristics, healthcare needs, and common clinical issues facing this population in general as well as subgroups within this group of clients. One subgroup is persons with RS, which we have used to show just one example of a syndrome in which treatment, support and intervention have resulted in these female children living into adulthood.

20.2 RS

The original observation of 6 girls with a peculiar disease, reported by Andreas Rett (1924–1997), was published in German in 1966 (6), but this syndrome gained international attention only when in 1983 when Hagberg and colleagues (7) published their findings on 35 cases. This author had in fact already observed his first such patient in 1960 (8).

RS is a neurological disease (9) affecting mainly females (10). It is characterized by the arrest of brain development (9) caused by an X chromosome mutation. RS is the first human disease found to be caused by defects in a protein involved in regulating gene expression through its interaction with methylated DNA (11) and has been traced to a defective gene on the X chromosome, called MECP2. This discovery was made by Ruthie Amir, who found the first mutations (11, 12) working at Baylor College of Medicine in Houston (USA).

RS typically presents at 6–18 months of age and is one of the most common causes of multiple disability among females. The disease incidence is 1 in 10,000–15,000 of live female births. There is a gradual reduction of speech and purposeful hand-use, seizures, autistic-like behavior, ataxia, intermittent hyperventilation and stereotypic hand movements. After initial regression, the condition stabilizes and patients usually survive into adulthood [8].

Although 50–75% of patients achieve independent mobility in early childhood, ~75% lose the ability to walk in later years and become wheelchair-bound (13). Some professionals recommend walking and/or other physical fitness programs as a preventive intervention that might hold back or diminish secondary regression (13–16). The debilitating disabilities common to this syndrome are scoliosis (appearing in up to 85% of affected individuals (14)), constipation and osteoporosis at a young age. All the medical conditions described above have been known to be affected positively by physical therapy and other intervention programs, suggesting that physical activity for this population may be beneficial.

20.2.1 RS stages

The stages of RS have been described as onset or pre-regression (stage 1); destructive, motor deterioration or regression (stage 2); essentially stable or *plateau* (stage 3) and in some cases the term fourth stage (late motor deterioration) has been used if an individual who achieved walking abilities at a young age becomes very handicapped and loses ambulation (17, 18) Development in females with RS proceeds in an apparently normal fashion *in utero* and during the first 6–18 months of life, at which point their development comes to a halt with regression and loss of many of their acquired skills (19). Thereafter, a rapid deterioration, with loss of acquired speech and purposeful hand use, ensues. A deceleration of head growth and jerky body movements of the trunk and limbs accompany the developmental deterioration in individuals with RS. Typically, they present with a broad-based gait and side-to side swaying movements of the shoulders when walking (20). Other physical problems such as seizures, scoliosis and breathing abnormalities may appear (21) which require constant care for the rest of the person's life (22). Scoliosis is a prominent feature in females with RS, but can vary from mild to severe (23). Apraxia (developmental dyspraxia), the inability to program the body to perform motor tasks, is the most fundamental and severely handicapping aspect of the syndrome. Apraxia can interfere with all body movement, including eye gaze and speech, making it difficult for individuals with RS to execute what they want to do. To sum up, the child adolescent and adult with RS is in need of an intensive and comprehensive management program throughout her lifespan (estimated life expectancy of individuals with RS in the past was ~50 years) (24).

20.2.2 Longitudinal follow-up of adults with RS

Studies conducted on aging and RS are scarce, with only a few casestudies available. We describe the longitudinal follow-up of adults with RS, thereby emphasizing the importance of such documentation. One casestudy (25) described a woman with RS from Norway who lived to the age of 60 years. That article provided no information about any genetic test, only a clinical diagnosis. The study was based on medical records, older and more recent videotapes and interviews with her sister and care-giving staff. After 21 years without being able to walk, after intensive physiotherapy, the woman regained that ability walking without support. A few years before she died, she also showed improvement in hand use. During the early regression of ambulation at around the age of ~20 years (which was due to moving from living at home to a residential facility) she appeared to lose social interest. The interest improved after some time but she remained wary of people whom she did not know.

Another casestudy was published from Denmark of a 77-year-old woman (26), born in 1923 after a normal pregnancy and delivery, who walked unsupported at the age of about 1 year. She deviated from normal development at 2 years of age. At 38 years of age, she had lost all purposeful hand use and constantlycarried out the hand mannerisms typicalof RS. She developed severe kyphosis and, at 41 years of age, ambulation was lost. At age 66 years, she was diagnosed as having RS with the following mutation in her MECP2 alleles: a C-to-P transition in exon 4 leading to a substitution of threonine by methionine at position 158, T158M in the conserved methyl binding domain of the corresponding gene product. The XCI showed a non-random pattern with an inactivation ratio of 10:90. This T158 mutation is a common mutation in RS and her skewed XCI may have resulted in her long survival. She died at the age of 79 from peritonitis caused by an abscess after the removal of anenlarged spleen.

Hagberg (27) described 3 cases to illustrate long-term clinical follow-up in RS. The first casestudy was of a girl born in 1957 who had developmental delay and was referred at $3^1/_2$ years of age but not diagnosed with RS until 19 years of age. At that time, the main problems were apraxia, general developmental retardation, and aggressive behavior. In addition, she was considerably growth-retarded, had developed a severe kyphosis and a more modest left convex C scoliosis. Her epileptiform symptomatology, which started at age 6 months, was under full control and no longer a problem. At the last follow-up (age, 47 years), she was a very small woman, 134-cm tall, weighing 50 kg, with an occipitofrontal head circumference (OFC) of 54 cm. She had short, thin, slightly distorted feet (only 34-cm long). She was still able to walk unsupported but showed some balance problems. She was less active in motorterms and had signs of excessively early gross motor-muscle aging of the legs. She had hand-finger stereotypes more or less continuously but a more subtle form of the regular hand stereotypic wringing and twisting carried out by females with RS. Her neurology was characterized by a complex gross motor dysfunction of the RS type. She had a complex MECP2 rearrangement with deletions of exon 3 and exon 4.

The second casestudy was of a female born in 1960, the second of three siblings, in a healthy family. Her pre- and peri-natal history was uneventful with birth at full term (weight, 3,590 g; length, 50 cm; OFC, 34 cm). Her first $1^{1}/_{4}$> years of life were reported to have been uneventful. At that age, she was able to walk with support, pincer-grasp and manipulated toys as expected. She had, however, never learned to crawl on all-fours. At that point a general stagnation occurred, followed rapidly by marked developmental regression. At the age of $1^{3}/_{4}$ years, she had stopped walking completely, had lost contact with her parents, had developed intense "hand-clapping" stereotypes (film documented) and showed "autistic-like" behaviors. In parallel, her head growth curve indicated a marked deceleration. At 23 years of age, she was diagnosed as a classic RS patient. At the last visit (44 years of age), she was extremely handicapped, very small and thin, with a small head (height, 130 cm; weight, 24 kg; OFC, 48.5 cm). She had a complex S-curved RS kyphoscoliosis and a markedly distended abdomen of the RS bloating type. Her feet were cold and sweaty, bluish in color, and extremely thin and small (length, 22 cm). Her examination was characterized by a dystonic-rigid syndrome of the advanced RS type with a right-sided dominance. She was reported to have repeated, unmotivated, long laughing attacks, as well as paroxysmal night screaming. She had never had epileptic seizures. She had a commonly found MECP2 mutation inaxon 4 (R270X).

The third case, born in 1965, was one of two siblings in a healthy family. Her perinatal and neo-natal histories were uneventful, as were her developmental abilities when she was born at full term (weight, 3,590 g; length, 50 cm; OFC, 34 cm). She developed normally but at a health check-up at 1 year, she was considered to be "late" but able to creep on her knees and sit up and walk with support and play with toys. She could say many single words. After $1^{1}/_{2}$ years of age, she slowly regressed, did not use her hands as before, was found socially detached from her parents and was more or less in her "own world". At the same time, she stopped crawling and talking and repeatedly had unmotivated screaming attacks. At the age of $2^{1}/_{2}$ years, her skull growth had stagnated significantly. She was slightly hypotonic and had some sort of ataxic movement patterns of the truncal ataxia type, as well as intention-tremor in her hands and stereotypic movement patterns. She did not develop seizures. Throughout the following three decades, she successively deteriorated neurologically into a generalized most severe dystonic-atrophic syndrome, with side-asymmetric secondary deformities, contractures and a collapsed scoliosis. She died at the age of 36 years in a deformed, growth-retarded and emaciated state.

20.2.3 Recent studies

A large North American cohort (N=1,928) examined the longevity of individuals with RS and found that ~80% of individuals diagnosed with atypical RS and 60% of individuals with typical RS survive to the age of 50 years (28). Nevertheless, the authors suggest that, given that clinical management has improved considerably from the time when RS was first recognized, improved survival among each successive cohort might be expected. Moreover, we believe that because the research was done only on people currently diagnosed with RS, institutionalized undiagnosed adults might change the data, suggesting even greater longevity in this population.

In another project conducted by researchers from Maastricht University in Holland in association with the Dutch Rett Syndrome Association, questionnaires were sent to families and caregivers of individuals with RS aged 16 years and older (29). It was found that, of the 53 responses to the questionnaire concerned with living conditions and use of care facilities, 36% of the research population resided with their parents and 71% in residential facilities.

Health of the individuals was assessed on a five-point scale ranging from very good [1] to very bad [5]. In general, the respondents valued the health of individuals with RS as good (mean, 2.15), but a significant relationship was found between health and apnea, breath-holding spells, mood changes, spasticity and joint deformities. In regards to weight status, 49% of the participants were underweight, 40% had a normal weight and 11% were overweight. In regards to communication, one-third of the participants with RS were able to express themselves sometimes by spoken language and/or signals. Communication was found considerably better in the older age groups. These findings support previous knowledge regarding adults with RS (30–32).

Cold feet were noted in 96% of participants with RS, and pressure sores and vesicles occurred in 46%. Half of the participants with RS showed sleeping problems on a nightly basis and the prevalence of sleeping problems was higher in older age groups. Daytime sleeping was reported in 85% of the research population. Apnea (38%), hyperventilation (39%), breath-holding spells (73%) and air swallowing (41%) were reported with a much lower prevalence in the oldest age group (in regards to apnea).

Night screaming was reported in 39%, prevalence of mood changes in 66% and abnormal agitation reported in 54%. Two-thirds of the research population showed anxiety. The prevalence of scoliosis in the study was 90%, of those 36% had undergone surgery, while the prevalence of kyphosis was found in 16%.

In contrast to other areas, gross motor function in the research population was found to slowly but continuously decline over the years, which has also been found by other researchers (17, 33–35). Ambulation and mobility were very limited in all agegroups, and no relationship with age was found. The prevalence of spasticity was 52%, mainly affecting the arms and legs. Joint deformities (mostly of the feet) were found in 60% of the research population. A history of epilepsy was present in 74%, of whom 95% used anti-convulsive treatment.

In general, in both research projects, better communication and autonomic function in the oldest age group was found compared with the younger age groups, which is in line with previous findings (35–37). This research demonstrated the potential for prolonged survival in this population, and suggested the need for careful planning for long-term care, as well as continued observation of the effects of improved clinical management on longevity.

20.2.4 Clinical manifestations of the aging person with RS

The person with RS presents some common clinical manifestations. Therefore specific acknowledgement, appropriate evaluation and specific intervention is required, as listed below.

- Scoliosis: 80–85% of individuals with RS (30, 38) are diagnosed with scoliosis. It has been found that intensive therapeutic intervention with adequate sensory (21) and physical (15) support can slow down deterioration of the scoliosis (15) and might even prevent the child from needing to undergo corrective surgery (21).

- Epilepsy: According to different studies, 30–90% of individuals with RS will be diagnosed with epilepsy (30, 36, 39–41). Individuals with RS show acute reactions to anti-epileptic medication and therefore the diagnostic procedure and medication prescription should be completed by physicians acquainted with this specific disorder (30). Moreover, many individuals with RS tend to have irregular night sleep (42) and excessive amounts of daytime sleep(43) so anti-epileptic medication should be introduced only if the seizures disturb the child's daily routine or functions. It has been found that 82% of individuals with RS show breathing abnormalities that might sometimes appear as epileptic-like attacks, so telemetry or electro-encephalography (video EEG) should be undertaken to avoid anti-epileptic over-medication. Many of this population show reduction in the severity and frequency of epileptic attacks in adulthood. Therefore, a slow reduction of anti-convulsive medication should be undertaken under the supervision of a Neurologist knowledgeable with adults with RS (30). Phenobarbitone and, to a lesser extent, benzodiazepines, display a severe effect on the level of alertness and responsiveness of the subject with RS, to a point of sudden pseudo-motor deterioration Therefore their use should be avoided as much as possible (31).
- Carnitine is a biological enhancer for the transport of fatty acids from the cytosol into the mitochondria during the breakdown of lipids. Reduction in carnitine level might cause muscle weakness, liverinsufficiency, neurological problems and hypotonia. All these behaviors might damage the functional ability of the individual with RS, yet they are masked by the fluctuating nature of the RS manifestation. Individuals with RS have been found in the past to show low levels of carnitine and, because the supply of carnitine has been found to contribute positively to the height, weight and motor function of these individuals (44, 45), carnitine level should be evaluated and supplied in cases of deficiency. Moreover, the combination of anti-convulsive medication (especially depakot) with carnitine has been found to be beneficial for this population.
- Constipation is common in individuals with RS (43). It is estimated that 85% of individuals with RS will experience severe constipation at least once in their life (46). Constipation in this population is derived from a lack of physical activity, low muscle tone, improper diet, medication, scoliosis and reduced liquid intake (47). Since all the above aspects contributing to constipation are treatable, their use should be examined prior to the use of laxatives and enemas (48).
- Nutrition: Intestinal problems are present in 74% of individuals with RS (41) and are a significant component of this syndrome. There is evidence that these symptoms worsen with age in connection to their functional/orthopedic situation (23, 32) and therefore constant and proper evaluation should be a part of the follow-up procedure of the adult with RS. Moreover, moderate-to-severe malnutrition is present in 85% of individuals with RS (49) and is aggravated with age (36, 47). However, many of the nutritional problems of this population are treatable (48) if properly diagnosed.
- Osteoporosis occurs frequently in females with RS and has been reported in very young girls (50–52). Patients with RS have been found to have decreased BMD compared with controls (53). These findings support the need for routine check-up from childhood of the bone density of individuals with RS and to commence

physical (such as intensive standing and walking programs (16, 54), nutritional (48) and medical intervention (50) as preventive intervention if the situation necessitates such courses of action (31).

- Dental treatment: Specific dental disorder-related problems have been identified in individuals with RS (55, 56). These problems include gum problems, teeth closure (56), bruxism, high risk of falling and facial trauma (32), teeth damage due to prolonged use of anti-convulsive medication and reflux (21). These accumulating problems require the acknowledged attention and care of a Dentist (57, 58).
- Functional improvements: a few studies have demonstrated that proper intervention can improve the function of children (16) and adults with RS, up to a point were walking was restored for a woman with RS who had stopped walking 20 years previously (25). Because of the possible lifespans of individuals with RS, it is suggested that proper and intensive care should be provided to clients with this syndrome at all ages in the hope of preventing (or at least reducing) the age-related deterioration that is typical in this population (59).

All the symptoms mentioned above are typical of adults with RS and can be treated with conventional intervention, thereby contributing to the longevity and QoL of this population. Therefore longitudinal follow-up for proper evaluation procedures and intervention implementation is needed for this population as it ages.

20.2.5 Adults with RS

Due to the fact that RS has been acknowledged by Western medicine only in the past 23 years, after the publication of the first English article on RS by Hagberg and his colleagues (7), most adults with RS are misdiagnosed and might therefore lack appropriate intervention.

The prevalence of RS in Israel is presented in ▶ Fig. 20.1. It is evident from the graph that many RS adults over the age of 15 years have not been located and diagnosed, and that older adults (25 years and older) have been scarcely detected.

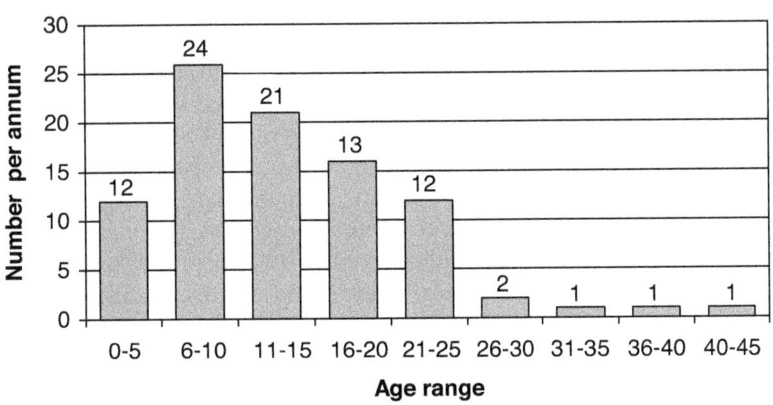

Fig. 20.1: Prevalence of individuals diagnosed with RS in Israel according to age.

Due to the specific medical challenges presented by adults with RS, the authors call for a widespread organized search for this population to detect, diagnose and implement intervention programs adapted for the specific needs of individuals with RS. Initial findings from an ongoing survey to detect undiagnosed adults with RS in residential care centers in Israel suggest that ~6% of all females in residential settings might be diagnosed with RS. Moreover, some of the typical characteristics of RS such as bruxism, bloating, sleep disorders, breathing abnormalities and sometimes even hand-mannerisms (reduced to subtle finger movements as described by Hagberg (30)) are less frequent in adulthood than in childhood within this population. Therefore, detection of these individuals requires a person who is highly experienced in RS.

20.2.6 Mortality

People with RS can survive into middle and old age, but life expectancy is reduced and the occurrence of sudden death is greater than in the general population. Longitudinal records of people with RS began in the United Kingdom in 1982 and developed into the British Survey in 1993. From this British Survey, the mortality for RS has been estimated to be 1.2% per annum (59), with 48% of deaths occurring in debilitated people, 13% from natural causes, 13% with prior severe seizures, and 26% due to sudden and unexpected causes (59–62). Respiratory dysrhythmias were usually present. Neuropathological studies confirmed reductions in cortical dendrites and, in one case, immaturity of cardiac conducting tissues (59). The possible causes of sudden death can include brainstem autonomic failure (respiratory failure, apnea, cardiac arrhythmias) (59–62).

20.3 Discussion

This chapter on the aging individuals with RS revealedvery few studies. We have to wait for additional, larger follow-up studies and large-cohort studies in the future.

The five casestudies from Norway, Denmark and Sweden showed deceleration of head growth appearing at an early stage that was associated with increased motor disability and with the appearance of epilepsy (27). The hand stereotypes, which are the trademark of RS from early childhood, usually change in adult middle-age toward frozen and stiff mal-positions or remain as finger movement. From childhood to young adulthood, some gross motor-functions appear to improve slightly with a temporary recovery and compensation, in contrast to the loss of fine motorabilities. In the long term, middle-aged women with RS lose a great deal of muscle volume, strength and power, and present with generally premature neuromuscular aging, necessitating the introduction of physical fitness intervention programs. The early general growth deceleration not only affects body and skull growth but also involves the overly thin, small, cold and sweaty feet and the insufficient, compressed, and curved spine (15, 27).

Epilepsy occurs in > 90% of cases with onset of clinical seizures at ~3–5 years of age. There is a peak frequency in adolescence, into young adulthood and successive decreases in early middle-age, with only rare and minor problems occurring after the age of 40 years (27, 63). Therefore, after 40 years of age, an attempt should be made to gradually withdraw anti-epileptic drugs (27, 63).

Many common characteristics of adults with RS are known. These include constipation, osteoporosis, potential for improvement in functional abilities, dental problems, nutritional needs, and orthopedic problems. All the above aspects necessitate special evaluation, which should lead to improved, more focused intervention for this population. Nevertheless, the novelty of this syndrome requires a search for undiagnosed adults with RS to enable the implementation of appropriate care.

The case studies presented here and recent findings showed that females with RS can live even to the age of 79 years and suggest significant longevity for this population. Due to the observed longevity of individuals with RS, it is suggested that appropriate, long-term and intensive care should be provided at all ages in the hope of preventing (or at least reducing) the age-related deterioration that is typical in this population.

References

1. Patja, K., Iivanainen, M., Vesala, H., Oksanen, H., Ruoppila, I. (2000) Life expectancy of people with intellectual disabilities: a 35-year follow-up study. J. Intellect. Disabil. Res. 44:591–599.
2. Maaskant, M. A., Gevers, J. P. M., Wierda, H. (2002) Mortality and live expectancy in Dutch residential centres for individuals with intellectual disabilities, 1991–1995. J. Appl. Res. Int. Dis. 15:200–212.
3. Fisher, K., Kettl, P. (2005) Aging with mental retardation: increasing population of older adults with MR require health interventions and prevention strategies. Geriatrics 60:26–29.
4. Heller, T., Janicki, M. P., Hammel, J., et al. Promoting healthy aging, family support, and age-friendly communities for persons aging with developmental disabilities: Report of the 2001 Invitational Research Symposium on Aging with Developmental Disabilities. http://www. uic. edu/orgs. rrtcamr/gsa. pdf. Accessed 17 Apr 2009.
5. Tyler, C. V. Jr., Noritz, G. (2009) Healthcare issues in aging adults with intellectual and other developmental disabilities. Clin. Geriatrics 17(8):30–35.
6. Rett, A. (1966) Uber ein eigenartiges hirnatrophisches Syndrom bei Hyperammonamie im Kindesalter. Wiener Medi-zinische Wochenschrift 116:723–738.
7. Hagberg, B., Aicardi, J., Dias, K., Ramos, O. (1983) A progressive syndrome of autism, dementia, ataxia and loss of purposeful hand use in girls: Rett's syndrome. Report of 35 cases. Ann. Neurol. 14:471–479.
8. Hagberg, B. (1985) Rett syndrome: Swedish approach to analysis of prevalence and cause. Brain Dev. 7:277–280.
9. Armstrong, D. D. (1995) The neuropathology of Rett syndrome overview 1994. Neuropediatrics 26:100–104.
10. Amir, R. E., van den Veyver, I. B., Schultz, R., Malicki, D. M., Tran, C. Q., Dahle, E. J., et al. (2000) Influence of mutation type and X chromosome inactivation on Rett syndrome phenotypes. Ann. Neurol. 47:670–679.
11. Amir, R. E., van den Veyer, I. B., Wan, M., Tran, C. Q., Francke, U., Zoghbi, H. Y. (1999) Rett syndrome is caused by mutations in X-linked MECP2, encoding methyl-CpG-binding protein 2. Nat. Genet 23:185–188.
12. Amir, R. E., Zoghbi, H. Y. (2000) Rett syndrome: Methyl-CpG-binding protein 2 mutations and phenotype-genotype correlations. Am. J. Med. Genet. 97:147–152.
13. Lotan, M., Hadar-Frumer, M. (2002) Hydrotherapy for Rett syndrome. Physiother Bull 4:23–28 [In Hebrew].
14. McClure, M. K., Battaglia, C., McClure, R. J. (1998) The relationship of cumulative motor asymmetries to scoliosis in Rett syndrome. Am. J. Occup. Ther. 52:488–493.

15. Lotan, M., Merrick, J., Carmeli, E. (2005) Managing scoliosis in a young child with Rett syndrome: a case study. Scientific World J. 5:264–273.
16. Lotan, M., Isakov, E., Merrick, J. (2004) Improving functional skills and physical fitness in children with Rett syndrome. J. Intellect. Disabil. Res. 48:730–735.
17. Kerr, A. M. (2002) Annotation: Rett syndrome: recent progress and implications for research and clinical practice. J. Child Psychol. Child Psychiatry 43:277–287.
18. Lotan, M., Merrick, J. (2004) Rett syndrome management with Snoezelen or controlled multi-sensory stimulation. A review. Int. J. Adolesc. Med. Health 16:5–12.
19. Graham, J. M. (1995) Rett syndrome. Information packet. Los Angeles, USA: Cedars-Sinai Medical Center.
20. Kerr, A. M., Stephenson, J. B. P. (1985) Rett syndrome in the West of Scotland. BMJ 291:579–582.
21. Budden, S. S. (1995) Management of Rett syndrome: a ten year experience. Neuropediatrics 26:75–77.
22. Leonard, H., Fyfe, S., Leonard, S., Msall, M. (2001) Functional status, medical impairments, and rehabilitation resources in 84 females with Rett syndrome: a snapshot across the world from the parental perspective. Disabil. Rehabil. 23(3–4):107–117.
23. Sponseller, P. Orthopedic update in Rett syndrome. IRSA-Int 'Rett Syndr Ass Inf Resources. www. rettsyndrome. org/main/orthopaedic-update. htm
24. Percy AK. International research review. IRSA-Int Rett Syndr Ass 12th Ann Conf, Boston, MA, 1996 May 24–27.
25. Jacobsen, K., Viken, A., von Tetzchner, S. (2001) Rett syndrome and ageing: a case study. Disabil. Rehabil. 23(3–4):160–166.
26. Nielsen, J. B., Ravn, K., Schwartz, M. (2001) A 77-year-old woman and a preserved speech variant among Danish Rett patients with mutations in MECP2. Brain Dev. 23:S230–S232.
27. Hagberg, B. (2005) Rett syndrome. Long-term clinical follow-up experiences over four decades. J. Child Neurol. 20:722–726.
28. Kirby, R. S., Lane, J. B., Childers, J., Skinner, S. A., Annese, F., Barrish, J. O., et al. (2010) Longevity in Rett syndrome: analysis of the North American database. J. Pediatr. 156:135–138.
29. Halbach, N. S. J., Smeets, E. E. J., Schrander-Stumpel, C. T. R. M., van Schrojensein Lantman De Valk, H. H. J., Maaskant, M. A., et al. (2008) Aging in people with specific genetic syndromes: Rett syndrome. Am. J. Med. Genet. A 146A:1925–1932.
30. Hagberg, B. (1993) Rett syndrome: clinical and biological aspects. London, UK: Mac Keith.
31. Lotan, M., Ben-Zeev, B. Rett syndrome. (2006) A review with emphasis on clinical characteristics and intervention Scientific World J. 6:1517–1541.
32. Lotan, M. (2006) Angels of silence: caring for Rett syndrome. Tel Aviv, Israel: Rotem [In Hebrew].
33. Steffenburg, U., Hagberg, G., Hagberg, B. (2001) Epilepsy in a representative series of Rett syndrome. Acta Paediatr. 90:34–39.
34. Hagberg, B. (2002) Clinical manifestations and stages of Rett syndrome. Ment. Retard. Dev. Disabil. Res. Rev. 8:61–65.
35. Williamson, S. L., Christodoulou, J. (2006) Rett syndrome: new clinical and molecular insights. Eur. J. Hum. Genet. 14:896–903.
36. Ellaway, C., Christodoulou, J. (2001) Rett syndrome: clinical characteristics and recent genetic advances. Disabil. Rehabil. 23:98–106.
37. Julu, P. O., Kerr, A. M., Apartopoulos, F., Al Rawas, S, Engerstrom, I. W., Engerstrom, L. et al. (2001) Characterization of breathing and associated central autonomic dysfunction in the Rett disorder. Arch. Dis. Child. 85:29–37.
38. Rossin, L. (1997) Effectiveness of therapeutic and surgical intervention in the treatment of scoliosis in Rett syndrome. A seminar work. Pittsburgh, USA: Universityof Duquesne, 1–19.
39. Nieto MA, Candau RS, Prieto P. Contribution to studies of seizures in Rett syndrome analysis of critical forms of four cases. Rev Neurol 1995; 23:1185-89.

40. Glaze D. Epilepsy. Presentation, IRSA 12th Ann Conf, Boston, MA, 1996 May 24–27, tape 622-18.
41. Leonard S. The Australian Rett Syndrome study inaugural report. Aust: Telethon Inst Child Health Res, 2002.
42. Nomura, Y. (2005) Early behavior characteristics and sleep disturbance in Rett syndrome. Brain Dev. 27(Suppl. 1):S35–S42.
43. Piazza, C. C., Fisher, W., Kiesewetter, B. S., Bowman, L., Moser, H. (1990) Aberrant sleep patterns in children with Rett syndrome. Brain Dev. 2:488–493.
44. Plioplys, A. V., Kasnicka, I. L. (1993) Carnitine as treatment for Rett syndrome. South Afr. Med. J. 86:1411–1412.
45. Glaze D. Research updates from Baylor College. IRSA Ann Conf, Las Vegas, NV, 2000 May 18–21, Tape RS 10.
46. Saavedra J. M. Gastrointestinal crises in Rett syndrome. Int Rett Syndr Assoc Newsletter 1997; Winter: 3–5.
47. Reilly, S., Cass, H. (2001) Growth and nutrition in Rett syndrome. Disabil. Rehabil. 23:118–128.
48. Lotan, M., Zysman, L. (2006) The digestive system and nutritional considerations for individuals with Rett syndrome. Scientific World J. 6:1737–1749.
49. Hunter, K. (1999) The Rett syndrome handbook. Washington, USA: International Rett Syndrome Association.
50. Zysman, L., Lotan, M., Ben-Zeev, B. (2006) Osteoporosis in Rett syndrome: a study on normal values. Scientific World J. 6:1619–1630.
51. Budden, S. S., Gunness, M. E. (2003) Possible mechanisms of osteopenia in Rett syndrome: bone histomorphometric studies. J. Child Neurol. 18:698–702.
52. Leonard, H., Thomson, M., Glasson, E., Fyfe, S., Leonard, S., Ellaway, C. (1999) Metacarpophalangeal pattern profile and bone age in Rett syndrome: further radiological clues to the diagnosis. Am. J. Med. Genet. 12:88–95.
53. Haas, R. H., Dixon, S. D., Sartoris, D. J., Hennessy, M. J. (1997) Osteopenia in Rett syndrome. J. Pediatr. 131:771–774.
54. Weeks L. Rett syndrome. Presentation, Sydney, 1997.
55. Tesini, D. A., Fenton-Sanford, J. (1994) Oral health needs of persons with physical or mental disabilities. Dent. Clin. North Am. 38:483–498.
56. Ribeiro, R. A., Romano, A. R., Birman-Goldenberg, E., Mayer, M. P. (1997) Oral manifestations in Rett syndrome: a study of 17 cases. Pediatr. Dent. 19:349–352.
57. Tenisi, D. A. (1988) Developing dental health education programs for persons with special needs. A training guide and reference text. Amherst, USA: Massachusetts Research Institute.
58. Tenisi, D. A. (1987) Providing dental services for citizens with handicaps: a prototype community program. Ment. Retard. 25:219–222.
59. Kerr, A. M., Armstrong, D. D., Prescott, R. J., Doyle, D., Kearney, D. L. (1997) Rett syndrome: analysis of deaths in the British Survey. Eur. Child Adolesc. Psychiatry 6(Suppl. 1):71–74.
60. Acampa, M., Guideri. (2006) Cardiac disease and Rett syndrome. Arch. Dis. Child. 91:440–443.
61. Ohya, T., Yamashita, Y., Matsuishi, T. Sudden death in Rett syndrome. Nippon Rinsho. 63:1178–1182 [In Japanese].
62. Byard, R. W. (2006) Forensic issues and possible mechanisms of sudden death in Rett syndrome. J. Clin. Forens. Med. 13:96–99.
63. Steffenburg, U., Hagberg, G., Hagberg, B. (2000) Epilepsy in a representative series of Rett syndrome. Acta Paediatr. 89:198–202.

Acknowledgements

21 About the editors

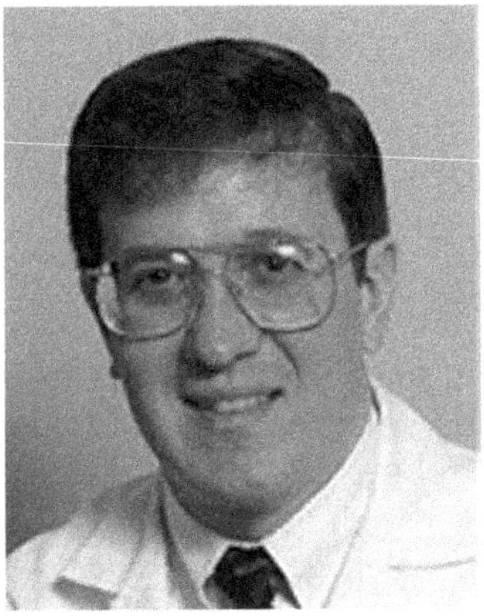

J. Timothy Bricker, MD, MBA, FACC, FAAP, is the Chairman of Pediatrics at the University of Kentucky and holds the Jacqueline A Noonan Endowed Pediatric Chair. He is also the Physician-in-Chief of the Kentucky Children's Hospital. Dr. Bricker's medical degree is from the Ohio State University College of Medicine. His MBA is from the University of Chicago. He was trained in pediatrics and pediatric cardiology at Baylor College of Medicine and Texas Children's Hospital, where he spent several years as Chief of Pediatric Cardiology before heading to chairmanship in Lexington in 2004. Scholarly work has included cardiac intensive care, pediatric aspects of coronary disease prevention, pediatric exercise physiology, pediatric cardiac transplantation, mechanical circulatory support and the cardiac effects of HIV infection in childhood. Dr. Bricker developed and staffs the Adult Congenital Heart Disease Program at the University of Kentucky. Email: tim.bricker@uky.edu; Website: http://ukhealthcare.uky.edu/education/KCH/chairmanwords. htm

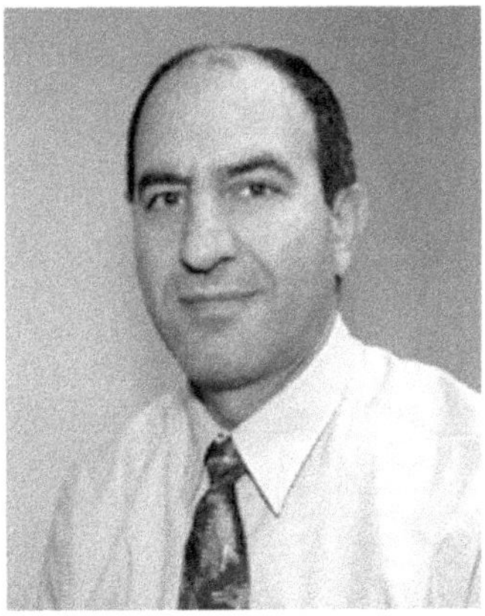

Hatim A. Omar, MD, FAAP, Professor of Pediatrics and Obstetrics and Gynecology and Director of the Section of Adolescent Medicine, Department of Pediatrics, University of Kentucky, Lexington. He is the holder of the Children's Miracle Network Endowed Chair in Pediatrics. Dr. Omar has completed residency training in obstetrics and gynecology as well as Pediatrics. He has also completed fellowships in vascular physiology and adolescent medicine. He is the recipient of the Commonwealth of Kentucky Governor's Award for Community Service and Volunteerism. He is the recipient of the Commonwealth of Kentucky Governor's Award for community service and volunteerism in 2000, KY teen Pregnancy Coalition Award for outstanding service 2002, Awards for suicide prevention from the Ohio Valley Society for Adolescent Medicine and Kentucky Pediatric Society in 2005 and 2007, Sexual Abuse Awareness Month Award for his work with sexual abuse victims from the KY Association of Sexual Assault Professionals in 2007, Special Achievement Award from the American Academy of Pediatrics 2007 and the Founders of Adolescent Medicine Award from the AAP in 2007. He is well known internationally with numerous publications in child health, pediatrics, adolescent medicine, pediatric and adolescent gynecology. Email: haomar2@uky. edu; Website: https://weblink.ukhealthcare.uky.edu/weblink/phyPro.do?poid=161106&ofid

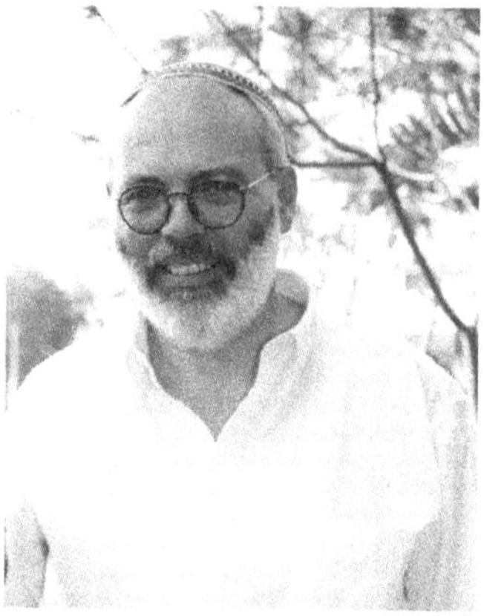

Joav Merrick, MD, MMedSci, DMSc, Professor of Pediatrics, Child Health and Human Development affiliated with Kentucky Children's Hospital, University of Kentucky, Lexington, USA and the Division of Pediatrics, Hadassah Hebrew University Medical Centers, Jerusalem, Israel, the Medical Director of the Health Services, Division for Intellectual and Developmental Disabilities, Ministry of Social Affairs and Social Services, Jerusalem, the founder and director of the National Institute of Child Health and Human Development in Israel. Numerous publications in the field of pediatrics, child health and human development, rehabilitation, intellectual disability, disability, health, welfare, abuse, advocacy, quality of life and prevention. Received the Peter Sabroe Child Award for outstanding work on behalf of Danish Children in 1985 and the International LEGOPrize ("Children's Nobel Prize") for an extraordinary contribution towards improvement in child welfare and well-being in 1987. E-Mail: jmerrick@zahav.net.il; Homepage: http://jmerrick50.googlepages.com/home

22 About the Kentucky Children's Hospital at the University of Kentucky, Lexington, Kentucky, USA

The Kentucky Children's Hospital is the only facility in central and eastern Kentucky dedicated to the expert medical and surgical care of infants, children and adolescents. The University of Kentucky has a proud and distinguished history of providing comprehensive programs and innovative care to the children of the region. Although patients are referred from every county of the Commonwealth of Kentucky and from every adjacent state, most patients are from the Bluegrass Region around Lexington and from Appalachian counties in the eastern part of Kentucky. The Department of Pediatrics has provided service and education from the opening of University of Kentucky College of Medicine in 1961.

The passion for teaching is palpable at the Kentucky Children's Hospital. In most years ~15% of our graduates choose to train in pediatrics. The University of Kentucky had one of the earliest combined Internal Medicine–Pediatrics residency programs with "med-peds" graduates very well represented throughout the faculty. This, in addition to a strong adolescent medicine program, is among factors which have led to a focus upon adolescent and adult graduates of pediatric care from Kentucky Children's Hospital.

The approach at the Kentucky Children's Hospital is focused on family-centered care. Full-time child life coverage, facilities for families to stay with children overnight, age-appropriate playrooms, children's library facilities, in-hospital school services, a dedicated television channel, a computer laboratory and many other features provide the special environment to provide the best of care for children. The Kentucky Children's Hospital includes a 12-bed Pediatric Intensive Care Unit, a 66-bed level-3 Neonatal Intensive Care Unit, 44 acute care pediatric beds, a 26-bed normal newborn nursery, and an 8-bed short-stay admissions/observation unit. Kentucky Children's Hospital has grown from ~3,750 discharges per year in 2004 to ~5,400 in 2009.

Pediatric medical and surgical outpatient facilities are primarily located in the Kentucky Clinic, which is attached to the hospital. Each year, the pediatric clinic has > 46, 000 patient visits. Of these, > 15,300 patient visits are in the general pediatric and continuity clinics, > 17,400 occur in the various subspecialty clinics. Kentucky Children's Twilight Clinic is open all but 2 days of the year in addition to the state-of-the-art pediatric emergency center.

Specialty care includes medical and surgical cardiac care, endocrinology, pediatric kidney disease, developmental pediatrics, pediatric allergy and immunology, solid-organ transplantation, behavioral pediatrics, pediatric emergency medicine, intensive care pediatrics, neonatology, gastroenterology and hepatology, dysmorphology, biochemical genetics, pediatric rheumatology, oncology, hematology, infectious diseases, hospitalist care, adolescent medicine, adolescent gynecology, child neurology, pediatric surgery, pediatric orthopedics, pediatric imaging, child psychiatry, pediatric anesthesiology, pediatric otorhinolaryngology, speech disorders, pediatric pathology, pediatric physical medicine, pediatric neurosurgery and many other fields. The Young

Parents Program is an innovative service of the Adolescent Medicine Division, which has been very successful. Many of these specialties cover outreach clinics throughout underserved Appalachian counties of Kentucky as well as in Lexington. New facilities are in preparation, because of the remarkable growth in clinical programs for children.

The growth of clinical programs and service capability has been matched by considerable growth in pediatric research at the University of Kentucky. Substantial programs in vascular biology and diabetes, pediatric inflammatory biology, molecular pediatrics, developmental biology, pediatric health policy research, epidemiology, prevention, cancer research and pediatric pharmacology are growing rapidly. The Kentucky Children's Hospital is located on the University of Kentuckycampus. Access to faculty in the other colleges, including social sciences and humanities, enhances the Kentucky Children's Hospital scholarly environment and provides unique opportunities for collaborative work.

As we approach our 50-year anniversary, we remain committed to improving the lives and health of young people of the Commonwealth and improving the future for their families.

Contact

J. Timothy Bricker, MD
Pediatric Cardiology
University of Texas Medical School
Children's Memorial Hermann Hospital
Houston, Texas
United States
John.T.Bricker@uth.tmc.edu

23 About the Division of Adolescent Medicine at the University of Kentucky, Lexington, Kentucky, USA

The Division of Adolescent Medicine was founded in 1998 to provide state-of-the-art care for adolescent patients from all areas of the commonwealth of Kentucky, to serve as a state-wide resource for education and training for local providers on adolescent issues, to study specific factors on the local level affecting youth in the state, to help teach medical students and residents, and to provide community service to help improve teen future in the commonwealth.

The division provides comprehensive, holistic team approach to adolescents, where teens receive all aspects for care from mental health to routine care from a team of professionals including Physicians, Mental Health Providers, Social Workers, Nutritionists and nursing staff. One unique program within the division is the Young Parent Program, where pregnant teens are cared for throughout pregnancy then they and their babies are cared for together in the program.

The division is active in research with > 10 peer-reviewed articles published each year as well as several books and special journal editions.

In the community, the program has founded several grassroot programs to help prevent youth suicide, teen pregnancy, accidental death and substance abuse among adolescents in Kentucky.

The division has provided > 300 lectures, workshops, media events and teaching for community providers, parents, teachers and school counselors. It also provides advocacy work on behalf of teens with active work at the state legislative and executive government as well as local governments to help improve the lives of teens.

23.1 Collaborations

The division collaborates locally with school boards, youth service centers, state and local governments, other universities and child advocacy centers as well as with regional adolescent medicine programs.

We have international links with the Institute for Child Health and Human Development in Jerusalem, Israel, the Division of Adolescent Medicine at Santa Casa University, Brazil, Quality of Life Research Center and Nordic School of Holistic Health, Copenhagen, Denmark, and the Department of Applied Social Sciences, Hong Kong Polytechnic University, Hong Kong.

23.2 The vision

The vision of the Division of Adolescent Medicine is to improve the health and long-term wellbeing of Kentucky youth to grow into productive adults. We also envision global work to help positive youth development worldwide.

23.3 Target areas of interests

The interest areas of the division are all aspects of youth development and adolescent health with focus on prevention and community involvement in collaboration on the local, national and global level, with programs having the same goal.

Contact

Hatim A. Omar, MD
Division of Adolescent Medicine
Kentucky Children's Hospital
University of Kentucky, Lexington
United States
haomar2@uky.edu

24 About the National Institute of Child Health and Human Development in Israel

The National Institute of Child Health and Human Development (NICHD) in Israel was established in 1998 as a "virtual institute" under the auspices of the Medical Director, Ministry of Social Affairs and Social Services to function as the research arm for the Office of the Medical Director. In 1998, the National Council for Child Health and Pediatrics, Ministry of Health and in 1999 the Director General and Deputy Director General of the Ministry of Health endorsed the establishment of the NICHD. In 2011 the NICHD became affiliated with the Division of Pediatrics, Hadassah Hebrew University Medical Centers in Jerusalem.

24.1 Mission

The mission of the NICHDin Israel is to provide an academic focal point for the scholarly interdisciplinary study of child life, health, public health, welfare, disability, rehabilitation, intellectual disability and related aspects of human development. This mission includes research, teaching, clinical work, information and public service activities in the field of child health and human development.

24.2 Service and academic activities

Over the years, many activities became focused in the south of Israel due to collaboration with various professionals at the Faculty of Health Sciences (FOHS) at the Ben Gurion University of the Negev (BGU). Since 2000, an affiliation with the Zusman Child Development Center at the Pediatric Division of Soroka University Medical Center has resulted in collaboration around the establishment of the Down Syndrome Clinic at that center. In 2002, a full course on "Disability" was established at the Recanati School for Allied Professions in the Community, FOHS, BGU, and in 2005 collaboration was started with the Primary Care Unit of the faculty and disability became part of the master of public health course on "Children and society". In the academic year 2005–2006, a one semester course on "Aging with disability" was started as part of the Master of Science program in gerontology in our collaboration with the Center for Multidisciplinary Research in Aging. In 2010, we had collaborations with the Division of Pediatrics, Hadassah Medical Centers, Hebrew University, Jerusalem, Israel.

24.3 Research activities

The affiliated staff has over the years published work from projects and research activities in this national and international collaboration. In year 2000, the *International*

Journal of Adolescent Medicine and Health and in 2005 the *International Journal on Disability and Human Development* of De Gruyter Publishing House (Berlin and New York), in 2003 the TSW-Child Health and Human Development and in 2006 the TSW-Holistic Health and Medicine of the *Scientific World Journal* (New York, USA, and Kirkkonummi, Finland), all peer-reviewed international journals were affiliated with the NICHD. From 2008 the *International Journal of Child Health and Human Development* (Nova Science, New York), the *International Journal of Child and Adolescent Health* (Nova Science) and the *Journal of Pain Management* (Nova Science) affiliated and from 2009 the *International Public Health Journal*(Nova Science) and *Journal of Alternative Medicine Research* (Nova Science).

24.4 National collaborations

Nationally the NICHD works in collaboration with the FOHsand BGU; Department of Physical Therapy, Sackler School of Medicine, Tel Aviv University; Autism Center, Assaf HaRofeh Medical Center; National Rett and PKU Centers at Chaim Sheba Medical Center, Tel HaShomer; Department of Physiotherapy, Haifa University; Department of Education, Bar Ilan University, Ramat Gan, Faculty of Social Sciences and Health Sciences; College of Judea and Samaria in Ariel and recently also collaborations have been established with the Division of Pediatrics at Hadassah, Center for Pediatric Chronic Illness, Har HaZofim in Jerusalem.

24.5 International collaborations

Internationally the NICHD works with the Department of Disability and Human Development, College of Applied Health Sciences, University of Illinois at Chicago; Strong Center for Developmental Disabilities, Golisano Children's Hospital at Strong, University of Rochester School of Medicine and Dentistry, New York; Centre on Intellectual Disabilities, University of Albany, New York; Centre for Chronic Disease Prevention and Control, Health Canada, Ottawa; Chandler Medical Center and Children's Hospital, Kentucky Children's Hospital, Section of Adolescent Medicine, University of Kentucky, Lexington; Chronic Disease Prevention and Control Research Center, Baylor College of Medicine, Houston, Texas; Division of Neuroscience, Department of Psychiatry, Columbia University, New York; Institute for the Study of Disadvantage and Disability, Atlanta; Center for Autism and Related Disorders, Department Psychiatry, Children's Hospital Boston, Boston; Department of Paediatrics, Child Health and Adolescent Medicine, Children's Hospital at Westmead, Westmead, Australia; International Centre for the Study of Occupational and Mental Health, Düsseldorf, Germany; Centre for Advanced Studies in Nursing, Department of General Practice and Primary Care, University of Aberdeen, Aberdeen, United Kingdom; Quality of Life Research Center, Copenhagen, Denmark; Nordic School of Public Health, Gottenburg, Sweden, Scandinavian Institute of Quality of Working Life, Oslo, Norway; Centre for Quality of Life of the Hong Kong Institute of Asia-Pacific Studies and School of Social Work, Chinese University, Hong Kong.

24.6 Targets

Our focus is on research, international collaborations, clinical work, teaching and policy in health, disability and human development and to establish the NICHD as a permanent institute at one of the residential care centers for persons with intellectual disability in Israel to conduct model research and together with the four university schools of public health/medicine in Israel establish a national master and doctoral program in disability and human development at the institute to secure the next generation of professionals working in this often non-prestigious/low-status field of work.

Contact

Joav Merrick, MD, MMedSc, DMSc
National Institute of Child Health and Human Development
Ministry of Social Affairs
Jerusalem
Israel
jmerrick@zahav.net.il

Index

www.ingramcontent.com/pod-product-compliance
Lightning Source LLC
Chambersburg PA
CBHW080938240926
51849CB00004BA/488
9783110255218